OXFORD HISTORICAL MONOGRAPHS

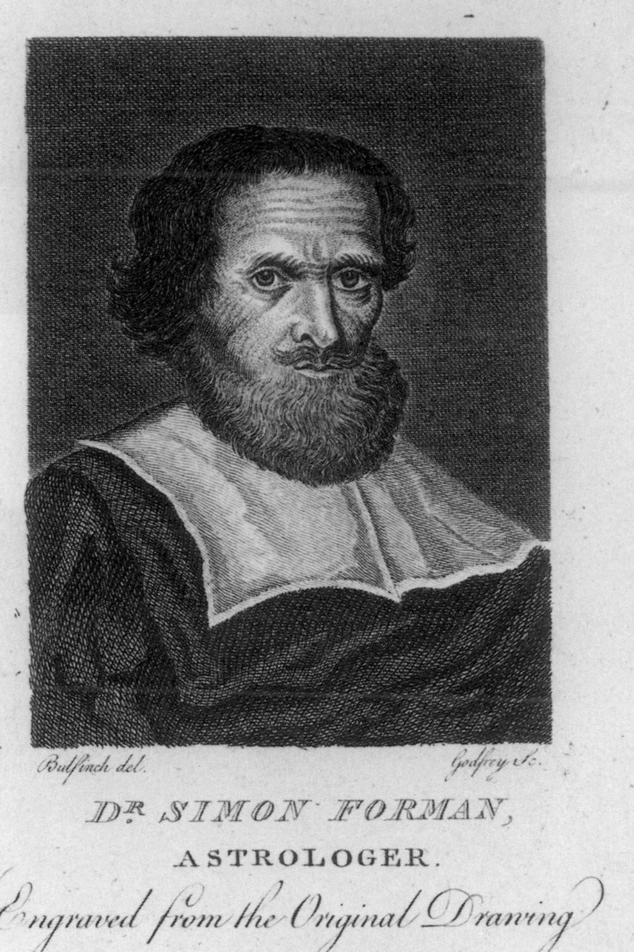
Bulfinch del.
Godfrey Sc.
Dr. SIMON FORMAN,
ASTROLOGER.
Engraved from the Original Drawing
in the Collection of the Right Honble
LORD MOUNTSTUART.
Publish'd July 1st 1776 by F. Blyth No. 87. Cornhill.

Portrait of Simon Forman by John Bulfinch (fl. 1680–1728), engraved by Richard Godfrey. By permission of the National Portrait Gallery, London.

Medicine and Magic in Elizabethan London

Simon Forman: Astrologer, Alchemist, and Physician

LAUREN KASSELL

CLARENDON PRESS · OXFORD

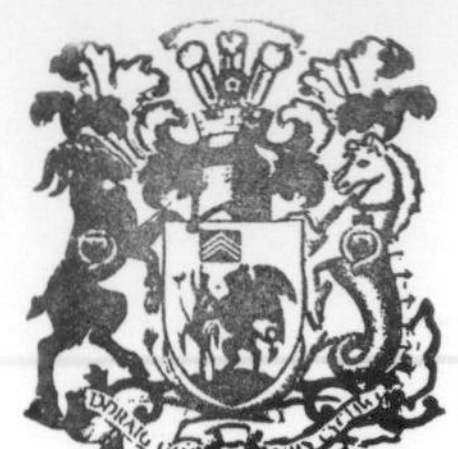

OXFORD
UNIVERSITY PRESS

Great Clarendon Street, Oxford OX2 6DP

Oxford University Press is a department of the University of Oxford.
It furthers the University's objective of excellence in research, scholarship,
and education by publishing worldwide in

Oxford New York

Auckland Cape Town Dar es Salaam Hong Kong Karachi
Kuala Lumpur Madrid Melbourne Mexico City Nairobi
New Delhi Shanghai Taipei Toronto

With offices in

Argentina Austria Brazil Chile Czech Republic France Greece
Guatemala Hungary Italy Japan South Korea Poland Portugal
Singapore Switzerland Thailand Turkey Ukraine Vietnam

Published in the United States
by Oxford University Press Inc., New York

First published 2005
First published in paperback 2007

British Library Cataloguing in Publication Data
Data available

Library of Congress Cataloging in Publication Data
Data available

ISBN 0–19–927905–5 978–0–19–927905–0
ISBN 0–19–921527–3 (Pbk.) 978–0–19–921527–0 (Pbk.)

1 3 5 7 9 10 8 6 4 2

Typeset by Graphicraft Ltd., Hong Kong
Printed in Great Britain
on acid-free paper by
Biddles Ltd.
King's Lynn, Norfolk

for Joad

ACKNOWLEDGEMENTS

Simon Forman had a habit of writing, Richard Napier preserved his papers, Elias Ashmole hoarded them for posterity, and William Black masterfully catalogued them. My first debt is to Forman, my second to those who saved and sorted his papers.

I have incurred countless other debts. Margaret Pelling has met many drafts with generous comments, fostering my understanding of early modern medicine and holding me to her scrupulous standards. Tony Grafton, Simon Schaffer, and Charles Webster have periodically read recensions of this book and shared their visions of Forman's world, confident that my archival prospecting would pay off. Jim Secord read a complete draft and made suggestions, such as the chronology, in the interests of the reader. Earlier Stuart Clark and Paul Slack suggested how to make the study broader and more coherent, and Paul has read subsequent drafts and shepherded the book through the press, trusting me to do what needed to be done. Versions of individual chapters have benefited from the comments of David Colclough, Marina Frasca Spada, Nick Jardine, Helen King, Bill Newman, Sophie Page, and anonymous readers. Often my mining and foraging turned to scrounging, and I am enormously grateful to the following for sharing their manuscript references and/or arcane expertise: Penny Bayer, Helen Brocklebank, Peter Forshaw, Peter Grund, Deborah Harkness, Susan Hitch, Martin Ingram, Mark Jenner, Peter Jones, David Katz, Giles Mandelbrote, Scott Mandelbrote, Sara Pennell, Max Satchell, and Bill Sherman. I have presented work on Forman to audiences in Oxford, Cambridge, Geneva, London, Manchester, and Princeton and I am grateful for their questions. I apologize to anyone I have forgotten. Many people have contributed to this book, and responsibility for its shortcomings and faults are wholly my own.

This project also has had enormous institutional support, direct and tacit. I began work on it in the 'old' Wellcome Unit, Oxford, a community that inspired rigour and independence. Two years of research and a trip to Jerusalem were funded by the Wellcome Trust. The Department of History, University of Aberdeen, briefly housed me. Pembroke College, Cambridge, supported me for two years as the R. A. Butler Research Fellow, and has provided a grant towards the illustrations. With fondness I remember the welcome I received in Pembroke and Cambridge from the late Mark Kaplanoff. The Department of

History and Philosophy of Science, University of Cambridge, home to some of the people listed above and many friends, has collectively willed me to completion. The Institute for Advanced Study, Princeton, has given me more time than I knew I needed. The Society for the Social History of Medicine awarded a much abbreviated and now revised version of Part III its 1997 Essay Prize, 'How to Read Simon Forman's Casebooks: Medicine, Astrology and Gender in Elizabethan London', *Social History of Medicine*, 12 (1999), 3–18, and I owe them gratitude for this award and Oxford University Press for permission to revisit that material in this book. Bill Newman and Tony Grafton nursed the germs of Part IV into print, '"The Food of Angels": Simon Forman's Alchemical Medicine', in Anthony Grafton and William Newman (eds.), *Secrets of Nature: Astrology and Alchemy in Early Modern Europe* (Cambridge, Mass., 2001), 345–84, and MIT Press has allowed me to include this material here. I am also indebted to the Bodleian Library, Oxford, the British Library, the Folger Shakespeare Library, Washington DC, the Provost and Fellows of King's College, Cambridge, the National Portrait Gallery, and the Master and Fellows of Pembroke College, Cambridge, for permission to reproduce images from their collections. I am grateful to the Royal Society for a grant towards the costs of the illustrations. Librarians and library staff throughout Britain and the United States have been more than accommodating. My dependence on the Bodleian Library, Oxford, is self-evident, and I am especially indebted to the staff in Duke Humphrey's Library, Alan Carter, Russell Edwards, Jean-Pierre Mialon, and William Hodges. Ashmole's volumes are big and heavy and only now am I learning not to want to look again at the ones I have just returned to the stacks.

Finally, in all of these places I have had many friends who bore with my talk of Forman and talked about other things. This book was begun when I stayed in England to be with Joad, and with him and for him it was written.

L.K.

June 2004

CONTENTS

LIST OF ILLUSTRATIONS

LIST OF TABLES

ABBREVIATIONS AND CONVENTIONS

Annals	London, Royal College of Physicians, Annals Bk. 2, 1581–1608, tr. J. Emberry and S. Heathcote (1953–5)
Ashm.	Oxford, Bodleian Library, Ashmole MS
'Astrologicalle judgmentes'	Simon Forman, 'The astrologicalle judgmentes of phisick and other questions', Ashm. 389, 363, 403
BL	London, British Library
Bodleian	Oxford, Bodleian Library
'Defenc'	Richard Napier, 'A treatise touching the defenc of astrologie', Ashm. 204, fos. 50–63, continued 240, fos. 137–8
DNB	*Dictionary of National Biography*, ed. L. Stephen and S. Lee, 63 vols. (1885–1900), with supplements
Folger	Washington, DC, Folger Shakespeare Library
'Grounds of arte'	Simon Forman, 'The grounds of arte gathered out of diverse authors', Ashm. 1495
'Heavens'	Simon Forman, 'The motion of the 3 superiour heavens', Ashm. 244, fos. 34–118
King's	Cambridge, King's College
'Life'	'Life of Adam and Eve', in H. F. D. Sparks (ed.), *The Apocryphal Old Testament* (Oxford, 1984), 141–67; Ashm. 802, ii
Longitude	Simon Forman, *The groundes of the longitude* (1591)
'Matrix'	Simon Forman, 'Matrix and paine therof', Ashm. 390, fos. 175–89; ed. Barbara Traister, '"Matrix and the pain thereof": A Sixteenth-Century Gynaecological Essay', *Medical History*, 35 (1991), 436–51
OED	*Oxford English Dictionary* <http://dictionary.oed.com/>
Sloane	London, British Library, Sloane MS

STC	A. W. Pollard and G. R. Redgrave, *A Short-Title Catalogue of Books Printed in England, Scotland, and Ireland*, 2nd edn. (1986)
Trinity	Cambridge, Trinity College

The place of publication is London unless otherwise noted.

All quotations are in the original spelling with i/j and u/v modernized and contractions expanded. Duplicate words and other minor copying errors have been silently corrected. Most first names have been standardized.

Forman wrote in a distinctive, often archaic fashion. Where necessary for clarity, punctuation has been added. Existing punctuation has been modernized, usually converting full stops into commas and slashes into full stops. The erratic use of capital letters has been retained when conveying emphasis. Red ink and different scripts are recorded in footnotes where relevant. The word 'wordle' for 'world' is a hallmark of his writings, and the letters have not been un-transposed. Forman's malapropisms remain.

Usually the most recent set of foliation or pagination in a manuscript is cited. Item numbers are omitted where citations are to a single set of numeration running throughout a volume. All folio and signature references are to the recto unless otherwise noted. Brackets indicate numbers that have been inferred.

Dates are given in Old Style, except the year is taken to begin on 1 January. References to the Annals include the page and date of the record. References to the casebooks include volume numbers and the name and date heading a consultation, omitting folio references unless the dated records are out of sequence.

LIST OF ASTROLOGICAL SYMBOLS

☉ Sun, gold, Sunday
☾ Moon, silver, Monday
♂ Mars, iron, Tuesday
☿ Mercury, mercury, Wednesday
♃ Jupiter, tin, Thursday
♀ Venus, copper, Friday
♄ Saturn, lead, Saturday

♈ Aries
♉ Taurus
♊ Gemini
♋ Cancer
♌ Leo
♍ Virgo
♎ Libra
♏ Scorpio
♐ Sagittarius
♑ Capricorn
♒ Aquarius
♓ Pisces

CHRONOLOGY

This list is designed to orient the reader, not to summarize the hundreds of dated events in Forman's life. All items in the list are mentioned in the text and included in the Index. Quotation marks designate Forman's words, italics his writings. The Bibliography contains full information about sources, and details of dates and dating are included there and in the text.

31 Dec. 1552	Born, Quidhampton, Wiltshire
1560–4	Attended school at St Giles Priory then in Salisbury
1 Jan. 1564	Father died
1566–*c.*1572	Apprenticed to Matthew Commin, hosier and grocer, Salisbury
May 1573	Went to Magdalen College, Oxford
*c.*1573	Began to study astrology, medicine, and magic
Sept. 1574	Returned to Quidhampton, taught school in Wilton
1575	Plague in Oxford, resulting in loss of books
June 1579–July 1580	Imprisoned in Salisbury; lost books a second time
1580	? Travelled in the Low Countries
*c.*1581	Began keeping a diary
1582	Reacquainted with Anne Walworth (née Young), his first love
1582–4	Tutor to John Penruddock's children
1584–9	Lived opposite St Thomas Church, Salisbury
*c.*1585	Began copying alchemical treatises and distilling strong waters
Mar. 1587	Caught with suspicious books in church in Salisbury and imprisoned; third loss of books
1588	Participated in a magic circle; first 'began to practice foiygomercy & to calle angells and sprites'
Jan. 1589	Left Salisbury, thereafter lived in many rooms in London and other places
*c.*1589?	*'The groundes of physique and chirurgerie', Sloane 2550, fos. 1–117ᵛ*
1589	*'De arte geomantica', Ashm. 354*
*c.*1590	*A treatise on geomancy, revised* c.*1611, Ashm. 392*

1590	'Wrote a bocke of nigromanti'
10 April 1591	'I put the longitude in question & that dai I rod to London & lai at Mullenaxes to teach him the longitude'
Aug. 1591	Moved to London
July 1591	Longitude *was printed*
22 Nov. 1591	'Mr Hoodes bock came out against me'
Feb. 1592	Took a chamber at Stone House, Philpot Lane
Summer 1592	Suffered from plague
1592	'This yere I did mani notable cuers and began to be knowen and com to credit'
1593	*'A disourse of the plague', Ashm. 208, fos. 110–35*
1593	'My knowledge in phisqu and in astronomy did encrease and I began to com to credit'
	First met Avis Allen, Forman's mistress until her death in 1597
Mar. 1594	Appeared before the College of Physicians for the first time, fined £5
Autumn 1594	Began to pursue the philosophers' stone
*c.*1594–5	*'Grounds of arte', Ashm. 1495*
Nov. 1595	Second appearance before the College of Physicians, fined £10 and imprisoned
*c.*1596–9	*'Astrologicalle judgmentes', Ashm. 403, revised 1600 (Ashm. 363), and 1606 (Ashm. 389)*
1596	*'Matrix', Ashm. 390, fos. 175–89*
3 Sept. 1596	Third interview with the College of Physicians, imprisoned
Mar. 1596–Feb. 1597	Casebooks vol. 1, Ashm. 234
1597+	*'Principles of philosofi', Ashm. 1472*
Feb. 1597–Feb. 1598	Casebooks vol. 2, Ashm. 226
20 Dec. 1597	Censors attempted, and failed, to arrest Forman
Dec. 1597	Rented house in Lambeth until June 1598; then back to Lambeth 1599
Feb. 1598–Feb. 1599	Casebooks vol. 3, Ashm. 195
Feb. 1599–Dec. 1599	Casebooks vol. 4, Ashm. 219
1599	'This yere I was quiete from the doctors from imprisonment but I condemned them in lawe, & put them to silence for a whole yer after & a half.'
1599	*Copied 'The life of Adam and Eve', Ashm. 802, ii*

22 July 1599	Married Jean Baker
19 Sept. 1599	Wrote to Napier about 'the bocke that I told you I mente to put in presse'
Jan. 1600–Dec. 1600	Casebooks vol. 5, Ashm. 236
1600	*'Liber juditiorum morborum', Ashm. 355*
Nov. 1600	College of Physicians summoned Forman, he sent a letter
23 Dec. 1600+	*'The bocke of the life and generation of Simon', Ashm. 208, fos. 136–42*
Dec. 1600–Nov. 1601	Casebooks vol. 6, Ashm. 411
June 1601	College of Physicians wrote to Whitgift about Forman
1600–1	Copied 'Ars notoria' three times
May 1602	Napier sent Forman his 'Defenc of astrologie'
May–Sept. 1603	Copies of casebooks in another hand, Ashm. 411, fos. 163–7
16 March 1603	Wrote to Napier asking for help against the College of Physicians
1603	*'Diary', Ashm. 208, fos. 1–74*
1603	Licensed to practise physic and astronomy by University of Cambridge
*c.*1603–7	*'Forman's treatise on the plague', Ashm. 1403*
1604	*'Forman his repetition of the troble he had with the doctors', a psalm, Ashm. 240, fos. 25–7ᵛ, cont. 802, fos. 131–3ᵛ*
Sept. 1605	Birth of daughter, Dority (d. 1 Jan. 1606)
Sept. 1605	*'Of the name of Forman', Ashm. fos. 214–19ᵛ*
*c.*1605–6	*'The firste of the Formans', Ashm. 802, fos. 211–15ᵛ*
Oct. 1606	Birth of son, Clement
1606+	*'The issue of Simon Forman', Ashm. 208, fos. 225–6*
*c.*1607	*'Heavens', Ashm. 244, fos. 34–118*
1607	*Untitled plague treatise, Ashm. 1436*
*c.*1607–10	*'Of appoticarie druges', Ashm. 1494, 1491*
*c.*1607	*Untitled alchemical commonplace book, Ashm. 1430*
Sept. 1611	Forman died, buried at St Mary's Church, Lambeth, 12 Sept.

INTRODUCTION

It was hard to summon the devil. On a stage in London in 1616 Fitz-dottrell lamented his inability to conjure the evil one. He had heard that even the most renowned astrologers and physicians, including Simon Forman, had failed 'to shew a man the Divell in true sort'. This was an opening scene of Ben Jonson's *The Devil is an Ass*, a satire recasting the story of Faust in which the devil visited London and found it so full of evil that there was no work for him to do.[1] Forman died in 1611 and in 1615 he was retrospectively implicated in the great Jacobean scandal: the trials of Frances Howard, countess of Essex, and her lover, Robert Carr, Viscount Rochester, earl of Somerset, for the poisoning of Sir Thomas Overbury.[2] In Forman's final decade, Howard had consulted Forman for assistance in winning the affections of Carr and further estranging her husband, Robert Devereux, third earl of Essex.[3] During the trial of Anne Turner, Howard's alleged accomplice, pieces of parchment and cloth with magical symbols and obscene figures in metals and wax were displayed as evidence of Forman's demonic activities. As the crowds moved forward to see these objects, the official report recorded, 'there was heard a crack from the scaffolds, which caused great fear, tumult, and confusion among the spectators, and throughout the hall, everyone fearing hurt, as if the Devil had been present, and grown angry to have his workmanship showed by such as were not his own scholars'.[4] Later, Sir Edward Coke, the presiding judge and great legal authority, denounced Turner as guilty of the seven deadly sins and concluded

[1] Ben Jonson, *The Devil is an Ass*, ed. C. H. Herford, P. Simpson, and E. Simpson, *Ben Jonson*, 11 vols. (Oxford, 1925–52), iv, I. ii; see also II. viii.

[2] A[nthony] W[eldon], *The court and character of King James* (1650), 110; [Arthur Wilson], *The five yeares of King James* (1643), 18–19; Alastair Bellany, *The Politics of Court Scandal in Early Modern England: News Culture and the Overbury Affair, 1603–1660* (Cambridge, 2003); David Lindley, *The Trials of Frances Howard: Fact and Fiction at the Court of King James* (1993); William McElwee, *The Murder of Sir Thomas Overbury* (1952); A. L. Rowse, *Simon Forman: Sex and Society in Shakespeare's Age* (1974), 255–8; Barbara Traister, *The Notorious Astrological Physician of London: Works and Days of Simon Forman* (Chicago, 2001), ch. 8; Beatrice White, *Cast of Ravens: The Strange Case of Sir Thomas Overbury* (1965).

[3] For a copy of a letter from Frances Howard to Forman which was shown during the trials see *Complete collection of state trials*, ed. T. B. Howell, (1816), 931–2. Manuscript copies of this and related letters circulated widely, e.g. Bodleian, Dowdson MS 58, fo. 158; see also Bellany, *Politics of Court Scandal*, 85, 95. During the public trial of Anne Turner, Jean Forman, Forman's widow, testified that on two occasions Turner came to her house to search for and burn letters and papers of Forman's: Rowse, *Forman*, 261; White, *Cast of Ravens*, 123.

[4] *State trials*, ed. Howell, ii. 934; see also Bellany, *Politics of Court Scandal*, 149, 151.

that she was 'the daughter of the devil Forman'.[5] Whatever his involvement in the Overbury affair, Forman was remembered on the stage of early modern London as a quack and a conjurer meddling in the affairs of women.[6]

Forman, however, was more than a stock character. He documented the thousands of clients who sought his astrological services, the complex rules of astrological physic, the texts he read and experiments he conducted in pursuit of the philosophers' stone, and his quarrels, romances, and dreams in 15,000 written pages.[7] After his death, Richard Napier (1559–1634), a cleric, astrologer-physician, and Forman's closest associate, acquired most of his papers.[8] He passed them along with the rest of his books and papers to his nephew, Sir Richard Napier (1607–76), in the early 1630s; and at his death his son, Thomas (b. 1646), offered the collection to the assiduous antiquarian Elias Ashmole (1617–92). Ashmole amassed thousands of astrological, alchemical, and other manuscripts, including the bulk of the Forman manuscripts that are now extant, and he bequeathed his collection to Oxford University, where it lay almost untouched until the nineteenth century.[9] While cataloguing Ashmole's manuscripts in the 1830s, William Black drew the attention of John Payne Collier, the Shakespearian scholar and notorious forger, to Forman's accounts of four plays by Shakespeare.[10] These accounts are the only 'discoveries' by Collier that have not been proved to be forgeries and, though their authenticity has been questioned, their contents and format are typical of Forman's writings

[5] *State trials*, ed. Howell, ii. 935. Coke had encountered Forman in 1596–7, in his capacity as Attorney General: Ashm. 234, fo. 132, 151v; *DNB*.

[6] In Jonson's *Epicoene*, Dauphine compares Truewit's powers to procure the love of women with those of Forman and Medea, the mythological enchantress: *Jonson*, ed. Herford *et al.*, v, IV. i. For the argument that there is a direct allusion to Forman in *The Alchemist*, and that Forman was the model for Christopher Marlowe's *Doctor Faustus* see Susan Cerasano, 'Philip Henslowe, Simon Forman, and the Theatrical Community of the 1590s', *Shakespeare Quarterly*, 44 (1993), 145–58. Nathaniel Hawthorne and other authors later used Forman as a demonic figure: Traister, *Forman*, 4, 188–9.

[7] A list of Forman's MSS, by subject, and with titles and dates, is provided in the Bibliography.

[8] Ashm. 227, fo. 85v, 103; 275, fos. 103, 108, 119, 171v, esp. 275, cited in Michael MacDonald, *Mystical Bedlam: Madness, Anxiety, and Healing in Seventeenth-Century England* (Cambridge, 1981), 290 n. Ashm. 227 is Napier's casebook for 1627 and records negotiations between Napier and Forman's son, Clement, about books and money. MacDonald's reference to Ashm. 275 should read 200. See also Ashm. 200, fos. 167v, 170, 172, cited in Traister, *Forman*, p. xiv.

[9] *Elias Ashmole, Autobiographical and Historical Notes, Correspondence, and Other Sources*, ed. C. H. Josten (Oxford, 1966), i. 210; iii. 1208; iv. 1454–5, 1809; *William Lilly's history of his life and times*, ed. C. Burman (1774), 23.

[10] These are *Macbeth*, *Cymbeline*, *The Winter's Tale*, and a play called *Richard II* which does not resemble the play by Shakespeare of that name. For the identification of Black as the person who brought the MSS to the attention of Collier see 'Dr Simon Forman's diary', ed. James Halliwell, *The Archæologist, and Journal of Antiquarian Science*, 1 (1841–2), 37. For interest in Forman's papers earlier in the 19th cent., see 'Extracts from a manuscript of Dr. Simon Forman', ed. Philip Bliss, *Censura literae*, 8 (1807), 409–13; Anthony Wood, *Athenae Oxonienses*, ed. Philip Bliss, 5 vols. (1813–20), ii. 98–105, 373–4; Joseph Ritson, *Bibliographia Poetica: A Catalogue of Engleish Poets* (1802), 5.

in his final years.[11] Another Shakespearian, James Halliwell, prepared an edition of Forman's life-writings for the Camden Society. Because these included details of Forman's sexual activities, the edition was stopped, and the appellation of philanderer once again adorned Forman's reputation.[12]

One historian has noted that Forman's 'life seems almost the invention of an intemperate romancer'.[13] A. L. Rowse capitalized on this reputation, christening Forman 'the Elizabethan Pepys'. Forman's casebooks, life-writings, and diary record the minutiae of his life, including his relations with women thinly guised in the phrase 'halek cum muher', meaning to have sexual intercourse with a woman.[14] Rowse focuses on Forman, the men with whom he dined, and the women with whom he was intimate, including Emilia Lanier, Shakespeare's alleged Dark Lady.[15] Finally, Barbara Traister portrays Forman's life and manuscripts, preserving the vivacity and complexity of his family, household, and career, but she stops short of recovering his voice for the histories of medicine and the occult sciences.[16] Forman would be delighted to have been remembered, and distressed to have been so enduringly misunderstood. Throughout this book as I document his tumultuous career he protests his importance. Despite his self-obsessed, humourless, and incoherent writings, he produced one of the most comprehensive archives of information about medicine, astrology, alchemy, and magic in early modern England. This is the subject of this book; it is not a biography. Forman was too twisted and

[11] The play accounts are Ashm. 208, fos. 200–2; James Halliwell, *Works of Shakespeare* (1859); Halliwell, *Outlines of the life of Shakespeare* (Brighton, 1881), 78; Rowse, *Forman*, 303–7. For discussions of whether they are forgeries see *The Tragedy of Macbeth*, ed. J. Q. Adams, (Boston, 1931), p. viii; J. Dover Wilson and R. W. Hunt, 'The Authenticity of Simon Forman's *Bocke of Plaies*', *Review of English Studies*, 23 (1947), 193–200; Katherine Duncan-Jones, *Ungentle Shakespeare: Scenes from his Life* (2001), xii–xiii; Dewey Ganzel, *Fortune and Men's Eyes: The Career of John Payne Collier* (Oxford, 1982), 61; Sydney Race, 'Simon Forman's "Bocke of Plaies" Examined', *Notes and Queries* (Jan. 1958), 9–14; Samuel Schoenbaum, *Shakespeare and Others* (Washington, DC, 1985), ch. 1; Samuel A. Tannenbaum, *Shakesperian Scraps, and other Elizabethan Fragments* (New York, 1933), ch. 1. This literature is surveyed and the MSS considered alongside Forman's other papers in my '"Remember Also the Storri of Cymbalin", or is Simon Forman's "Bocke of Plaies" a Forgery?' (forthcoming).

[12] One hundred copies were printed privately, *The autobiography and personal diary of Dr Simon Forman*, ed. James Halliwell, (1849). See also 'Forman's diary', ed. Halliwell, 34–7. Rowse, *Forman*, 267–302, includes these texts and part of a family history, Ashm. 208, fos. 218–23. I have relied on the MSS.

[13] D. C. Allen, *The Star-Crossed Renaissance: The Quarrel about Astrology and its Influence in England* (New York, 1973 [1951]), 105.

[14] The full phrase was 'halekekeros harescum tauro cum muher', but Forman almost always abbreviated it.

[15] Judith Cook, *Dr Simon Foreman, a Most Notorious Physician* (2001) follows Rowse. Emilia Lanier has received more attention than Forman's other patients, e.g. Germaine Greer, Jeslyn Medoff, Melinda Sansone, and Susan Hastings (eds.), *Kissing the Rod: An Anthology of Seventeenth Century Women's Verse* (1988), 44–6; Diane Purkiss (ed.), *Renaissance Women: The Plays of Elizabeth Carey; the Poems of Aemelia Lanyer* (1994).

[16] Traister, *Forman.*

self-absorbed to act as a lens; instead his papers are a cornucopia, offering up the histories of medicine and magic in London. Before saying more about the methods that guided my reading of Forman's papers and the organization of this book, I will reflect on the disciplines that have informed this work.

In the past three decades the social history of medicine has burgeoned. Histories of institutions and physicians have been augmented with accounts of the full medical hierarchy, including unauthorized, or irregular, medical practitioners.[17] The notion of a medical marketplace has been used to explore the dynamics in the exchange between medical practitioners and their clients; popular notions of healing and health have been reconstructed through surveys of vernacular, printed, medical works; and experiences of healing have been retrieved from diaries and life-writings.[18] Questions of gender, representations, and the life-cycle have been considered, often through non-textual sources.[19] Elizabethan and Jacobean England holds a pivotal place in these histories. Calls for new, reformed natural philosophy, mechanical arts, and medicine could be heard during this period, but are drowned out in the later, raucous programmes to implement Baconian reforms in London beginning in the 1630s.[20] Nonetheless, the promotion of alchemical and Paracelsian medicine in the sixteenth century has been teased from prefaces to cheap treatises

[17] Margaret Pelling and Charles Webster, 'Medical Practitioners', in Charles Webster (ed.), *Health, Medicine and Mortality in the Sixteenth Century* (Cambridge, 1979), 165–235; Margaret Pelling, *The Common Lot: Sickness, Medical Occupations and the Urban Poor in Early Modern England* (1998); Margaret Pelling, *Medical Conflicts in Early Modern London: Patronage, Physicians, and Irregular Practitioners 1550–1640* (Oxford, 2003); Charles Webster, *The Great Instauration: Science, Medicine and Reform 1626–1660* (1975). For the impact of Pelling and Webster's 1979 essay see, for instance, Laurence Brockliss and Colin Jones, *The Medical World of Early Modern France* (Oxford, 1997); Michael McVaugh, *Medicine before the Plague: Practitioners and their Patients in the Crown of Aragon, 1285–1345* (Cambridge, 1993); Katharine Park, *Doctors and Medicine in Early Renaissance Florence* (Princeton, 1985).

[18] For the medical marketplace, see Harold Cook, *The Decline of the Old Medical Regime in Stuart London* (Ithaca, NY, 1986); David Gentilcore, *Healers and Healing in Early Modern Italy* (Manchester, 1998); Roy Porter, *Health for Sale: Quackery in England 1660–1850* (Manchester, 1989). For medical texts see Paul Slack, 'Mirrors of Health and Treasures of Poor Men: The Uses of the Vernacular Medical Literature of Tudor England', in Webster (ed.), *Health, Medicine and Mortality*, 237–73; Mary Fissell, 'Readers, Texts, and Contexts: Vernacular Medical Works in Early Modern England', in Roy Porter (ed.), *The Popularisation of Medicine, 1650–1850* (1992), 72–96. For studies that focus on the patient see Lucinda McCray Beier, *Sufferers and Healers: The Experience of Illness in Seventeenth-Century England* (1987); Barbara Duden, *The Woman beneath the Skin: A Doctor's Patients in Eighteenth-Century Germany*, tr. Thomas Dunlap (Cambridge, Mass., 1991); Mary Fissell, *Patients, Power and the Poor in Eighteenth-Century Bristol* (Cambridge, 1991); Gianna Pomata, *Contracting a Cure: Patients, Healers, and the Law in Early Modern Bologna* (Baltimore, Md., 1998); Dorothy and Roy Porter, *In Sickness and in Health: The British Experience, 1650–1850* (1988).

[19] For instance, see Helen King, *Hippocrates' Woman: Reading the Female Body in Ancient Greece* (1998), esp. chs. 10, 11; Pelling, *Common Lot*, chs. 5–8.

[20] Christopher Hill, *Intellectual Origins of the English Revolution* (1972 [1965]); Webster, *Great Instauration.*

and manuscript collections.[21] Projects to improve and reform natural philosophy and the mathematical and mechanical arts have also been recovered.[22] Forman's papers provide an exceptional record of medical practices, ideas, and conflicts in London from his arrival there around 1590 to his death in 1611. But Forman's medicine is itself extraordinary. He was self-taught, he espoused a radical astrology, he thought himself destined to discover the philosophers' stone and other secrets of nature, and he formulated, articulated, and defended his credentials as an astrologer-physician in opposition to the College of Physicians of London. He was not a reformer, but he undermined the principles of humanist medicine at the same time as aspiring to the status of a physician.

In theory most medical practitioners in European urban centres were regulated according to a tripartite hierarchy. Physicians were schooled in the theory of medicine, or physic, and diagnosed diseases and prescribed courses of therapy. Surgeons were concerned with the surface of the body and performed manual operations, such as bleeding or setting broken bones. Apothecaries prepared medicines according to physicians' prescriptions. The art of physic was taught at the universities in England and abroad, while the manual skills of the surgeons and apothecaries were learned through apprenticeships. In London the practice of physic was regulated by the College of Physicians, surgery by the Barber-Surgeons' Company, and until 1618 the apothecaries were included within the Grocers' Company.[23] This was an ideal structure of authority and knowledge, not the medical reality; in practice, the boundaries between physic, surgery, and the preparation of medicines were often traversed despite regulatory mechanisms. Irregular medical practitioners represented all ranges of learning, from those trained at universities to those who were illiterate, and

[21] Allen Debus, *The English Paracelsians* (1965); Paul Kocher, 'Paracelsian Medicine in England: The First Thirty Years', *Journal of the History of Medicine*, 2 (1947), 451–80; Charles Webster, 'Alchemical and Paracelsian Medicine', in Webster (ed.), *Health, Medicine and Mortality*, 301–34.

[22] See for instance Eric H. Ash, *Power, Knowledge, and Expertise in Elizabethan England* (Baltimore, Md., 2004); James A. Bennett, 'The Mechanics' Philosophy and the Mechanical Philosophy', *History of Science*, 24 (1986), 1–28; Mordechai Feingold, *The Mathematicians' Apprenticeship: Science, Universities and Society in England 1560–1640* (Cambridge, 1984); Deborah Harkness, '"Strange" Ideas and "English" Knowledge: Natural Science Exchange in Elizabethan London', in Pamela H. Smith and Paula Findlen (eds.), *Merchants and Marvels: Commerce, Science, and Art in Early Modern Europe* (New York and London, 2002), 137–60. For work focusing on John Dee see esp. Nicholas Clulee, *John Dee's Natural Philosophy: Between Science and Religion* (1988); Deborah Harkness, *John Dee's Conversations with Angels: Cabala, Alchemy, and the End of Nature* (Cambridge, 1999); William Sherman, *John Dee: The Politics of Reading and Writing in the English Renaissance* (Amherst, Mass., 1995).

[23] R. S. Roberts, 'The Personnel and Practice of Medicine in Tudor and Stuart England: Part 2, London', *Medical History*, 8 (1964), 217–29; Patrick Wallis, 'Medicines for London: The trade, regulations and life-cycle of London apothecaries, *c.*1610–*c.*1670', D.Phil. thesis, University of Oxford, 2002.

from those who earned substantial fees to those who might practise medicine occasionally, for little or no payment. Like other practitioners, Forman disregarded the strictures of this ideal; unlike them he kept records of his defiance of the College of Physicians, study of astrological and alchemical medicine, and consultations with thousands of patients.[24]

Forman's activities have previously been made to conform to the hierarchical model of medical practitioners. He has been dismissed either as a member of the popular legions of unlettered medical practitioners or as an anomalous astrologer who appealed to the whims of the gullible masses and fanciful gentlewomen alike. Neither of these descriptions accurately reflects Forman's position in the medical world of Elizabethan and early Jacobean London. He was unusual in the numbers of patients who consulted him and in the detailed records that he kept. He stood apart from the medical elite because he was not formally educated and because he represented, and boldly asserted, medical ideas that were antithetical to those held by most learned physicians. Like many people who became irregular medical practitioners, he had been apprenticed to a grocer-apothecary. Unlike them he styled himself as an astrologer-physician, not a provider of specific remedies. He saw himself as divinely chosen to be a practitioner of the true physic and a nemesis of the College of Physicians, portraying himself as singularly accomplished in the medical applications of alchemy, astrology, and magic. He speaks for the shadowy figures in the history of medicine who were interested in hermeticism and Paracelsianism and with his voice this study reassesses the model of the medical world and the status of the occult arts in early modern England.

In sixteenth-century Europe the Galenic theory of disease was integral to medical cosmology, as taught at the universities and articulated in humanist books. According to the teachings of Galen, a person's temperament depended on the balance of the humours, varied according to sex, and changed over time. People with an abundance of hot and moist humours were sanguine, those with hot and dry were choleric, those with cold and moist were phlegmatic, and cold and dry were melancholic. Women were generally colder and moister than men, and people became colder and dryer with age. The temperament also fluctuated with the seasons. Disease occurred when the balance of the humours was disrupted and this balance could be maintained or restored by evacuating the body with purges, vomits, or blood-letting in accordance with a person's temperament and the time of year.[25]

[24] Pelling and Webster, 'Medical Practitioners', 165–89; Pelling, *Medical Conflicts*, 228 and *passim.*

[25] Oswei Temkin, *Galenism: Rise and Decline of a Medical Philosophy* (Ithaca, NY, 1973). For an Elizabethan account see e.g. William Bullein, *The governement of healthe* (1595).

The Swiss reformer and physician, Theophrast von Hohenheim, known as Paracelsus (1493–1541), challenged the humoral theory of disease and the teachings of Galen. He outlined what amounts to a philosophy of medicine which combined the late fifteenth-century revival of hermeticism by the Florentine Neoplatonists with a call for the value of experience above bookish learning. Galenism, he argued, was a corruption of the medicine that Adam had practised after the Fall; the true and ancient medicine needed to be recovered from the secrets of nature. Like the Neoplatonists he outlined a cosmology in which the macrocosm (the universe) and the microcosm (man) were analogous. Instead of the elements of earth, air, fire, and water, he described all things as made from salt, sulphur, and mercury and he outlined analogies between each of these substances and, for instance, the body, soul, and spirit and the liver, heart, and brain. Disease was not the result of an imbalance of humours but was caused by damage to or impediment of the spirit (*archeus*) when a malevolent influence penetrated a part of the body. Paracelsus' ideas were codified and promoted by his followers in the second half of the sixteenth century. Throughout this and the next century Paracelsian notions of infection and Galenic theories of occult diseases overlapped with one another, a shared territory where Galenists and Paracelsians defined their doctrines in opposition to one another.[26]

In practice Paracelsian and traditional learned practitioners used different methods, though there was not always a direct correlation between a practitioner's methods of diagnosis, repertory of treatments, and philosophy of medicine. Conventionally a physician heeded the positions of the stars and planets, checked the speed of the pulse, and examined the colour, smell, and taste of the urine to assess the state of the humours and to recommend a diet and evacuations to maintain and restore health. According to a Paracelsian cosmology the malevolent influences of the stars and planets might actively cause disease and a practitioner versed in the complex skills of astrology could identify these causes and determine the best type and timing of a remedy. While Galenic teachings defined remedies according to a principle of opposites, Paracelsian remedies were governed by the doctrine of signatures, according to which a plant, mineral, or animal with characteristics similar to those of the

[26] Stuart Clark, 'Demons and Disease: The Disenchantment of the Sick (1500–1700)', in Marijke Gijswijt-Hofstra, Hilary Marland, and Hans de Waardt (eds.), *Illness and Healing Alternatives in Western Europe* (1997), 38–55, esp. 42–4; Clark, *Thinking with Demons: The Idea of Witchcraft in Early Modern Europe* (Oxford, 1997), 226–7; Brian Copenhaver, 'Scholastic Philosophy and Renaissance Magic in the *De vita* of Marsilio Ficino', *Renaissance Quarterly*, 37 (1984), 523–54; Linda Deer Richardson, 'The Generation of Disease: Occult Causes and Diseases of the Total Substance', in Andrew Wear, Roger K. French, and I. M. Lonie (eds.), *The Medical Renaissance of the Sixteenth Century* (Cambridge, 1985), 175–94, esp. 184, 188–93. The revival of the Hippocratic tradition is another component of this story.

afflicted part of the body had healing properties. Strong waters and other substances, alchemically prepared to release vital mineral properties, could be used to fortify health or to open obstructions through vomiting, purging, urination, or sweating. Amulets harnessing astral or sympathetic powers might also be used to enhance health or counter disease.[27]

Forman was an untutored, irregular medical practitioner, more concerned with the complexities of medical practices than the intricacies of doctrinal positions. Occasionally he opposed Galenic medicine and promoted a Paracelsian cosmology. He never articulated a clear philosophy of medicine, though in his final decade he came close, prompted by his conflicts with the College of Physicians. Mostly he expounded the virtues of the astrologer-physician and protested his divinely imparted gifts to read the stars and heal disease. He called himself a physician and a gentleman, and, without affixing a label to his activities, he presented himself as a philosopher, adept, prophet, and magus, heir to the wisdom of Adam, Moses, Hermes Trismegistus, and Solomon. Forman's medical ideas and practices cannot be separated from his pursuit of astrology, alchemy, and magic. This study is as much about the occult, or hermetic sciences as it is about the history of medicine.

Throughout this book I will dwell on the fates of diverse astrological and alchemical traditions. Various sorts of magic also feature in my account, but unlike astrology and alchemy, magic has a plurality of meanings and requires some words here. Magic is often defined in opposition to science, religion, and rationality; it is unsystematic, unorthodox, irrational.[28] In medieval Europe it was defined as a perversion of religion. Demons invented it, taught it to men, and were the vehicles through which man could effect the unnatural. It might be used to create amusing illusions, to bind the will of another person, or to divine the future. From the thirteenth century, following Albertus Magnus' taxonomy of magic, scholars differentiated between magic effected through rituals to invoke demons or spirits, and natural magic, operating through the occult forces in nature. At the same time increasingly elaborate ritual magic from Arabic and Jewish sources was imported to Europe.[29]

[27] Owen Hannaway, *The Chemists and the Word: The Didactic Origins of Chemistry* (Baltimore, Md., 1975); Walter Pagel, *Paracelsus: An Introduction to Philosophical Medicine in the Age of the Renaissance* (Basel, 1982); D. P. Walker, *Spiritual and Demonic Magic from Ficino to Campanella* (1958); Charles Webster, *From Paracelsus to Newton: Magic and the Making of Modern Science* (Cambridge, 1980). For a clear contemporary account of Paracelsian medicine, see Oswald Croll, *Philosophy Reformed and Improved*, tr. Henry Pinnell (1657).

[28] Stanley Tambiah, *Magic, Science, Religion, and the Scope of Rationality* (Cambridge, 1990).

[29] Richard Kieckhefer, *Magic in the Middle Ages* (Cambridge, 1989), chs. 1, 4, 6; Sophie Page, 'Magic at St. Augustine's, Canterbury, in the Late Middle Ages', Ph.D. thesis, Warburg Institute, University of London, 2000.

Astrology, alchemy, and the varieties of magic hold a central yet shifting place in the history of early modern science. Together they are the pre-sciences or pseudo-sciences, the domain of the occult, itself brought into the remit of the natural philosopher in the seventeenth century.[30] Separately they each have detailed histories, technical, social, and political.[31] In the late fifteenth century Marsilio Ficino combined astrological medicine and Neoplatonic philosophy and articulated a comprehensive and influential theory of magic. He explicated the notion of a *spiritus mundi*, beamed to the earth by the stars and planets, potentially understood and controlled by magic. Stones and metals with stellar characteristics could be positioned on one's body; medicine infused with appropriate properties ingested; words and songs could invoke heavenly powers. Magic was not a perversion of religion but a perfection of it. This is what Frances Yates refers to as the hermetic tradition, following Ficino's exposition of the writings attributed to Hermes Trismegistus, the mythical ancient Egyptian sage. Yates posits a bold thesis about hermetic magic as the beginning of man's cosmological relocation from being a subject of God to an agent capable of altering his own destiny: wherein lie the seeds of modern science.[32] Numerous scholars have queried such a general and determined definition of hermeticism. There was not a unified theory of the occult, a singular tradition of natural magic, nor a notion of a hermetic philosophy.[33]

I have used each of these terms, following Forman in meaning if not in terminology. Where he presented himself as heir to the knowledge of Hermes, I refer to hermeticism and call him a magus; where he explicated a wild cosmology drawn from a pseudo-Paracelsian text, I refer to Paracelsianism; where he referred to hidden powers, I might use the term occult, though if these powers came from the stars, they were also astral; where he stressed the importance of knowing the natural, demonic, or divine causes of a disease and specified the astral properties necessary to treat it, I refer to his drawing on vitalist, Paracelsian, hermetic, or occult principles, depending on his sources and

[30] John Henry, 'Occult Qualities and the Experimental Philosophy: Active Principles in Pre-Newtonian Matter Theory', *History of Science*, 24 (1986), 335–81; Keith Hutchison, 'What Happened to Occult Qualities in the Scientific Revolution?', *Isis*, 73 (1982), 233–53.

[31] For a discussion of the historiographies of alchemy and astrology, see William Newman and Anthony Grafton, 'Introduction: The Problematic Status of Astrology and Alchemy in Premodern Europe', in Newman and Grafton (eds.), *Secrets of Nature: Astrology and Alchemy in Early Modern Europe* (Cambridge, Mass., 2001), 1–37. For an example of the merits of an eclectic approach see Michael Hunter, 'Alchemy, Magic and Moralism in the Thought of Robert Boyle', *British Journal for the History of Science*, 23 (1990), 387–410.

[32] Frances Yates, *Giordano Bruno and the Hermetic Tradition* (Chicago, 1964), esp. p. 116 and ch. 22.

[33] For criticisms of the Yates thesis see esp. Clulee, *John Dee's Natural Philosophy*, ch. 1; Brian Vickers (ed.), *Occult and Scientific Mentalities in the Renaissance* (Cambridge, 1984), introduction.

exposition; where he called himself a necromancer, so do I. Across the subjects that he studied and practised, Forman brought together many traditions, ancient, medieval, modern; pagan, Jewish, Arabic, and Christian. In the title of this book magic encompasses all of these things, the hidden powers, dangerous knowledge, and particular arts to control such powers and acquire such knowledge, whether natural, demonic, or divine.

These fluid and specific definitions are in part necessary because Forman was not a rigorous scholar. They have allowed me to identify instances in which Forman associated occult, hermetic, Paracelsian, astral, and vitalist traditions, and guarded against my essentializing his studies and practices into an reified, coherent philosophy. Despite, or perhaps because of the Yates thesis, grand narratives of the occult sciences in the scientific revolution have subsided in favour of histories of the astrological or alchemical pursuits of individual practitioners, thus recovering the expertise necessary to study such a subject, but at the same time imposing artificial disciplinary boundaries on the endeavour. Medicine is especially problematic. For instance, although Yates describes Ficino's medicine as inextricably bound to astrology and natural magic, she presents it as a personal quest, the by-product of something bigger.[34] Similarly, although John Dee has prompted scholars to consider his interests in the round, medicine has not figured in accounts of the religious and national motives of his studies.[35] Finally, historians increasingly interested in the preternatural have demonstrated the centrality of medicine to understanding the pursuit of strange and wondrous things in nature; curiosity itself prompting eclectic history.[36]

With the exception of a pamphlet on longitude, nothing that Forman wrote was printed. He did not engage with the community of Latin scholars in which there was a forum for treatises on the occult. He did not have the book-learning or linguistic expertise of Dee, Giordano Bruno, or Robert Fludd. But

[34] Yates, *Giordano Bruno*, 60–1. See also Lynn Thorndike, *A History of Magic and Experimental Science*, 8 vols. (New York, 1923–41), iv. 562–3; Brian Copenhaver, 'A Tale of Two Fishes: Magical Objects in Natural History from Antiquity through the Scientific Revolution', *Journal of the History of Ideas*, 52 (1991), 373–89, esp. 384–5; Copenhaver, 'Natural Magic, Hermetism, and Occultism in Early Modern Science', in D. Lindberg and R. Westman (eds.), *Reappraisals of the Scientific Revolution* (Cambridge, 1990), 261–301, esp. 272–5; Copenhaver, 'Astrology and Magic', in Charles Schmitt (ed.), *The Cambridge History of Renaissance Philosophy* (Cambridge, 1988), 264–300, esp. 283–4.

[35] Dee's library was an indispensable resource for Elizabethans seeking alchemical and Paracelsian texts: Penny Bayer, 'Lady Margaret Clifford's Alchemical Recipe Book and the John Dee Circle', *Ambix*, 52 (2005), 271–84; David Harley, 'Rychard Bostok of Tanridge, Surrey (*c*.1530–1605), M.P., Paracelsian Propagandist and Friend of John Dee', *Ambix*, 47 (2000), 29–36; Webster, 'Alchemical and Paracelsian Medicine'.

[36] Clark, *Thinking with Demons*; Lorraine Daston and Katharine Park, *Wonders and the Order of Nature 1150–1750* (New York, 1998); Lyndal Roper, *Oedipus and the Devil: Witchcraft, Sexuality and Religion in Early Modern Europe* (1994); Simon Schaffer, 'Piety, Physic and Prodigious Abstinence', in Ole Peter Grell and Andrew Cunningham (eds.), *Religio Medici: Religion and Medicine in Seventeenth Century England* (Aldershot, 1996), 171–203; and many of the essays in Smith and Findlen (eds.), *Merchants and Marvels*.

he read, magpie-like, through all of the books that he could, depositing the fruits of his reading in his notes and treatises. Precedents for studying Forman lie in the histories of reading and in microhistories of other untutored readers.[37] Like Nehemiah Wallington, a London wood turner, Forman filled dozens of notebooks, though Forman was keen to act as an agent of God while Wallington chronicled His judgements.[38] Like Menocchio, an Italian miller, Forman boldly and incoherently asserted a controversial cosmology, though he was curiously, and perhaps prudently, almost silent on the subject of religion.[39] Indeed the handful of clues about Forman's religion are heterodox and inconsistent, like so much about him. He gestured to Roman Catholic doctrines, pursued pre-Reformation legends about creation, and deployed Protestant language; many of his friends were recusants, others Protestant clerics, and he served as a vestryman in Lambeth in 1610.[40] I have tried to allow for the possibility that Forman's religion was more evident in his life than in his papers, and for the impact that his Catholic tendencies had on his studies and reputation.

While this has become a study that engages with the history of medicine and the history of science, from the outset it has been an anthropology of the medical world of early modern London.[41] Naïve, in part deliberately, with William Black's catalogue of the Ashmole collection as my guide, I escaped into the thousands of Forman's pages bound in well-tooled and brass-clasped leather, anticipating that they would generate questions about history, mythology, politics, ritual, economics, sociology, kinship, and culture.[42] Forman paraded his

[37] On the history of reading, see for instance Roger Chartier, *The Order of Books: Readers, Authors and Libraries in Europe between the Fourteenth and the Eighteenth Centuries*, tr. Lydia Cochraine (Cambridge, 1994); Anthony Grafton and Lisa Jardine, '"Studied for Action": How Gabriel Harvey Read his Livy', *Past and Present*, 129 (1990), 30–78; Grafton, *Commerce with the Classics: Ancient Books and Renaissance Readers* (Ann Arbor, 1997); Kevin Sharpe, *Reading Revolutions: The Politics of Reading in Early Modern England* (New Haven, 2000); Sherman, *Dee*. On microhistory see Edward Muir, 'Introduction: Observing Trifles', in Edward Muir and Guido Ruggiero (eds.), *Microhistory and the Lost Peoples of Europe*, tr. Eren Branch (Baltimore, 1991), pp. vii–xxviii.

[38] Paul Seaver, *Wallington's World: A Puritan Artisan in Seventeenth-Century London* (1985).

[39] Carlo Ginzburg, *The Cheese and the Worms: The Cosmos of a Sixteenth-Century Miller*, tr. John and Anne Tedeschi (1980). See also Wolfgang Behringer, *Shaman of Oberstdorf: Chonrad Stoeckhlin and the Phantoms of the Night*, tr. Erik Midelfort (Charlottesville, Va., 1998).

[40] See Ch. 11 below.

[41] This research was inspired by Michael MacDonald's *Mystical Bedlam* and prompted in reaction to Keith Thomas's *Religion and the Decline of Magic*. For a discussion of anthropology and history, see Thomas's exchange with Hildred Geertz: 'An Anthropology of Religion and Magic', parts 1 and 2, *Journal of Interdisciplinary History*, 6 (1975), 71–89, 91–109. See also Jonathan Barry, 'Keith Thomas and the Problem of Witchcraft', in Jonathan Barry, Marianne Hester, and Gareth Roberts (eds.), *Witchcraft in Early Modern Europe: Studies in Culture and Belief* (Cambridge, 1996), 1–45.

[42] William Black, *A descriptive, analytical and critical catalogue of the manuscripts bequeathed unto the University of Oxford by Elias Ashmole* (Oxford, 1845); W. D. Macray, *Index to the catalogue of manuscripts of Elias Ashmole* (Oxford, 1866). For Black's experience of working with these papers, see R. W. Hunt, 'The Cataloguing of the Ashmolean Collection of Books and Manuscripts', *Bodleian Library Record*, 4 (1952–3), 161–70.

treatises on astrological physic and the stories of his life; he assiduously logged thousands of consultations in his casebooks; he refused to explain the magical and cosmological underpinnings of his interest in the lives of Adam and Eve, burying them in an incoherent set of essays on the motions of the heavens. I indulged him, then sought the voices of others. But although he was always with people, few of them are known to us through the historical record, and Forman seldom provided introductions.[43] Unlike Girolamo Cardano, for instance, whose interest in anatomy led him to examine Leonardo da Vinci's drawings and to calculate Vesalius' horoscope, there is no evidence that Forman knew notable scholars of his time.[44] He did not comment on the new astronomy, nor had he any contact with John Dee or the Sidney Circle.[45] Nostradamus was a celebrity, Forman was not.[46] He was a creature of the city, not the court.[47] He fought with the College of Physicians and mathematical practitioners of London, and though he seldom cited them he probably read countless books by his contemporaries on plague, creation, alchemy, astrology, astronomy, medicine, and other subjects.

Forman lived with and through his papers, constantly shifting passages, copying and recopying, never completing; mercifully naming and dating most of his notes and writings in a hand that became larger and looser as his eyes troubled him and he could afford more paper. I have generated a superabundance of bibliographical evidence, mostly relegated to the notes and Bibliography. My method is ingenuous and forensic, assuming nothing, recovering the value and meaning of each event and text through close analysis and association. Forman has rewarded my efforts with the vivid stories that

[43] Although many of the associates whom Forman mentioned were identified by Rowse, more work needs to be done on, for instance, Forman's involvement with the recusant community and numerous legal cases: Rowse, *Forman*, esp. chs. 7–10; Traister, *Forman*, ch. 7.

[44] Nancy Siraisi, *The Clock and the Mirror: Girolamo Cardano and Renaissance Medicine* (Princeton, 1997), 99.

[45] On Forman's astronomy, see Ch. 2 below. It would not be surprising if Forman, a native of Wiltshire, had sought patronage from Mary Herbert, countess of Pembroke, and in 1602 he had a dream about meeting the Herberts in Wiltshire: Ashm. 1472, p. 810. Perhaps though he shunned them, since he noted in 1605 that his grandfather, Richard, had a dispute with William Herbert, earl of Pembroke, over some land: Ashm. 208, fos. 214–27. John Aubrey speculated on Forman's dealing with the Herberts: John Aubrey, *The natural history of Wiltshire*, ed. John Britton (1847), 79. Richard Napier seems to have known Dee from at least 1602, though there is no indication that he introduced Forman to him: Ashm. 338, fos. 7, 43; 221, fo. 56. For the possibility that Forman knew Robert Burton, see Ch. 3 n. 74 below. For the suggestion that Fludd copied a book of Forman's see Lilly, *Life*, 17–18: 'for I have seen the same word for word in an English manuscript formerly belonging to Dr Willoughby of Gloucestershire'.

[46] Pierre Brind'Amour, *Nostradamus astrophile: Les Astres et l'astrologie dans la vie et l'oeuvre de Nostradamus* (Paris, 1993).

[47] Cf. Bruce Moran, *The Alchemical World of the German Court: Occult Philosophy and Chemical Medicine in the Circle of Moritz of Hessen (1572–1632)* (Stuttgart, 1991); Hugh Trevor-Roper, 'The Court Physician and Paracelsianism', in Vivien Nutton (ed.), *Medicine at the Courts of Europe* (1990), 79–94.

this book tells about the circulation of esoteric texts, the politics of medicine, the popularity of astrology, the vagaries of Paracelsianism, and the powers of magic.

The book is in four parts, each thematic and to some extent chronological. It begins with knowledge, writing, secrecy, and print, tracing Forman's portrayal of himself as a magus from his portentous dreams as a child and uncanny passion for learning as a youth; through his engagement with the mathematical practitioners in London in his sole printed publication, a pamphlet advertising, but not disclosing, a hermetic method for calculating longitude; to his drafting and redrafting a major treatise on astrological medicine that circulated in manuscript. These episodes introduce Forman's habits of writing and the troubles that punctuated his life and proved his divine authority, themes that recur throughout the book. The second part considers Forman's identity as an astrologer-physician and singularly well-documented opponent of traditional learned medicine, focusing on two trials that he overcame in the 1590s: he survived the plague and defied the efforts of the College of Physicians to stop him from practising medicine. Spurred by his divine prerogative to heal, and indignant that outmoded physicians might brand him a quack, he articulated his medical and cosmological ideas in a series of treatises on astrological physic and plague. These in turn unwittingly document Forman's engagement with other traditions of unorthodox and occult medicine in Elizabethan London. Part III turns from theory and conflict to Forman's practices, as recorded in his astrological casebooks. These are formulaic records of thousands of medical and other consultations, each mapping the positions of the heavens at the time a question was asked and listing, in general, the age, sex, complaint, and occasionally a therapy or outcome of a case. The structured format of these documents, however, masks the dynamics of authority and gender at work in the consulting room. Understanding the complexities of the casebooks allows the voices of Forman and his patients to begin to be heard. Throughout the book I consider Forman's engagement with hermetic and Paracelsian texts and practices, and I address alchemy and magic directly in the final part. This plots a course through thousands of pages, retracing Forman's reading and writing across several decades and hundreds of texts, a process through which he defined a practice of 'chymical and hermetical physic'; pursued the secrets of creation, life, and death known to Adam; and elicited the help of spirits and angels to improve his fortune, alter his destiny, and learn the secrets of medicine. In the conclusion I reflect on Forman's reputation as a quack, conjurer, and womanizer and consider his legacy as a source of occult knowledge through the seventeenth century. Despite himself,

Forman set a standard against which future generations of astrologers, alchemists, diviners, and necromancers were defined.

It is said that if you must sup with the devil you should eat with a long spoon. Fitz-dottrell's lamentation that Forman failed to conjure the devil is double-edged: Forman had demonic intentions but was not powerful enough to summon the evil one. Jonson mocks those who aspired to consort with demons, questioning the plausibility of such actions. If the devil did not appear it was either because those who summoned him lacked the requisite powers, or because such actions were impossible. This was a world in which man's relationship with nature and God was uncertain, but unlike Jonson, Forman never jests about this matter or any other. He was serious about his divine imperative to read the stars, to find the philosophers' stone, and to receive angelic wisdom. He had a knack for a good story and a tendency to tragic escapades and his life and writings provide a vivid account of the medical and magical worlds of early modern London hitherto obscured.

I

THE MAKING OF AN ASTROLOGER-PHYSICIAN

When Simon Forman was 6 years old he began to have recurring dreams about mountains and hills rolling over him and water swallowing him up. Bruised and battered, he always scaled the heights and crossed the rivers. These dreams lasted until Forman was 9 or 10, and many years later he interpreted them as portents of 'his trobles in his riper years. For the mightie mountaines mighte signifie the great & mightie potentates that he had controversy with after wards. And the waters mighte signifie the greate councells that were houlden againste hime to overthrowe hime.'[1] As he triumphed in his dreams, so he triumphed in his life. His 'first troubles' were with the Wiltshire authorities, particularly the Salisbury sheriff, Giles Estcourt, and later he was hounded by the College of Physicians of London. At the peak of his life, aged 48, having established himself as the self-styled astrologer-physician of Lambeth, residing in a house surrounded by an orchard, Forman sat in his study amidst his books, large and small, old and new, printed and manuscript, bound and unbound, heaps of papers, loose and folded into notebooks, pots of brown and red ink and a clock on the table, bottled potions on a ledge near the hearth, bits of silk and velvet clothing and trinkets held in pawn for his astrological services, and the tools and debris of his life as an astrologer-physician and gentleman of London. He might have worn his purple velvet gown and his eagle stone ring and he certainly held a pen in his hand. He was writing the book of his life, documenting his ancestry, his early life, and the trials that he had foreseen in his childhood dreams. The books and papers in his room and the events of his life were his credentials as a magus.

On any day Forman might have been found putting pen to paper, though the room, its furniture and his attire had only recently become so fine. On this occasion, 23 December 1600, Forman was writing about himself. This was

[1] Ashm. 208, fo. 137.

probably the first time that he had written such a narrative, though he had habitually recorded the minutiae of his life. He had noted everything: the names of the thousands of people who consulted him with medical complaints and questions about missing property, procedures for distilling strong waters, locations of buried treasure, visits to the playhouses, a burning sensation when he urinated. He took notes on and transcribed alchemical and magical, astrological and astronomical, and literary and historical treatises, printed and in manuscript, and he scribbled in the margins of the books he owned. He wrote and rewrote his own treatises on astrological medicine. He wrote constantly. All of this writing was the product of Forman's pursuit of knowledge and his definition of himself as chosen by God to possess this knowledge. He scratched his experiences, his authority, and his name onto the thousands of pages of paper in his study. Almost all of these papers are now preserved, bulging from the over full brass-clasped leather bindings that hold them in the Bodleian Library, Oxford. Yet Forman lived with and through his papers, projecting the changing tenor of his voice across three decades as he announced his knowledge, proclaimed his wisdom, charted his life, and concealed his secrets; his life and papers were part of the same enterprise, an enterprise that did not produce a corpus of finished books.

The following three chapters explore Forman's acquisition of arcane knowledge through printed and manuscript books and his own use of print, manuscript, and shifting authorial registers to convey his ideas and practices. I begin not with his ancestors or portentous dreams but with the life-writings from his final decade. Through these he introduces himself as a bookish youth, thirsting for knowledge, then a young man both feckless and righteous, unable to keep hold of the books that he so cherished and defiant of those who confiscated them. He then delved into mystery and silence in his thirties, leaving only a thin trail of details about his study of medicine and the occult arts. Occult books and hermetic knowledge here upstage Forman as the heroes of the story. They are joined by the twin sisters print and manuscript in Chapter 2 which centres on Forman's publication, in print, of a pamphlet advertising a method for calculating longitude, without saying anything more about the method except that it was God-given. No longer feckless, Forman in his early forties has become a righteous, humourless maverick. The longitude episode would be incomplete without details of Forman's secret method, but neither he nor his opponents described it. I have found the secret, or at least the beginnings of it, in Forman's astronomical and magical writings from the 1600s. Finally, Chapter 3 charts Forman's changing authorial voice throughout his treatises, and reflects on his attitude to print and publication in an account of his plans to print an astrological manual around 1600, plans that were never realized. These were the voices of the man who would become the astrologer-physician of Lambeth, dressed in purple in his cluttered room, duly anxious about his place in histories of medicine, astrology, and magic.

I
Early Life and Learning

Forman's story begins on 23 December 1600 because this is the day that he dated the first and most extensive version of his life. He would write at least five more accounts during the next decade, though writing about oneself was not a commonplace activity. Biography and autobiography became codified genres in the eighteenth century. Before that, writings about the events of one's own or someone else's life took various forms, and historians and literary scholars recently have tackled these nimble species of texts armed with the generic and cumbersome labels life-writing, self-writing, and ego-writing.[1]

Forman's accounts of his life have held a place in the history of life-writing in England since James Halliwell edited two of them in the nineteenth century.[2] The texts which Halliwell edited have been singled out as marking a new spirit, 'amusing and flamboyant', in self-presentation, though Forman does not feature in more recent studies of life-writing.[3] Social historians have harvested episodes from Forman's childhood, adolescence, and amorous life, but his possible motives, models, and inspiration for writing these documents remain obscure.[4] He does not fit the mould of the English seventeenth-century Puritan diarist, tallying up and scrutinizing his acts before God, nor does his self-obsession figure in the history of modern individualism. Forman represents different sorts of life-writings. He wrote about himself in the traditions of physicians and surgeons, astrologers, and alchemists before and after him, noting the importance of timing, the authority of experience, the sanctity

[1] See esp. the introduction to Thomas F. Mayer and D. R. Woolf (eds.), *The Rhetoric of Life-Writing in Early Modern Europe: Forms of Biography from Cassandra Fédèle to Louis XIV* (Ann Arbor, 1995). See also Kaspar von Greyerz, 'Religion in the Life of German and Swiss Autobiographers (Sixteenth and Early Seventeenth Centuries)', in von Greyerz (ed.), *Religion and Society in Early Modern Europe 1500–1800* (1984), 223–41; Michael Mascuch, *Origins of the Individualist Self: Autobiography and Self-Identity in England, 1591–1791* (Cambridge, 1997).

[2] *The autobiography and personal diary of Dr Simon Forman*, ed. James Halliwell (1849). These texts are Ashm. 208, fos. 136–42, 1–74.

[3] Paul Delany, *British Autobiography in the Seventeenth Century* (1969), 16.

[4] Ilana Krausman Ben-Amos, *Adolescence and Youth in Early Modern England* (New Haven, 1994), 41, 54, 101, 112, 126, 154, 173, 196, 201, 205, 212; Paul Griffiths, *Youth and Authority: Formative Experiences in England 1560–1640* (Oxford, 1996), 184, 297; Lawrence Stone, *The Family, Sex and Marriage in England 1500–1800* (1977), 95–6, 167, 547–51.

1.1. 'The bocke of the life of and generation of Simon', Ashm. 208, fo. 136. By permission of the Bodleian Library, University of Oxford.

of his privileged knowledge, and the need for the record itself to vindicate its author in the eyes of posterity against his enemies.[5]

Forman's life-writings narrate his first forty years, the period for which few papers survive. During these years Forman outfitted himself with the skills and attitudes with which he was equipped when he settled in London in 1591 and embarked on his career as a notorious astrologer-physician. In order to tell the story of Forman's childhood thirst for knowledge, ill-fated possession of books, and study of the occult, I first need to establish the dates and contents of each of the six texts which Forman devoted solely to his own life.

Forman wrote his most extensive account of his life, 'The bocke of the life and generation of Simon . . .' towards the end of his forty-eighth year, not long after he had married and perhaps while anticipating the births of legitimate children.[6] He began with his ancestry and the visions of mountains and hills noted above, then recounted episodes from his early years, including the death of his father, a fight with a servant when he was an apprentice, his first love, and the details of his schooling and studies. This narrative is in the third person and it reports Forman's life as though he were a character cavorting through a combination of the Bible, the Golden Legend, and an Elizabethan romance.[7]

In 1604 Forman composed a psalm charting his troubles with the College of Physicians that was to be sung to the tune of 'Ye children which doe serve the Lord'.[8] In September 1605, just after the birth of a daughter, Dority, Forman constructed a family genealogy and wrote a family history, beginning in the year 1028 with a Norman soldier who served in the Roman army against the Hungarians. The soldier pleased the Roman emperor, Conrad, and 'bye reason of his true service forwardnes and faithfullnes and valiantnes, he [the emperor]

[5] Delany classifies Forman along with William Lilly and Goodwin Wharton as 'déclassé opportunists and adventurers', exploiting 'astrology, necromancy, and kindred arts' in their secular autobiographies: *British Autobiography*, 133. There are parallels between Forman's life-writings and Cardano's, about whom there is an extensive literature. See esp. Anthony Grafton, *Cardano's Cosmos: The Worlds and Works of a Renaissance Astrologer* (Cambridge, Mass., 1999), ch. 10; Siraisi, *Cardano*, 175–6; Grafton and Siraisi, 'Between the Election and my Hopes: Girolamo Cardano and Medical Astrology', in Grafton and Newman (eds.), *Secrets of Nature*, 69–131. For stories of alchemists in the 17th cent., termed 'transmutation histories', see William Newman, *Gehennical Fire: The Lives of George Starkey, an American Alchemist in the Scientific Revolution* (Cambridge, Mass., 1994), 3–10; Lawrence Principe, *The Aspiring Adept: Robert Boyle and his Alchemical Quest* (Princeton, 1998), 93–8.

[6] Ashm. 208, fos. 136–42. In 1599 Forman married Jean Baker, 'Sir Edward Monninges sisters daughter'. She was then 16, and he sometimes refers to her as Ann, but more often as 'Tronco'.

[7] Delany, *British Autobiography*, 133–4.

[8] The pages of this psalm were at some point separated, and are now bound in Ashm. 240, fos. 25–7^{v} and 802, fos. 131–3^{v}. For a bowdlerized edn. see James Halliwell, *A brief description of the ancient and modern manuscripts preserved in the Public Library, Plymouth* (1853). Earlier in 1604 Forman had composed a psalm to be sung at his burial: Ashm. 802, fos. 135–40^{v}. For other psalms on his troubles, see Ashm. 802, fos. 121–7.

called him forman, for that he was for every man, more then for him selfe.'[9] Dority died on New Year's Day 1606, and a son, Clement, was born in October that year. He lived to be an adult, but little is known about him.[10] Around this time Forman also wrote a very brief account of his life, again in the third person, containing the same themes as the version he wrote in 1600, with a few marked differences in detail.[11]

Around 1603 Forman wrote the text that has become known as his diary. It is renowned for the intimate details that it records.[12] This is not an annual diary in the modern sense, as Halliwell's and Rowse's printed editions imply. It is a series of astrological figures mapping the positions of the planets, beginning with Forman's birth on 31 December 1552, then continuing from 1562 to 1601 with an astrological figure for the first or second day of January of each year. On pages flanking each figure Forman recorded an annual list of the details, or 'accidents', of his life, creating for himself a retrospective version of a luxury horoscope with yearly revolutions. The information is uneven. In general, both sides of a page are devoted to a single year. An exception is the entry for 1567, where Forman covered the events in his life from the age of 15 to 25, the period that is most vividly described in his life-writings. Up to 1581 many entries have the words 'proved true' or 'verified' noted in the margins. After 1581 the entries often contain minute details, followed by a general summary of the year. Forman probably calculated annual nativities for himself from the early 1580s, and perhaps he also, as was conventional, recorded events in an ephemeris, almanac, or one of his notebooks.[13]

Wherever these details were recorded, the diary is the product of Forman's retrospective use of them as the foundation for a series of astrological experiments, hence the notes of verification. He compiled this document in order to study the influences of the motions of the stars and planets on his life and he recycled examples here and in notes on how to read astrological figures. These

[9] Ashm. 208, fo. 214ᵛ. The genealogy, 'The firste of the Formans', is Ashm. 802, fos. 211–16. The family history, 'Of the name Forman', is Ashm. 208, fos. 214–24; cf. Rowse, *Forman*, 300–2, for a partial transcription of Ashm. 208, fos. 218–23.

[10] Clement wrote to Richard Napier, 20 Aug. 1628, Ashm. 174, fo. 479. For evidence that Clement planned to train as a lawyer, see Traister, *Forman*, pp. xiv–xv.

[11] 'The issue of Simon Forman', Ashm. 208, fos. 225–6.

[12] Ashm. 208, fos. 11ᵛ–67.

[13] For Forman's calculations of his own nativity for 9.45 p.m., 31 Dec. 1552, see Ashm. 206, fos. 76ᵛ–7, 216–25; 208, fo. 12; 195, fos. 69–72; cf. 219, fo. 135, the annual calculation for his 47th year. For notes on Forman's nativity, perhaps in Napier's hand, calculated for 2.00 a.m., 1 Jan. 1553, see Ashm. 205, fo. 286ʳ⁻ᵛ. For Dee's diaries see Ashm. 487 and 488; cf. *The private diary of Dr. John Dee, and the catalogue of his library and manuscripts*, ed. James Halliwell, Camden Society, 19 (1842). *The Diaries of John Dee*, ed. Edward Fenton (Charlbury, 1998) constructs a seamless narrative from many of Dee's life-writings. For interleaved English almanacs see Mascuch, *Origins of the Individualist*, 72.

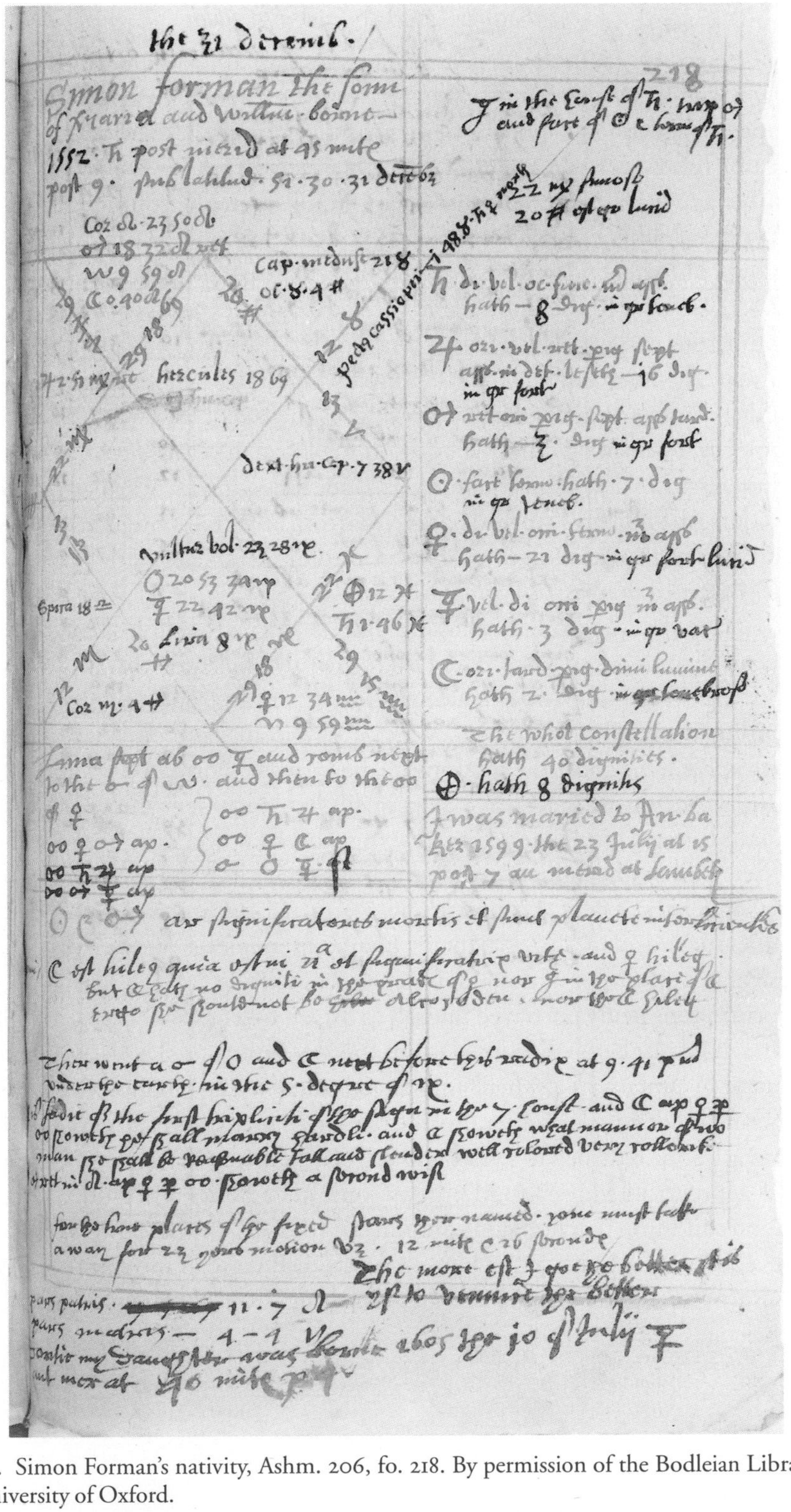

1.2. Simon Forman's nativity, Ashm. 206, fo. 218. By permission of the Bodleian Library, University of Oxford.

are organized thematically, and in some cases contain more detail than the diary, evidence perhaps that they were drawn from a parent set of records.[14] For instance, in a section on determining a propitious moment to move into a new house or room, Forman recorded that on 6 April 1590 he 'entered first my chamber at Mr Dales & tok it absolutely'. While there, he continues, '[I] had many privi enimies but I gote reasonable & many fair women cam to me', and he moved out after two months.[15] In the diary Forman simply noted, 'I cam to lie at Mr Dalles'.[16] Reading the diary as an astrological experiment also explains the numerous passages which Forman has crossed through, only some of which then appear under different years. Rowse's and Halliwell's editions do not include Forman's omissions and neglect the vagueness of, and frequent contradictions in, Forman's dating. One reason for Forman's (mis)dating is that he was interested in astrological influences, and, following standard astrological procedures, he probably worked backwards from an astral configuration to calculate the specific date and time of an event. For the sake of clarity I will continue to refer to this text as Forman's diary.

These are the six accounts of his life that Forman wrote in his final decade. Three of them focus to some extent on his family and the events, both major and trivial, of his life (two of these are in the third person); one is a psalm describing his conflict with the College of Physicians; and one maps a list of events in his life against the motions of the heavens. Forman does not tell us why he wrote any of these texts. Separately they document the credibility of Forman's lineage; his divine prerogative to study, heal, and overcome adversity in order to do so; the influences of the heavens on his life, and his ability to read these influences. These accounts allow me to tell the story of how Forman became the astrologer-physician of Lambeth, nemesis of the College of Physicians, and author of thousands of pages of writing.

Forman repeatedly portrayed himself as driven by a passion for learning. He began school just before he turned 8, but this was interrupted with the death of his father in January 1564, when Simon had just turned 11. His mother kept him home and made him look after the sheep, plough fields, and gather wood, but within a year he returned to school and learned to write.[17] Two years later, aged 14, he apprenticed himself to Matthew Commin, a hosier and grocer in Salisbury, on condition that he could continue his studies. Forman borrowed books from a boy who boarded in the house, and studied these in the evenings.[18] He also 'learned the knowledge of all wares and drugs' from his master.[19] After five

[14] Ashm. 390. [15] Ashm. 390, fo. 59v. [16] Ashm. 208, fo. 46v.
[17] Ashm. 208, fos. 137v–8v; 208, fos. 15–17. [18] Ashm. 208, fos. 20v, 140.
[19] Ashm. 208, fo. 138v.

to seven years he left Commin (*c.*1572), visited the Isle of Wight, returned to his mother in Quidhampton, and studied under one Anthony Nicholas for eight weeks until himself becoming a schoolmaster.[20] In a description of this period he wrote,

This yere I had that gret desier to my bock that when I was at scolle with Antoni Nicolas I wold wepe when he gave us leave to plaie, and when he wold not beate me when I could not saie my lesson. And I wold saie I should never be a good scollar yet he wold not beate me. Yt was hell for me to go to plaie or to goe from my bock, and yet I had noe maintenaunce but did shifte for lerninge & then becam a scolmaster at michelmas my selfe.[21]

In the spring of 1573, at age 20, Forman went to Oxford and became a poor scholar in the service of two Wiltshire gentlemen: Robert Pinckney, who would return to Wiltshire as a cleric, and John Thornborough, who would ultimately become bishop of Worcester.[22] Forman's intellectual expectations were not fulfilled. He recalled, 'And this yere with them I began to learn to goe on hunting for deare & hare & all evill & could not imploi my bocke to my desier.'[23] Forman left Oxford in autumn 1574. His disappointment there is the final event in the longest of his life-writings.

In two accounts that continued into the 1580s, the story of Forman's education did not end here. In June 1579 he was committed to prison and stayed there for sixty weeks, and on his release in July 1580 he travelled to London where 'a cosening quen professed her self to be my sister', then on to the Low Countries.[24] As he noted in his diary, 'The 4 of September I went over with Henry Jonson into the Lowe countries into Sealand & Holland and we lay at the Hage som fortnight & the 3 of October I cam to London again'. He also recorded going to sea with one Robert Grey in 1582 and being captured by pirates.[25] In another account, in the third person, Forman suggested that he made several trips abroad: 'he travailed moch in to the Estern countries to seke for arte and knowledge, and was often at Sea'.[26] These texts are William Lilly's primary source of information about Forman, and hence his statement that Forman 'traveled into Holland for a month in 1580, purposely to be instructed in Astrology, and other more occult Sciences, as also in Physick, taking his degree of Doctor beyond Seas' is an overstatement.[27] If Forman's records were

20 Ashm. 208, fo. 25^{v}.

21 Ashm. 208, fo. 26^{v}. This passage is crossed out and a version of it appears in Ashm. 208, fo. 141^{v}.

22 Ashm. 208, fos. 20^{v}, 26^{v}, 27^{v}.

23 Ashm. 208, fo. 27^{v}, crossed out.

24 Ashm. 208, fo. 34^{v}.

25 Ashm. 208, fos. 34^{v}, 37^{v}.

26 Ashm. 208, fo. 225^{r-v}.

27 Lilly, *Life*, 17. These papers are also perhaps the source for an alchemical poem, perhaps in Napier's hand, in which Forman features as the hero: Trinity O.8.1, fos. 95–113.

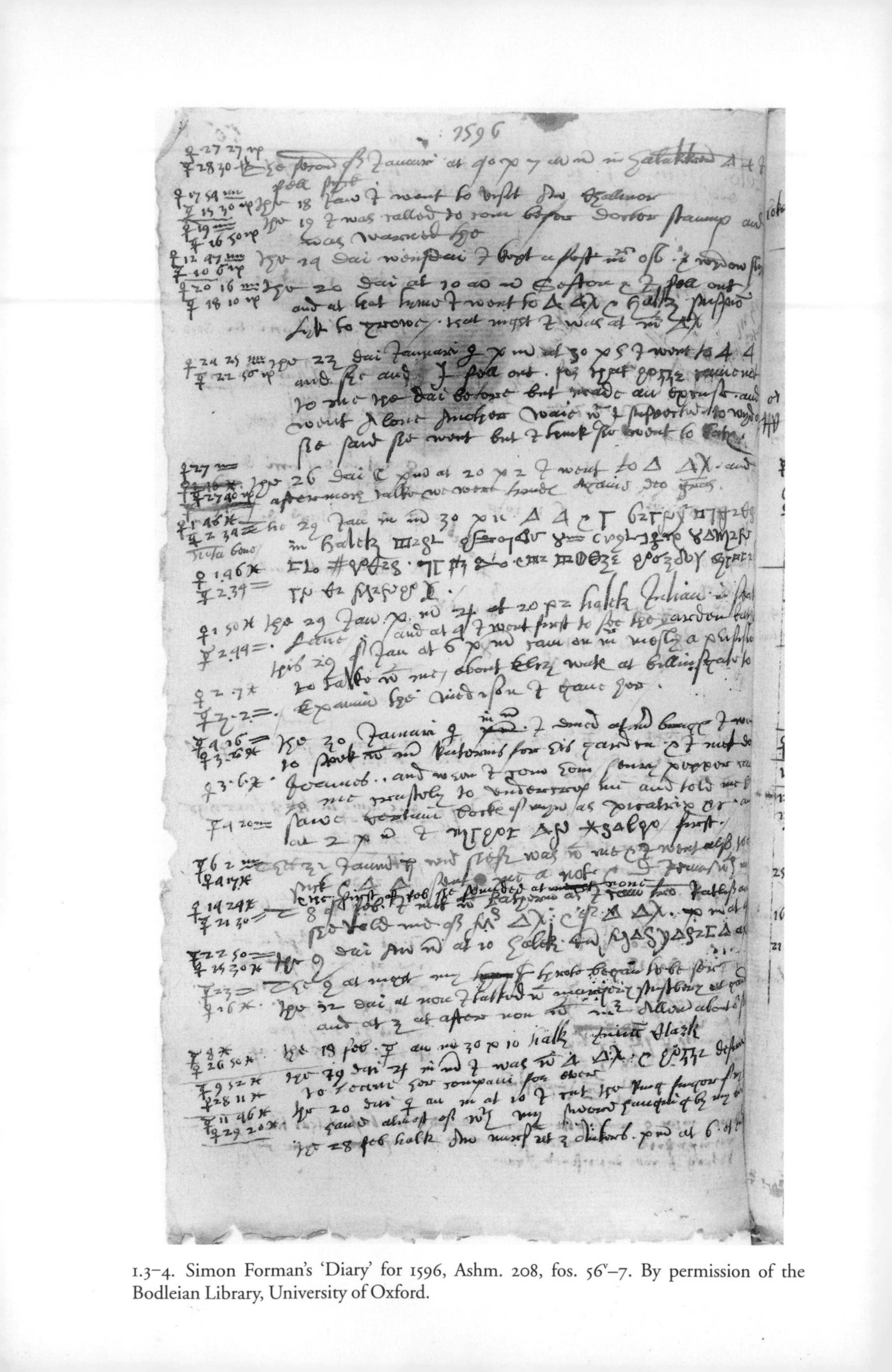

1.3–4. Simon Forman's 'Diary' for 1596, Ashm. 208, fos. 56v–7. By permission of the Bodleian Library, University of Oxford.

1596 the 2 of January ♀ Ante m(eridiem) at 33 minute p(ast) 2 Revolucio mei natalis Annorum 44. 57

1579 11 3.

♂ [illegible] in domo [illegible] j [illegible]

☉ [illegible] j

♄ [illegible] j

♃ [illegible] domo 20

♀ [illegible]

☿ [illegible] o

☾ [illegible]

☊ 2

☋ 2

Luna sep a ♄ ap ♃ □.

✶ ♃ ♀.

♂ [illegible] Anni in ♉

♂ [illegible] ♃ [illegible]

This is the [illegible] figure [illegible] the dimissions [illegible] dimissions. [illegible] is ye 22 ♉

♀	☿		
			~~This is a d[illegible] of a man child the 26 of June named alexander that died shortly after~~
♉	♓		
12	0 30		first march [illegible] with pepy about words
13	2	.	2 march [illegible]
			the 12 march ♀ p m at 30 p 5 I went to garden where I found
			Δ ΔX & we became friends again and [illegible]
25 42	20	30	I did [illegible]
16 40.7		30	the 5 of march ♀ I put on my new [illegible] gowne [illegible]
			the 9 march I put on my velvet jerkin and [illegible]
21 40	24	59	the 29 of march Δ Δλ gave me in the morning [illegible]
			[illegible]
			the 5 of April ☾ Δ ΔX [illegible] me by the [illegible]
			the 6 of April [illegible] I rode out to [illegible]
			the 10 day I came home from [illegible]
			the 27 [illegible] all my [illegible] was lost [illegible]
			the 30 of April ♀ [illegible] at 5 [illegible]
			[illegible]

intended to establish his credentials as a man of learning and expertise, they succeeded: Lilly's account was the basis for the Oxford antiquarian Anthony Wood's notes on Forman's life, then Sidney Lee's article on Forman in the *Dictionary of National Biography* which has perpetuated this error.[28]

Whether or not he travelled abroad in the early 1580s, the young Forman was schooled like many Elizabethans of the lower gentry or merchant class.[29] His passion for learning in his early years was eccentric, and it matured into an adult quest for scholarly and arcane texts. Books, lost and found, played a role in the misfortunes that his childhood dreams had foreshown, and Forman thought that his contemporaries deprived him of his books out of jealousy of his learning and success. In 'The issue of Simon Forman' (1606+) he wrote: 'at 20 years he becam a scolmaster again, and begain to studdie astronomy & phisicke magick & philosophie, wherin he profited & prospered mightily, and in chirurgerie and other artes, for the which he suffered moch troble afterwards, and loste all his goods and bocks 3 tymes'.[30] Unfortunately Forman did not record the titles of the books that would have surrounded him as he worked in his study in Lambeth, nor how he came to possess them. He may have acquired some texts while he was in Salisbury, but books and manuscripts were readily available in Oxford, and while he was there he bought a pair of fifteenth-century medical treatises bound together. This is one of the nine manuscripts which can today be identified as having belonged to Forman.[31] In his diary Forman recorded that the plague came to Oxford around 1575, and he 'loste all that ever I had ther, bocks and all'.[32] This was the first loss of his books. Later that year or the next, when Forman had moved to Ashgrow, Wiltshire, the parson was brought to inspect his books. This appears to have been at the instigation of a Mr Cox, apparently a former employer whom Forman had offended.[33] It is not clear why these books were considered suspicious and they seem not to have been confiscated. By the summer of 1579 Forman was in trouble with the law in Salisbury, and either just before, or in the process

[28] Wood, *Athenae Oxonienses*, ii. 98–105 (Forman), 373–4 (John Davies), though Wood did not include Forman in the original edn. of this work; *DNB*. For Wood's notes on Forman's life, see Bodleian, Rawlinson MS D.912, fo. 643. For the impact of Lilly's account in the 18th cent. see e.g. Daniel Lyson, *The environs of London*, i (1792), 301–3.

[29] Felicity Heal and Clive Holmes, *The Gentry in England and Wales, 1500–1700* (Basingstoke, 1994), ch. 7; Rosemary O'Day, *Education and Society, 1500–1800* (1982).

[30] Ashm. 208, fo. 225.

[31] King's MS 16. The extant books and MSS that Forman owned and copied are listed in the Bibliography.

[32] Ashm. 208, fo. 28^{v}. Forman seems to have left Oxford in 1594, and the inconsistencies in these dates may explain why Forman crossed out the account of the plague in Oxford in 1575, though not why he did not include it under another year.

[33] Ashm. 208, fo. 28^{v}.

of his being arrested, his goods were spoiled and his books stolen. Thus Forman lost his books a second time and had his first experience of prison, remaining gaoled for more than a year.[34] Although Forman recorded that he was released by a warrant signed by the queen and six of her councillors, no official record of the charge against Forman or the royal intervention has been located.

Eight years later Forman lost his books for the third time. In March 1587 he was arrested in Salisbury for bringing a book containing 'bad and fond prayers and devises' to morning prayer. 'Fond' probably meant foolish, and the unorthodox prayers and diagrams or images suggest that this was a book of magic.[35] Forman's house was searched and four 'paper books' and three parchment rolls were found and sent to the Privy Council for inspection. Forman denied that the writing in the margins of the book and an inserted page of notes were his.[36] He was imprisoned for a few weeks, and in the months following his release he recorded various obscure squabbles, book-buying expeditions, and magical activities.[37] Later that year his books, perhaps the ones confiscated on this occasion or 'stolen' on the previous one, were deposited with Sir John Penruddock, a Wiltshire gentleman and lawyer of Gray's Inn whose children Forman had tutored in 1582–4. Forman did not recover them until 1592 by which time many had been lost.[38]

I will add a fourth episode to the tale of the stolen books. Perhaps because he had learnt that his books could get him into trouble, while living in London Forman kept some of them in a house in Lambeth.[39] On 10 March 1598 three men broke into his study there and stole five astrological texts and a gilt-bound Bible.[40] Forman pursued the culprits for a year, identifying them as three students from Cambridge, William Grange, Thomas Russell, and George Nicolas, the last of whom later moved to the continent and entered a seminary. One of Forman's sources was his friend, George Coney, who had also encountered the wayward students when they first attempted to sell him some books, then stole some of his. According to Coney, who had heard it from a Master Napier (presumably Richard or his brother, Robert, a London merchant), the

34 Ashm. 208, fo. 32^{v}; 390, fo. 65. Elsewhere these events are dated 1576: Ashm. 802, fo. 113.

35 *OED.*

36 *The Complete State Papers Domestic, 1/5. 1547–1625* (Brighton, 1978), reel 81 (10 Mar. 1587); Ashm. 208, fo. 42^{v}; 390, fo. 125.

37 Ashm. 390, fos. 109^{v}, 159^{r-v}; 208, fo. 42^{v}.

38 Ashm. 208, fos. 42^{v}, 48. Rowse mistranscribes Forman's record that he did not recover his books for 14 years as 24 years: *Forman*, 287. On Forman's employment with the Penruddock's see Ashm. 208, fos. 37^{v}, 39^{v}. Forman's details, and perhaps his memory, about the dates of the losses and recoveries of his books are here confused; cf. Traister, *Forman*, 17.

39 Traister suggests that Forman commonly kept his books and occult equipment in a separate house in the 1590s: *Forman*, 161.

40 Ashm. 390, fo. 61; 195, fos. 9, 72, 95, 151^{v}; 219, fo. 229^{v}.

Cambridge men also had shown the books to a Master Gressam, probably Edward Gresham (1565–1613), an astrologer-physician.[41] Forman had lost his books because he did not have a secure place to keep them, because he was arrested for an unnamed offence, because their contents were suspect, and finally because they could be sold on the underground book market. These misfortunes, Forman thought, were signs of God's design for him.

Forman chronicled the impediments to his studies and his triumphs over them through the mid-1580s as evidence of the divine imperative behind his medical and astrological activities. At this point the details in his narrative life-writings become thin, though his diary continues with incidental details through 1602. These narratives establish Forman's credentials as a magus, yet do not document his activities in this role. Where the life-writing dwindles, the other writings increase, tagged with Forman's name and the date and littered with astrological figures, timed to the minute, which allow me to trace his studies, practices, and personal life through the following decades.

Forman's earliest extant, datable writings are some poems from the late 1570s.[42] His datable medical, astrological, and geomantical texts date from after 1588. Perhaps, as he later claimed, he began to practise medicine in the mid-1570s.[43] In 1581, at the age of 29, he cast an astrological figure, the earliest extant record of his mastery of the rudiments of astrology.[44] This year also

[41] Ashm. 195, fo. 151ᵛ; 219, fo. 54. Coney appears in Forman's notes several times. He asked Forman questions, was imprisoned for trespassing, and Forman considered but decided against raising bail for him. See for instance Ashm. 390, fos. 70ʳ⁻ᵛ; 234, fos. 84ᵛ–5, 119ᵛ; 236, fo. 138ᵛ (28 July, 4 and 6 Aug., and 27 Oct. 1596 and 7 June 1600). For his nativity, which provides a lively character sketch see Ashm. 206, fo. 312; this passage is quoted by Rowse, *Forman*, 213. In a magical treatise, Forman notes that he copied some prayers out of a paper book that Coney had brought him: Trinity MS O.9.7, fo. 107ᵛ. In addition to the gilt-bound Bible, which had been a gift to Forman from Anne Young, his first love and the mother of his son, Joshua Walworth, the stolen books included astrological treatises by Albubater, Ricardus Anglicus, and Alcabitius, with John of Saxony's commentary. For Forman's beginning of a translation of the final text in 1601, see Ashm. 206, fos. 1–3. For extant astronomical and astrological texts owned by Forman, see Ashm. 360, iii–v; Trinity, O.8.23, O.9.7; Bodleian, Rawlinson MS C. 269. On Gresham, see *DNB, Missing Persons.*

[42] For a notebook of poems, including one dated 1578, see Ashm. 208, fos. 250–64. This contains verses for the queen which may relate to Forman's record of giving an oration before her in Wilton in 1574: Ashm. 208, fo. 27ᵛ. She was on progress in Wilton in August of that year: John Dasent (ed.), *Acts of the Privy Council of England*, xi (1897), 280. A magical MS from 1567 has been misattributed to Forman: BL Additional MS 36674, fos. 47ᵛ–58.

[43] In Mar. 1584 he told the Censors of the College of Physicians that he had practised medicine for sixteen years (i.e. since 1578): Annals, 8 Mar. 1593/4, pp. 84–5. In his 1607 plague tract he said that he had practised for thirty-four years (i.e. since 1573): Ashm. 1436, fo. 139. In his latest account of his life he said that he began studying medical arts when he was 20: Ashm. 208, fo. 225. Elsewhere he specified that he had practised since 1570: Ashm. 363, fo. 132. In a note *c.*1607–10 he specified that he had practised astrological medicine for thirty years: Ashm. 1491, p. 1275.

[44] Ashm. 205, fo. 121. It concerned the location of lost goods. For Forman's possible early reading of a number of 15th-cent. introductions to astronomy see Ashm. 360, iii–v. On learning astrology, cf. Michael Hunter and Annabel Gregory (eds.), *An Astrological Diary of the Seventeenth Century: Samuel Jeake of Rye 1652–1699* (Oxford, 1988), 4.

marks a point at which Forman's life began to improve; 'this year I began to live again', he noted.[45] He 'dwelte practising phisick & surgery' in a leased house on the ditch near the skinner in Salisbury.[46] Perhaps preparing for the conjunction of Jupiter and Saturn in 1583, in 1582 he recorded the configurations of the planets at the moments of changes in the weather, and used these notes towards a general prognostication and perhaps an almanac.[47] In 1583 he recorded 'profit by my pen', perhaps indicating that he published a prophecy or almanac or was employed as a scribe.[48] In the summer of the same year he was reported to the ecclesiastical authorities in Salisbury for illicitly practising physic.[49]

Evidence for Forman's involvement in and practice of more explicitly dangerous arts such as alchemy and magic dates from the mid-1580s, though he probably began these activities along with the study of astrology and medicine in the 1570s. Perhaps he became interested in alchemy when he was in Oxford in 1573–4, meeting with, talking to, or borrowing books from scholars at the university such as John Case or the recently arrived Thomas Allen. But Forman did not record such encounters and members of the university have left scant traces of explorations of the occult arts during these decades.[50] John Thornborough, Forman's master while in Oxford, published an obscure alchemical book in 1621, but he and Forman are equally silent about whether they shared an interest in alchemy while students or had any contact with each other thereafter.[51]

Further circumstantial evidence connects Forman with people who were interested in alchemy and astrology in Oxford at a later date. He visited Oxford in 1578, and again in 1590 and 1591, though he did not record whom he saw or what he did while there.[52] Ashmole told Anthony Wood, the great recorder of people's lives, that Forman had taught astrology to Sir John Davies, who had been taught by Thomas Allen, when Davies moved to London after taking his

45 Ashm. 208, fo. 34ᵛ. 46 Ashm. 208, fo. 36ᵛ. 47 Ashm. 384, fos. 116–87.

48 Ashm. 208, fo. 38ᵛ. There are parts of one or more almanacs amongst Forman's papers, Ashm. 384, fos. 187–8; King's MS 16, fos. 146g–k. These may be copied from printed almanacs, though such texts have a low survival rate and no positive match has been made. They may also be fragments of a draft of an almanac which Forman intended to publish; cf. Bernard Capp, *Astrology and the Popular Press: English Almanacs 1500–1800* (1979), 26.

49 Ashm. 208, fo. 38ᵛ.

50 Feingold, *Mathematicians' Apprenticeship*, 111, 157; Feingold, 'The Occult Tradition in the English Universities', in Brian Vickers (ed.), *Occult and Scientific Mentalities in the Renaissance* (Cambridge, 1984), 73–94, esp. 84–7.

51 John Thornborough, *Lithotheorikos, sive, nihil, aliquid, omnia, antiquorum sapientum vivis coloribus depicta, philosophico-theologice* (Oxford, 1621). For the suggestion that it is not a coincidence that Forman, like Thornborough, pursued alchemy see William Huffman, *Robert Fludd and the End of the Renaissance* (1988), 32, 170–1.

52 Ashm. 208, fos. 31ᵛ, 46ᵛ, 47ᵛ.

MA at Oxford in 1581.[53] Forman was in Salisbury for most of 1581 and 1582, but he spent the first quarter of 1583 in London, where he 'spent moch & got nothing' while he worked 'in business' in the service of Mrs Penruddock, whose children he was schooling.[54] The identities of at least three men called John Davies are often confused. Sir John Davies (1569–1626) is distinguished by his title, John Davies of Hereford (1565?–1618) is known for his poetry, and John Davis (1552–1605) was a prominent navigator.[55] Whether Forman taught one of these men, he knew at least one John Davies. In 1595 Avis Allen, a married woman with whom Forman was romantically involved, told him that John Davies had spoken ill of him to her husband.[56] In 1596 Forman dreamt about meeting a John Davies and his brother, and that evening he again discussed Davies with Avis Allen.[57] Here Forman allows us a whisper of the conversations that his papers muffle and glimpses of his friends and enemies.

Without recording who facilitated or encouraged his study of various arts and sciences, Forman specified that he began to study astronomy, physic, magic and philosophy after he left Oxford in the mid-1570s.[58] He tells us nothing more about his studies until the end of the decade, when his diary records that he prophesied correctly and 'the sprites were subject unto me'.[59] Then the silence lasts another five years, probably masking magical and medical pursuits.

By the mid-1580s Forman was collecting alchemical and related texts and distilling medicines. He went on book-buying expeditions through the 1580s and filled at least two notebooks with copies of texts on the philosophers' stone.[60] On 31 December 1584 he completed a transcript of 'The compound of alchemy' by George Ripley, the fifteenth-century English alchemist; on 2 February 1585 he completed notes on mercury that he described as 'following' the thirteenth-century physician, Arnald of Villanova; and on the first of March he began distilling *aqua vitae*.[61] In August he took notes on several medieval alchemical works, and on the first of October he finished copying and correcting a translation of a text by the late fourteenth-century physician,

[53] Wood, *Athenae Oxonienses*, ii. 373–4; *Ashmole*, ed. Josten iv. 1809. Wood concluded that this was probably the John Davis who eventually entered the service of the earl of Essex. One John Davis, probably the navigator, skried for Gabriel Harvey: Webster, 'Alchemical and Paracelsian Medicine', 312. Davis the navigator was associated with John Dee and might have stolen some of his books: Julian Roberts and Andrew Watson (eds.), *John Dee's Library Catalogue* (1990), 32, 34.

[54] Ashm. 208, fos. 37^{v}, 39^{v}. [55] *DNB*. [56] Ashm. 208, fo. 53^{v}.

[57] Ashm. 234, fo. 123^{v} (28 Oct. 1596). [58] Ashm. 208, fo. 225. [59] Ashm. 208, fo. 32^{v}.

[60] Ashm. 390, fos. 157, 159^{v}. Forman filled twelve notebooks with transcriptions of alchemical texts. These are now bound in Ashm. 1490, 1433, and 208.

[61] Ashm. 1490, fos. 114–36^{v}; 143^{v}–9^{v}; 208, fo. 40^{v}. See *George Ripley's Compound of Alchemy*, ed. Stanton J. Linden (Aldershot, 2001). For Villanova see Thorndike, *Magic and Experimental Science*, ii, ch. 68; iii, ch. 4.

Bernard of Trier.[62] In 1585 he copied 'A dialogue between a scholler and master' and took a few notes in English on a printed, Latin text attributed to the great Arabic philosopher and physician, Avicenna.[63] He also made notes of a dozen recipes for chemical waters, ranging in attribution from the unknown 'William Fraunces' to the thirteenth-century Franciscan friar and alchemist Roger Bacon; two years later, in May 1587, he noted that he 'began to distill many waters'.[64] In November 1587 Forman dreamt that he met a boy and a woman who were discussing how to make the philosophers' stone.[65] In 1587 he began to call angels.[66] In 1588 he and his 'special friends' embarked on a 'learned matter' when Saturn was inauspiciously placed, and had an argument.[67]

Throughout this period Forman lived in Salisbury. When things went well he made money from practising medicine or tutoring children, when they went poorly he had little money or was imprisoned. He occasionally travelled in the south of England to buy books or flee his enemies and he was often involved in legal cases, sometimes as the plaintiff, sometimes as the defendant. In 1582 he became reacquainted with Anne Young, the A.Y. who fell in love with Forman when he was an apprentice, and though she was now married to John Walworth they became romantically involved, resulting, on 27 March 1585 at 7.10 a.m., in the birth of Forman's first son, Joshua Walworth.[68] Later that year Forman seems to have been gravely ill, occasioning him to write a poem, 'The argumente between Forman and deathe in his sickness'.[69] In January 1589 he planned to bring a legal case against someone, in his terms to 'arrest' the person, and when he went to find an officer he was impressed to serve in the 'Portugal voyage'. Two hours later he had left Salisbury and would never again reside there.[70] Evidently he protested against his conscription and in February he spent two nights in prison in 'Hampton', but was soon released.[71] He returned to Salisbury, within a week travelled to Newbury, then

[62] Ashm. 1490, fo. 87; fos. 221–36ᵛ. On the origin and impact of the texts attributed to Bernard of Trier see Thorndike, *Magic and Experimental Science*, iii. 618–27; Newman, *Gehennical Fire*, 103–6 and *passim*. For further English copies see Ashm. 1487, fos. 182–96 and Robert M. Schuler (ed.), *Alchemical Poetry 1575–1700 from Previously Unpublished Manuscripts* (New York, 1995), 446–63.

[63] Ashm. 1490, fos. 81–6ᵛ. Other versions of the dialogue have not been identified. That Forman was using a printed, Latin text by Avicenna is clear from his reference to 'fo. 458, primus ordo est'. For Avicenna see Nancy Siraisi, *Avicenna in Renaissance Italy: The Canon and Medical Teaching in Italian Universities after 1500* (Princeton, 1987).

[64] Ashm. 1490, fos. 90–2; 208, fo. 42ᵛ. For basic details about Bacon see Thorndike, *Magic and Experimental Science*, ii, ch. 61.

[65] Ashm. 1472, p. 813.

[66] Ashm. 208, fos. 42ᵛ, 43ᵛ.

[67] Ashm. 390, fos. 120, 157ᵛ; 208, fo. 43ᵛ.

[68] Ashm. 208, fo. 40ᵛ. For full details of Walworth's life, including the moment of his conception on 25 June 1584, see Ashm. 206, fos. 102–3; 240, fo. 31.

[69] Ashm. 208, fos. 232–48. This is dated 4 Sept. 1585.

[70] Ashm. 390, fo. 117; 208, fo. 45ᵛ.

[71] Ashm. 208, fo. 45ᵛ.

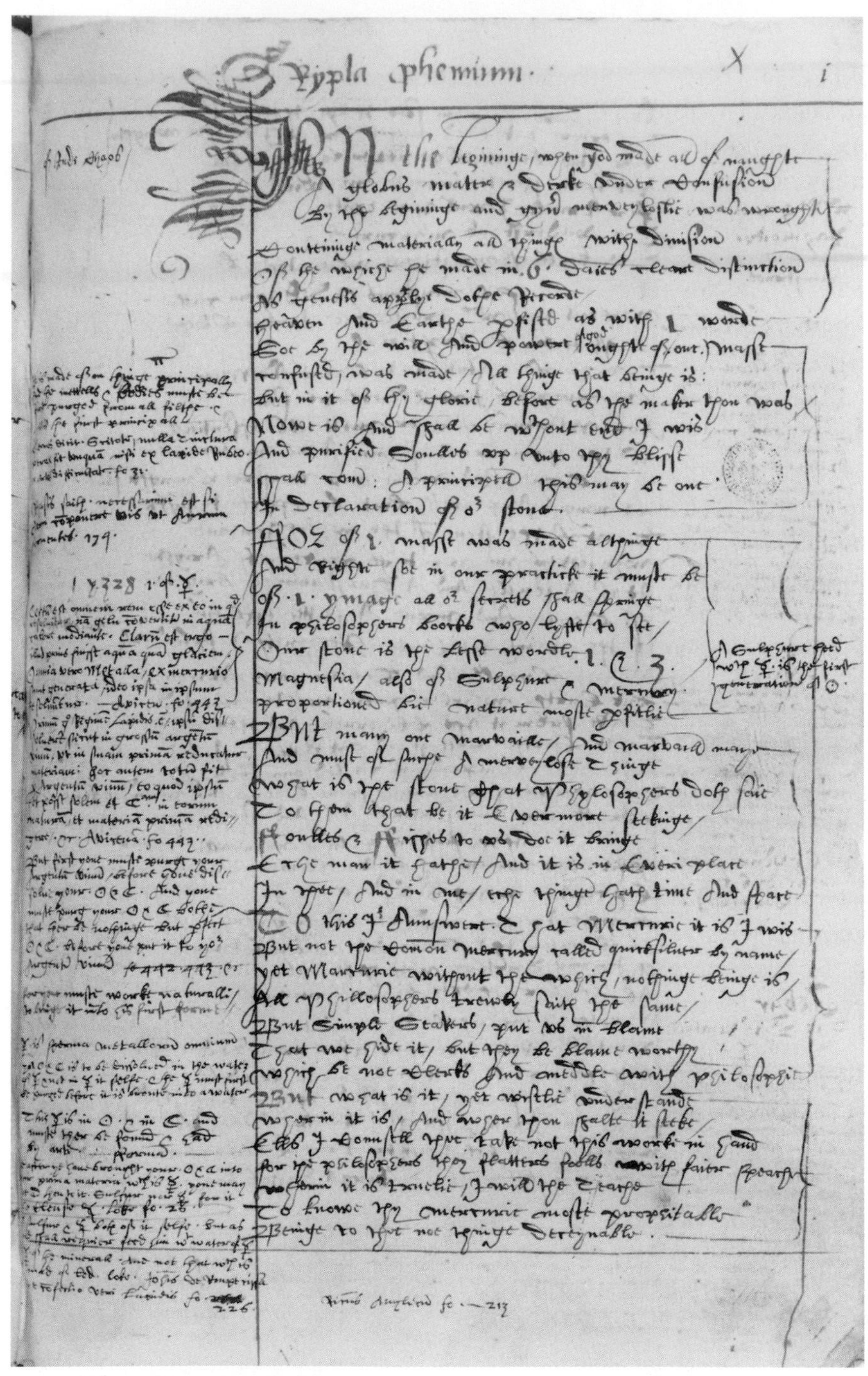

1.5. Simon Forman's copy of George Ripley's 'The compound of alchemy', Ashm. 1490, fo. 116. By permission of the Bodleian Library, University of Oxford.

within a fortnight back to Quidhampton, then back to Newbury almost immediately, and after a month there on to Ash in Surrey and so forth until he moved to London in August.[72] There he lived in five different rooms in the course of a year.[73] He was fleeing his enemies. He did not record their names, but a case of slander in Salisbury in May 1589 reveals a facet of his reputation in his home town.

William Young, Anne Young's father, accused Markes Fareland of slander. Fareland was reputed to have said that he had seen Young's wife, Alice, and his daughter Anne (or Agnes) Walworth in St Thomas's Church with Simon Forman. This was two years earlier, in 1587, on the morning of the funeral of Giles Estcourt, the sheriff who had imprisoned Forman in 1578. Fareland then reported that he had seen Forman and Anne Young go to the aisle of the church containing Estcourt's recently laid tomb and there they 'had their pleasure one of thother and had carnall knowledge eche of others bodie'. Alice, Anne's mother, was present as a 'bawd', and Fareland added a final detail to lend credibility to his story: 'he then saw the said Simon Forman shortly thereupon to go up in the belfry there carring his breetches in his hands'.[74] Forman and Anne had had previous troubles. In January 1587 their affair was almost discovered, in June 1588 they had an argument, and in November that year the constable came to arrest her.[75] In May 1589 Forman noted that 'a slander was raised' against him. Two years had passed since the event was reputed to have occurred, and the depositions note that this story had 'blowen abrode into the eares of many' and 'very evell speeches geeven of & by the said Agnys & the said Simon Forman', stressing that it was unclear whether the couple's reputation came before or after Fareland's story.[76] Thereafter, whether Forman found Salisbury particularly inhospitable or London enticing, he made London his home.

Wherever he was living, Forman continued to collect books and to pursue medicine and magic. In 1590–1 he filled at least another three notebooks with copies of alchemical tracts.[77] He probably borrowed these treatises from friends with whom he stayed and their neighbours. In June 1590, while staying with a 'Mr Dalles' he copied a long and unusual treatise written by Humfrey

72 Ashm. 208, fo. 45^{v}; 390, fos. 158^{v}, 160^{v}.

73 Ashm. 208, fos. 45^{v}, 46^{v}; 390, fo. 59^{r-v}.

74 Salisbury record office, Bishop of Salisbury deposition books no. 10, fo. 46^{r-v}. For full details of this case see deposition books no. 10, fos. 46^{r-v}, 57; no. 11, fos. 17^{r-v}, 25^{v}, 26. I am indebted to Martin Ingram for these references.

75 Ashm. 208, fos. 42^{v}, 43^{v}.

76 Ashm. 208, fo. 45^{v}; Bishop of Salisbury deposition book no. 10, fo. 46^{r-v}.

77 In chronological order: Ashm. 1490, fos. 294–325, 181–96, 199–216, 154–7^{v}, 217–20, 277–89, 165–6, 167–8, 42–5, 28–36; 1433, fos. 10^{v}, 34. For details of these treatises see Bibliography.

Lock while he was in exile in Russia and dedicated to William Cecil, Lord Burghley.[78] In June and again in July Forman went to stay with Robert Parkes, a merchant.[79] In September Forman visited a 'Mr Cumbers' in Lewes, Sussex, who employed him for a year and gave him a house in Wickham, though the details of this arrangement are unclear.[80] In October Forman copied a fifteenth-century manuscript of a treatise on the transmutation of the five essences by John of Rupescissa (fl. 1345).[81] In December he borrowed an English manuscript translation of Paracelsus' 'De natura rerum' and 'De natura hominis' from one John Fallowfield and he finished copying it in February 1591.[82] In March he made a transcript of the well-known 'Ordinal of Alchemy' of Thomas Norton (*c.*1433–1513 or 1514).[83] In August Forman went to stay with the merchant Parkes again, and copied Sir Robert Greene's (1467?–1538+) treatise on the philosophers' stone, the work that is known as 'Blomfild's Blossoms' by William Blomfild, Forman's near contemporary, and prophecies found carved in Paris, translated from Portuguese into English the previous month.[84] In September he began a transcription of the Emerald Tablet, an alchemical treatise attributed to Hermes Trismegistus, with the fourteenth-century commentary by Hortulanus.[85] During this period Forman participated in a magical society and 'wrote' a book of necromancy, probably meaning that he copied a magical text.[86]

While swarming with detail, Forman's notes are deceptively incomplete. He portrayed himself as a self-sustaining intellectual steeled against his enemies. But he seldom wrote about the people with whom he lived, travelled, worked,

[78] Ashm. 1490, fos. 291–325; for a study of this text, see Peter Grund, 'In Search of Gold: Towards a Text Edition of an Alchemical Treatise', in Peter J. Lucas and Angela M. Lucas (eds.), *Middle English from Tongue to Text: Selected Papers from the Third International Conference on Middle English* (Frankfurt, 2002), 265–79.

[79] Ashm. 390, fo. 59ᵛ; 208, fo. 46ᵛ.

[80] Ashm. 390, fo. 158. This might be Wickham near Newbury.

[81] Ashm. 1490, fos. 181–96.

[82] Ashm. 1490, fos. 199–220, 'The 7 bookes . . . toching the nature of thinges' and 'Two bockes . . . concerninge the nature of man'. These had been printed together in German in 1573. Charles Webster has identified this text as Karl Sudhoff, *Bibliographia Paracelsica*, i (Berlin, 1894), no. 145. Five years later Forman noted that he rode through William Fallowfield's woods on his way from London to Salisbury, Ashm. 208, fo. 54ᵛ.

[83] Ashm. 1490, fos. 277–89. For a critical edn. of this text see *Thomas Norton's Ordinal of Alchemy*, ed. John Reidy, Early English Text Society (Oxford, 1975).

[84] Ashm. 1490, fos. 165–6, 167–8, 106. Blomfild's verses are printed in Elias Ashmole (ed.), *Theatrum chemicum Britannicum* (1652), 305–23. On Blomfild see Robert M. Schuler, 'William Blomfild, Elizabethan Alchemist', *Ambix*, 20 (1973), 75–87.

[85] Ashm. 1433, ii, fos. 4ᵛ–10ᵛ. The date is recorded in the colophon. A translation of this text was soon issued with Roger Bacon, *The mirror of alchemy* (1597).

[86] Ashm. 208, fos. 46ᵛ, 47ᵛ. I do not think that Forman was referring to 'De arte geomantic', a manual on geomancy that he wrote in 1589 (Ashm. 354), though Ashm. 366 is an undated geomantical text written on parchment like a magical treatise.

spoke, or called angels. Occasional comments reveal that Forman was not a lone scholar ensconced in his library. A network of people with whom he shared interests and aspirations in the 1580s supported his activities, enabling him to study both printed and manuscript books, practise a variety of 'arts', many either dangerous or, like surgery, officially regulated, and write one, and possibly two or three or more, substantial treatises.[87] By the age of 38, with a constantly changing address and little money, Forman had invented himself as a medical practitioner, magician, astrologer, and alchemist. This was only the beginning. His studies continued, his aspirations increased, and new enemies opposed him. By 1591 Forman and Robert Parkes, the merchant in whose house he had stayed the previous year, had devised a method for calculating the longitude while at sea. In April Forman rode to London and stayed with the globe maker, Emery Molyneux, in order to teach him this method. In early June Forman was in Oxford and in July he advertised the method in a pamphlet, *The groundes of the longitude*.[88] This was Forman's first and last foray into print and it signals the beginning of his career in London.

[87] 'De arte geomantic', 1589 (Ashm. 354) is his earliest dated treatise. He probably wrote 'The groundes of physique and chirurgerie gathered out of the sayinges of dyvers auncient philosofers', *c.*1589 (Sloane 2550, fos. 1–117^{v}), though it is undated, see Ch. 3 n. 32. Ashm. 1429 has been misattributed to Forman by Black, probably because it is inscribed, perhaps by Napier, 'September 1611 Docter Formans booke reserved for the use of Clement his sonne'.

[88] Ashm. 208, fo. 47^{v}.

2

Astronomy, Magic, and the Mathematical Practitioners of London

On 6 July 1591 Forman sent to press his pamphlet, *The groundes of the longitude: with an admonition to all those that are incredulous* (hereafter *Longitude*).[1] It does not contain information about how to calculate longitude. It announces that the author, Simon Forman, has a secret method for doing these calculations, and it defends his method against those who had doubted its veracity. Like many of Forman's writings, its style is incoherent and self-aggrandizing. This chapter will document Forman's engagement with the mathematical practitioners of London in the months preceding and following the printing of this pamphlet; begin to explain Forman's reluctance to venture into print thereafter; and situate this episode amidst accounts by historians of science of the place of the occult in natural philosophy.

In his papers Forman does not record how he learnt astrology, medicine, magic, or any of the subjects that he pursued as an adult. He does tell us how he learnt his method for finding longitude. Robert Parkes (also described as Parker), merchant of London, had 'never thought of such a thing, nor never had indevoured himselfe there abouts, nor applied any parte of his studie to that intent', but one day God put an idea into his head. Parkes approached Forman, and,

> intreated me to take some paines therein, at whose earnest request I bestowed some part of my studie & endevour therein. And by the grace and helpe of God have brought it to that passe, which any man that is desirous of the knowledge thereof, may learne the trueth thereof at the Authors handes if he repayre unto him, or else if he or they repaire to *Master Robart Parkes* in pudding lane.[2]

[1] Ashm. 208, fo. 46^{v}. The Stationers' Company granted Thomas Dawson a licence to publish it on 12 July, Edward Arber (ed.), *A transcript of the registers of the Company of Stationers of London*, ii (1875), 277b. Forman used the formula 'the grounds of' in the titles of two other works, 'The grounds of arte', *c.*1594 (Ashm. 1495), a guide to astrology, and 'The groundes of physique and chirurgerie', *c.*1589? (Sloane 2550, fos. 1–117^{v}). The phrase was used for a variety of moral and mathematical primers, most notably Robert Recorde's oft-reprinted *The grounde of artes* (1543). Four copies of Forman's pamphlet are known to survive: one bound with his papers in the Ashmole collection, one in Salisbury Cathedral Library, one in the Pepys Library, Magdalen College, Cambridge, and one at Pembroke College, Cambridge.

[2] *Longitude*, sigs. A3^{v}–4.

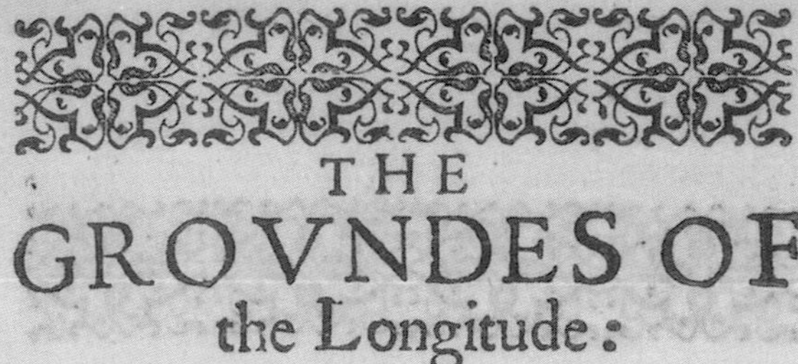

THE

GROVNDES OF

the Longitude:

With an Admonition to all those that are Incredulous and be- *leeue not the Trueth of* the same.

VVritten by Simon Forman, *student in* Astronomie and Phisique. 1591.

Nihil Impossibile Deo
Nil tam difficile quod non solertia vincat
Veritas filia Temporis.

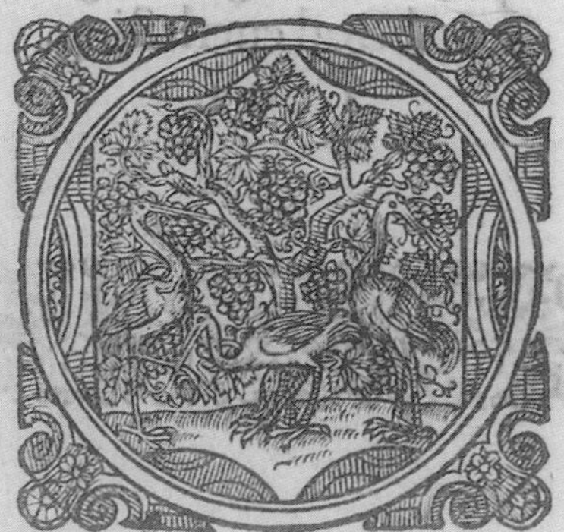

Imprinted at London by Thomas Dawson. 1591.

2.1. Simon Forman, *The groundes of the longitude* (1591), title-page. By permission of the Master and Fellows of Pembroke College, Cambridge. Shelfmark: 11.17.92(6).

Parkes and Forman had been friends since at least 1590 when Parkes had helped Forman: 'I ran into debt moch and had not Mr Parke bin I could not have told what to doe'.[3] Forman stayed with him in July 1590, and would stay with him again in August 1591. He probably advertised Parkes's address in the pamphlet because he did not have one of his own. It seems that they were a team: Parkes had the inspiration and an income, and Forman the astronomical expertise and audacity to launch the project.

As an astronomical pamphlet, *Longitude* was unremarkable. Numerous vernacular astronomical and navigational tracts had been printed in London since the 1550s, when Robert Recorde and John Dee had lauded the benefits to the commonwealth of providing mathematical instruction to craftsmen.[4] By the 1580s the city housed a thriving community of mathematical practitioners who made instruments, wrote books, and provided technical services and instruction.[5] Forman's involvement with this community was brief, and his contribution to it is considered negligible.[6] He opened *Longitude* with a survey of the instruments available in London and the books that described how to use them:

> Forasmuch as there hath beene diverse Bookes written heretofor, by diverse and sundrie learned men of the arte of Navigation and Cosmografical science, the invention & helpe of the Compasse: the making and use of the Astralabie, the practise of the Crosse staffe, and Ballestile, and divers other instruments aswell profitable as necessarie for those that use and practise the arte of Navigation . . .[7]

Forman's method, he explained, would make these instruments and their companion manuals redundant. Like these books, Forman's adopted the rhetoric of

[3] Ashm. 208, fo. 46v. E. G. R. Taylor compares Parkes with William Sanderson, a patron to John Davis (the navigator) and Emery Molyneux. She suggests that he may be the Robert Parke, a merchant, who translated Juan González de Mendoza, *The historie of the great and mightie kingdome of China* (1588): *The Mathematical Practitioners of Tudor and Stuart England* (Cambridge, 1967 [1954]), 190.

[4] On books, see H. S. Bennett, *English Books and Readers*, ii (Cambridge, 1965), 196–205; Francis R. Johnson, *Astronomical Thought in Renaissance England* (Baltimore, Md., 1937), ch. 5. On instruction, see Bennett, 'Mathematicians' Apprenticeship'; Feingold, *Mathematicians' Apprenticeship*; Hill, *Intellectual Origins*; Geoffrey Howson, *A History of Mathematical Education in England* (Cambridge, 1982), ch. 1.

[5] On the mathematical practitioners, see Ash, *Power, Knowledge, and Expertise*; Bennett, 'The Mechanics' Philosophy'; Feingold, *Mathematicians' Apprenticeship*; Harkness, '"Strange" Ideas'; Stephen Johnston, 'Mathematical Practitioners and Instruments in Elizabethan England', *Annals of Science*, 48 (1991), 319–44; Nick Popper, 'The English Polydaedali: How Gabriel Harvey Read Late Tudor London', *Journal of the History of Ideas*, 66 (2005), 351–81; Taylor, *Mathematical Practitioners*. On instrument makers specifically, see Gerard L'E. Turner, 'Mathematical Instrument-Making in London in the Sixteenth Century', in Turner, *Scientific Instruments and Experimental Philosophy 1550–1850* (Aldershot, 1990), 93–106; Turner, *Elizabethan Instrument Makers: The Origins of the London Trade in Precision Instrument Making* (Oxford, 2000).

[6] Johnston, 'Mathematical Practitioners', 319. Taylor dismisses Forman's pamphlet as vacuous: *Mathematical Practitioners*, 330.

[7] *Longitude*, sig. A2.

the availability of knowledge, was intended for a local audience, and was a quarto in the vernacular printed by Thomas Dawson, who had a line in navigational and related books.[8] Unlike these tracts, Forman's pamphlet was short (two quarto sheets), had no illustrations, and protested the privilege and secrecy of knowledge. He used a public medium to advertise *arcana imperii*; his profit depended on his discretion.[9]

Calculating longitude while at sea was an enduring problem.[10] Having dismissed conventional astronomical methods and new instruments alike, Forman advertised his solution. By his method,

> Masters and Sailers, that entend any long voyages, here shall you finde one of the chiefe pillers of your Arte, here shall you find a Pilate to direct you in a dangerous passage, being driven with a storme be it never so long, here shall you find a Load starre, that shall shewe you where you shall goe forth or backe, East or West. Yea you shall finde such a practise and knowledge that shall prove, or disprove all your Maps, Cardes, Globes, and Bookes that here before have beene written thereof and further it resolveth and discovereth all the doubts here before had in Navigation.[11]

Forman promised that the sailor would find a pilot, a polestar, and a 'practise and knowledge' that would test instruments. It is not clear, however, whether this was a literal or metaphoric description of his method. In either case, he provided no substance for the bold claims that, were they true, would have put the fate of nations in his hands.

Forman's audience, however, was not primarily the queen, not her advisers, not even the merchants who sought new routes to the riches of the new world. His audience was 'the travailers aswell by land as Sea, for the discoverie of straunge Places', the ship's captains and sailors whom he beckoned in the above passage along with the cosmographers and astronomers who had doubted him, attempted to steal his method, and would write books against it.[12] Forman

[8] H. G. Aldis *et al.* (eds.), *A Dictionary of Printers and Booksellers in England, Scotland and Ireland, and of Foreign Printers of English Books 1557–1640* (London, 1910), 86. See *STC* for Dawson's full publications. These include Thomas Hood, *The use of both the globes, celestiall, and terrestriall* (1592), Robert Hues, *Tractatus de globuset eorum usu* (1594), John Davis, *The seaman's secreats* (1595) and *The world's hydrographical description* (1595), and Pedro de Medina, *Arte of navigation*, tr. John Frampton (1581, 1595). Dawson also printed John Blagrave's *A mathematical jewel* (1585), a folio describing an instrument beyond all others. Cf. Feingold, *Mathematicians' Apprenticeship*, 181.

[9] Cf. Hugh Plat, *The jewell house of art and nature* (1594), sigs. B1–B4^{v}; pt. 2, pp. 69–76.

[10] See James A. Bennett, 'The Longitude and the New Science', *Vistas in Astronomy*, 28 (1985), 219–25; Bennett, 'The Mechanics' Philosophy'; David W. Waters, 'Nautical Astronomy and the Problem of Longitude', in John G. Burke (ed.), *The Uses of Science in the Age of Newton* (Berkeley, 1983), 144–69.

[11] *Longitude*, sig. A4^{v}; see also sig. A2. For a text that Forman might have echoed in this passage, see Medina, *Arte of navigation*, sig. ¶3^{v}.

[12] *Longitude*, sigs. A1^{v}, A4^{v}.

addressed locals and experts, and his reputation amongst the mathematical practitioners was at stake. Perhaps Forman was referring to this audience when he noted in his papers that 'vexations and evil speeches were used against me privily' in June of that year.[13]

Longitude was the product of a series of events in London. In a somewhat muddled passage Forman indicated that he had demonstrated the method, without revealing its secret, to a group of people: 'those to whom my selfe here before have shewed it upon the request of some which were very incredulous therof, and yet remaine because themselves as yet do not know the waie of dooing it'.[14] These were the cosmographers and astronomers who had accused Forman of being ignorant and his method illicit, and *Longitude* was a defence of his credit. Moreover, Forman had witnesses to and proponents of his methods:

> And as there hath beene heretofore diverse proffers made in the absence and behalfe of the Author, by Maister *Emery Mulleneux* & others, for the trueth and triall hereof and hath not beene accepted hetherto: because some have thought it eyther to be doone upon presumption, or on a Bravado, &c. But whatsoever they before have offered in the premises, I the Author hereof am ready at all times to performe the same God willing.[15]

Emery Molyneux was on Forman's side.[16]

Forman had stayed at Molyneux's house in Lambeth and taught his method for finding longitude only several months before, in the spring of 1591.[17] Molyneux was a compass and sandglass maker and the first English globe maker, but little is known about his life. In 1588 he had begun plans for the celestial and terrestrial globes that he would present to the queen in 1592, and he also made smaller versions of these for students of astronomy.[18] It is not clear how well Molyneux knew Forman or Parkes nor when or for how long this association lasted. In 1595 Forman recorded a list of substances, including various kinds of coal, saltpetre, pitch, oils, and waxes, which Parkes was supposed to buy for Molyneux, and several years later he described how Molyneux made perfect plaster casts of flowers.[19] Parkes was inspired with the knowledge of the secret method to discover longitude, Forman had perfected it, he had taught it to Molyneux and others, and they had 'sworne by a sacred othe not to manifest

13 Ashm. 390, fo. 127. 14 *Longitude*, sig. A2^{r-v}. 15 Ibid., sig. B3.

16 This passage has conventionally been read as indicating that Molyneux had spoken against Forman, and I am indebted to Traister for encouraging me to reread it: *Forman*, 224.

17 Ashm. 208, fo. 47^{v}.

18 For details of Molyneux's globes and further references see Gloria Clifton, *Directory of British Scientific Instrument Makers 1550–1851* (1995), 191 and Peter von der Krogt, *Globi Neerlandici: The Production of Globes in the Low Countries* (Utrecht, 1993), 107–12.

19 Ashm. 1490, fo. 350^{v}; 1494, fo. 324.

or teach the same to any' without Forman's permission. Some people voiced disbelief, Molyneux had offered either to demonstrate the method himself or to ask Forman to do it, and these offers had been declined.[20]

Longitude advertised and defended Forman's method. To the argument that someone as ill-educated as he could not discover a solution to a problem that had eluded scholars of previous generations, he replied that God had chosen this moment to reveal the secret to someone unlearned.[21] To the argument that his method was the work of the devil, he replied with fifteen grounds drawn from Genesis, Aristotle, and Ptolemy (for example, God created the sun and moon; the sun rises and falls and never stays put; there is fire in a flint stone). To challenge his method, he postured, was to challenge these truths.[22]

Forman left the cosmographers and astronomers who doubted him unnamed, but Thomas Hood, a Cambridge-trained astronomer and physician who had been mathematical lecturer to the City of London since 1588, identified himself.[23] He was writing *The use of both the globes, celestiall, and terrestriall* (1592), a treatise on how to apply Molyneux's globes, and he replied to Forman with a pamphlet which is now lost. Forman knew about it, noting in his diary that Hood's book against him came out on 22 November.[24] Thomas Harriot, the great mathematician, also read Hood's attack, and included it and Forman's *Longitude* in a list of works mentioning himself, though he did not specify whether he sided with Forman or Hood.[25] Hood it seems, either witnessed Forman's initial demonstration of his method to calculate longitude and remained incredulous, or refused to accept Molyneux's offers of another demonstration; Forman denounced him (and others unnamed) in his pamphlet; and Hood replied in kind. Hood's feud with Forman continued into the following year with the publication of his book on the use of Molyneux's globes. This included a loosely veiled reference to Forman in the preface: 'I am

20 *Longitude*, sig. A2^{v}. 21 Ibid., sig. A4^{r-v}.

22 Ibid., sigs. B1^{r-v}. He concluded, 'Too Groundes more I haue left out, because as they are most true so they give plain evidence, and too much understanding to a subtill witte.' Cf. the fourteen precepts in Hermes's 'Emerald tablet', printed in Roger Bacon, *Mirror of alchimy*, 16–17, and others in the Hermetic corpus, *Hermetica: The Greek* Corpus Hermeticum *and the Latin* Ascelpius *in a New English Translation with Notes and Introduction*, ed. Brian Copenhaver (Cambridge, 1992). On Copernicanism in England see Johnson, *Astronomical Thought.* Late in his life Forman recorded an isolated note about Copernicus' calculations for how long it took the fixed stars to move one degree: Ashm. 244, fo. 102^{v}.

23 *DNB*; Francis R. Johnson, 'Thomas Hood's Inaugural Address as a Mathematical Lecturer of the City of London (1588)', *Journal of the History of Ideas*, 3 (1942), 94–106; Johnston, 'Mathematical practitioners'; Taylor, *Mathematical Practitioners*, 178.

24 Ashm. 208, fo. 47^{v}. Rowse mistranscribes Hood as 'Good': *Forman*, 287.

25 For the identification of Forman's numerous references to 'doubting Thomas' as attacks on Thomas Hariot, see David B. Quinn and John W. Shirley, 'A Contemporary List of Hariot References', *Renaissance Quarterly*, 22 (1969), 9–26, esp. 22. But these also could be read as allusions to Thomas Hood. See also Johnston, 'Mathematical Practitioners', 335 n.

credible informed of late that certaine men, whereof one (how profoundly soever hee thinketh of his learning) not being hable ether to write true English, or Latine, hath gone about to *form an* outrageous, and most imprudent pamphlet to my disgrace, & to commit it to the presse' (Hood's italics). Hood then recriminated against one Kendell who could not read or write at all and ran up and down the court and city attempting to discredit Hood and others, thus showing that Forman was not a lone lunatic.[26] The animosity between the mathematical lecturer to the City of London and an impoverished, quasi-itinerant astrologer is evidence both of the lack of structure in the mathematical community in Elizabethan London and the possible rifts within it. Hood declaimed Forman's inability to write in English, let alone Latin, not because he objected to the pursuit of longitude by someone ill-educated, but because despite his lack of education Forman was so bold.[27] Hood probably also objected to the premisses of Forman's secret method.

Forman's engagement with the mathematical practitioners was short-lived and ill-fated, like many of his ventures in the previous years. He blamed Mars. In some notes relating to his diary he records that from 1586 until November 1595 the location of Mars meant that any matter that he spoke about failed. If he talked about plans for a trip, he was unable to go. If he told someone that he was owed money, it was not paid to him. But if he determined to do something and did it 'privily & secretly', then he prevailed.[28] Forman's concerns about the position of Mars reflect his tendency to indiscretion, and in part explain the hostility with which his method for calculating longitude was met. He was arrogant and secretive about his skills as an astrologer and alchemist. Towards the end of *Longitude* he promised that if his method for calculating longitude was duly rewarded (he hinted that he would sell it to the Spanish if it was not), he would 'perhaps make declaration, of the principles of another science, as much desired as this, of some other sortes of men, who labour continually for the knowledge thereof, and wander in darknesse, in a thing more mysticall and of greater importaunce then this'.[29] He was probably describing the secret of

[26] Hood identified Kendell in a pun: 'these men ... have gone about to Kendell a most vile conceit against me in your mindes'. Hood, *Use of both the globes*, sigs. A3^{v}–4. In 1594 Robert Hues also wrote a treatise on Molyneux's globes, and he similarly complained that although many methods for finding the longitude had been discredited, including measuring the equinoctal hours between the meridians of two places by using sun dials, clocks, or hour glasses, 'there are a kind of trifling Impostors, that make publike sale of these toyes or worse, and that with great ostentation or boasting; to the great abuse and expense of some men of good note and quality, who are perhaps better stored with money, then either learning or judgement.' *A learned treatise of globes*, tr. John Chimead (1639), 171–2. For a possible dismissal of Forman's 'great obscuritie, in finding the longitudes' see Robert Tanner, *A briefe treatise for the ready use of the sphere* (1592), 84.

[27] Cf. Francis Cooke's dedication of *The principles of geometrie, astronomie, and geographie* (Dec. 1591) to Hood.

[28] Ashm. 208, fo. 70; see also fo. 49^{r-v}.

[29] *Longitude*, sig. B3.

the philosophers' stone. This had been known to the ancients, then lost; but the secret of longitude had never before been known to any man. After tempting the reader with the divulgence of this secret, Forman concluded *Longitude* with a list of books that he planned to publish. These included a freshly calculated ephemeris and other books on astrology and astronomy.[30]

None of these books materialized and Forman never again succeeded in venturing into print. This is not to say that he ceased to write. By 1591 he had written at least one and perhaps two or more treatises. Over the next twenty years he composed no less than a dozen works and filled many notebooks with writings on subjects including plague, astrology, alchemy, cosmology, geomancy, magic, and Cabala. These writings mark Forman's pursuit of astronomy and astrology through the 1590s and his rekindled interest in alchemy and magic after 1600. With the exception of a guide to astrology that he planned and failed to have printed, Forman shunned or neglected the possibility of having his manuscripts printed, manuscripts that contained his methods for discerning the secrets of the heavens and the earth, the past and the future, life and death, and perhaps even one's longitude while at sea.

Here is Forman's description of the books that he planned to publish if *Longitude* was well received:

> certaine other Bookes of Astronomie and Astrologie, as the Booke of the three sortes of houres, Naturall, Artificiall and Magicall, with all the doubtes of Astronomie, and alterations and significations of the Planets, the mooving of the eight Sphere, and the way to errect a figure both by the Eccliptike line, as also by the oblique ascention, wherein the misterie of Arte lieth hid, with divers other Bookes God willing if they may be permitted.[31]

The items in this list do not match the extant notes on prognostications or treatises on geomancy that Forman had written by 1591, though some notes on the eighth sphere probably date from this period.[32] Fifteen years later he drafted a

30 Ibid., sig. B3ᵛ. There are some tables headed 'longitude' in Ashm. 205, fos. 213–20.

31 *Longitude*, sig. B3ᵛ.

32 The treatises on geomancy are Ashm. 354, dated 1589; 392, *c.*1590, revised *c.*1611. Astronomical notes in Forman's small and tidy hand typical of *c.*1590 (see the dated items in Ashm. 1490) now are bound with the 1589 treatise on geomancy. These discuss the motions of the eighth sphere, the moon, and the sun, perhaps following Sacrobosco's 'Spheres': Ashm. 354, fos. 178–82, 187ᵛ–8, 189–97. His later treatise on geomancy also included astronomical information, e.g. Ashm. 354, fo. 190. Ashm. 366, a parchment book of geomancy which included longitudinal tables, probably relates to Forman's methods in the early 1590s, though the hand is more typical of his later years. For notes attributed to Forman and copied in a strangely antiquated hand on 'ye syns of planets and … ye degress of ye clock' see Trinity MS O.2.13, fo. 236. For eclipses and the weather see Ashm. 384 throughout, esp. fos. 116–87 for early notes and fos. 38–80 for 'Of the eclipses of the sonne and moone' dated 1592 and added to later. It is possible that Forman had written 'The groundes of physique and chirurgerie' (Sloane 2550, fos. 1–117ᵛ) *c.*1589, see Ch. 3 n. 32.

set of essays that included discussions of at least three of the promised subjects, 'the three sortes of hours', 'the mooving of the eight Sphere', and 'the way to errect a figure both by the Eccliptike line, as also by the oblique ascention'. Although many years had passed between the promised list in *Longitude* and these writings, they are a key to understanding Forman's method for calculating longitude and the controversy that it provoked.

These essays are grouped under the heading 'The motion of the 3 superiour heavens' (hereafter 'Heavens') and Forman drafted them between 1606 and 1608, probably intending them to form a coherent treatise.[33] For most Renaissance astronomers the cosmos was divided into ten celestial, crystalline spheres or heavens (some authors argued that there were nine). The earth was fixed at the centre of the cosmos, surrounded by the spheres of the five known planets (Mercury, Venus, Mars, Jupiter, and Saturn) plus the moon and the sun. Beyond these were three superior spheres, known as the eighth, ninth, and tenth heavens, and these were the subject of Forman's essays. The tenth sphere was the *primum mobile*, the first mover, and the source of all of the motion in the cosmos; the ninth sphere was an immobile zodiac; the eighth sphere was a mobile zodiac of fixed stars. This scheme was outlined in astronomical primers and at the outset of treatises on navigation, and Forman's account describes the same details and draws on the same authors as, for instance, Pedro de Medina's *Arte of navigation*.[34] Forman's 'Heavens', however, departed from the typical scheme in two ways. He drew analogies between the motions of the heavens, the divine Trinity, and man's body, and he described the relationship between the motions of the heavens and magical operations.

'Heavens' begins with the motions of the three superior, celestial heavens, and their analogies with the supercelestial Trinity of the Father, Son, and Holy Spirit, analogies drawing on varieties of Neoplatonic and Christian cosmology.[35] The tenth heaven was the first mover, God's first work of creation. It moved naturally from east to west, and carried all of the spheres 'against their own proper and naturalle motions'. It was analogous to God in

[33] Ashm. 244, fos. 34–117. Distinguishing between the different sets of papers now bound together in this volume is difficult. This is a set of papers probably grouped together by Forman, beginning with 'The account of the years of the wordle gathered by my self out of the wordle 1610 the 8 octob' (fos. 25–33). The sections beginning with 'the motion of the 3 superiour heavens' (fos. 34–118) seem to have been stitched together previously, date from 1606 to 1608, and include multiple drafts of some of the headings. For related, and damaged, pages on the ninth heaven, see Ashm. 802, fos. 169–70^v.

[34] e.g. William Cunningham, *The cosmographical glasse* (1559); Medina, *Arte of navigation*; Martin Cortes, *The arte of navigation*, tr. Richard Eden (1561). Cf. Robert Recorde, *Castle of knowledge* (1556), 7–10. On the traditions on which these tracts drew, see Edward Grant, *Planets, Stars, and Orbs: The Medieval Cosmos, 1200–1687* (Cambridge, 1994); S. K. Heninger, *The Cosmographical Glass: Renaissance Diagrams of the Universe* (San Marino, Calif., 1977), chs. 1, 2, 4; Johnson, *Astronomical Thought*, chs. 1, 2.

[35] Grant, *Planets, Stars, and Orbs*, chs. 13, 18, esp. pp. 315–23; Heninger, *Cosmographical Glass*, chs. 3, 4.

purity, eternity, and constancy of motion; and to the spirit of man.[36] The ninth sphere, or second mover, was the 'watrie firmamente or glasse heaven'. It had no natural motion of its own, was analogous to Christ in stability, similitude, power, and virtue, and it contained the souls of men; the soul obeyed the spirit as the ninth heaven followed the tenth heaven.[37] The eighth heaven was the third mover and the 'starry firmament'. It contained the fixed stars, the 'immobile zodiac', and had two motions, one 'natural', one 'unnatural'. The 'unnatural' motion was from east to west, carried by the tenth heaven, but the eight degrees of variation of its equinoxes observed by astronomers were caused by its 'natural' motion. Finally, the eighth heaven was assigned to the Holy Ghost and the spiritual body of man.[38] Forman added a Paracelsian dimension to this scheme: as the three spheres corresponded to the Trinity and to the spirit, soul, and body, so they were analogous to mercury, sulphur, and salt.[39]

The motions of the eighth and ninth spheres, Forman explained, factored in astrological calculations and magical operations. The ninth heaven was filled with souls and symbols, the 'sigils, signs and characters of all the angels and sprites and of every particular man and all the stars and planets and every creature of god celestiall, terrestrial, and infernal'.[40] Symbols and angels resided in the ninth heaven, and its motions governed the powers of symbols and angelic revelations, but 'the influences operations and effectes magicalle are in and don by the 8 heaven and not by the 9 heaven and primo mobile'.[41] This is why Forman's earlier distinction between the natural and unnatural motions of the eighth heaven was important: 'all influences naturall & operations naturalle doe com from and procead from the 8 heaven and from ye fixed stars therin, and from the plannetes movinge under the 8 heaven accordinge to nature and naturalle workinge'.[42] More specifically, the access and recess of the eighth heaven.

> doe make and cause the alteration of all thinge more and lesse in the wordle and in the cause of putrifaction and corruption, of encrease and decrease, of strength and weknes, of good and bad, of rising and fallinge, of pride and humblenes and plainnes, and of the alteration of countries places states lawes religion & nations, of autorities and dignities, of drith heat moisture and cold, of barraines & plenty, of artes labors industries and conninge skille, & all other things & tymes what somever.[43]

The good magician worked with the natural motions of the planets and needed to know his astronomy and his astrology. Magic and astrology motivated Forman's study of astronomy.

[36] Ashm. 244, fo. 35^{r-v}. [37] Ashm. 244, fos. 36–41^{v}. [38] Ashm. 244, fos. 44–7.
[39] Ashm. 244, fos. 35^{v}, 46^{v}–7. [40] Ashm. 244, fo. 40^{v}. [41] Ashm. 244, fo. 44.
[42] Ashm. 244, fo. 46. [43] Ibid.; see also fo. 45^{v}.

He studied the differences between the motions of the three superior heavens, particularly between the eighth and the ninth. Such calculations determined the times to make a variety of magical objects (rings, images, sigils, swords) that could be used to cure diseases, expel vermin, dogs, and wolves, vanquish one's enemies, and improve or hinder a man's fortune. These had to be made according to the positions of the eighth heaven because the eighth heaven governed all things that changed with time.[44] When Forman noted at the end of *Longitude* that he would print an astronomical and astrological book that discussed the motions of the eighth sphere, this was probably what he had in mind.

The eighth sphere, Forman explained in the 'Heavens', was also essential in calculating the three sorts of hours, natural, artificial, and magical, another topic promised in *Longitude*. 'Natural hours' were measured by a clock, according to which the day always began at midnight. These were the units used for measuring all natural causes and calculating a nativity. 'Artificial hours' were measured by dividing the period between sunrise and sunset into twelve, and the same for the period between sunset and sunrise, and thus they varied in length throughout the year. This sort of hour was used for calculating the timing of ordinary actions, known as elections, such as the beginning of a journey, setting sail, praying, or administering medicines. 'Magical hours' determined the times to make magical amulets, for instance, and were measured according to the ascension of the ecliptic line of the eighth heaven.[45] Illustrating how to make such a calculation, Forman set an astrological figure for the ninth heaven then adjusted it according to his stellar tables.[46] These notes probably related to 'the way to errect a figure both by the Eccliptike line, as also by the oblique ascention', a third topic that Forman promised at the conclusion of *Longitude*. This was the secret of Forman's method for calculating longitude, 'wherein the misterie of Arte lieth hid'; perhaps these were calculations to divine one's longitude.[47]

In *Longitude* Forman implied that his astronomy was linked to occult subjects. Fifteen years later in the 'Heavens' he articulated an analogy between the

44 Ashm. 244, fo. 48.

45 Ashm. 244, fos. 91–2. Cf. Heinrich Cornelius Agrippa von Nettesheim, *De occulta philosophia*, (Paris, 1567), bk. 2, ch. 34 on natural and artificial hours. Forman cited this and ch. 29 in his discussion of how the eighth heaven governs magical operations: Ashm. 244, fo. 48^{r-v}.

46 Ashm. 244, fo. 96^{r-v}. There are further notes about setting figures and references to a number of ephemerides throughout this volume. For tables to calculate the motions of the eighth sphere, see fos. 54^{v}–60, 109–14. See also Forman's tables for calculating nativities throughout Ashm. 206.

47 *Longitude*, sig. $B3^{v}$. 'Heavens' did not include a discussion of the 'alterations and significations of the Planets', though one of Forman's guides to astrological physic had a section 'Of the natures and alterations of the plannets accordinge to ye signes they are in': Ashm. 355, pp. 201–404.

A table of the motion of the 8 heaven that I found in an old parchment booke. In the which booke yt was thus writen. In knowing to make an instrument to know the beginnings and endings of the 28 mansions. The said

Mansiones sphere 8a sunt 28 que incipiunt a principio signis None sphere. propter quod inde tabulam equationis motus 8e sphere a Nona sphera

Ista tabula est tabula Equationis 8 sphere super 9 annis Christi est 2 signa 17 gradus 50 minuta ad Annum domini 23.

Anni Collecti	Tabula Equationis motus 8e sphere		
Radix	gr	minute	2a
1300	9	27	50
1310	9	31	42
1320	9	36	3
1330	9	40	29
1340	9	44	49
1350	9	49	3
1360	9	53	11
1370	9	57	13
1380	10	1	10
1390	10	50	0
1400	10	51	25
1410	10	55	17
1420	10	59	9
1430	11	3	1
1440	11	6	53
1450	11	10	45
1460	11	14	37
1470	11	18	29
1480	11	22	21
1490	11	26	13
1500	11	26	5
1510	11	26	57
1520	11	30	49
1530	11	34	41
1540	11	38	33
1550	11	42	27

so farr — this following I have added

Anni collecti	Tabula motus equationis 8e sphere		
	gr	m	2a
1560	11	46	19
1570	11	50	11
1580	11	54	3
1590	11	57	55
1600	12	1	47
1610	12	5	39
1620	12	9	31
1630	12	13	23
1640	12	17	15
1650	12	21	7
1660	12	24	59
1670	12	28	51
1680	12	32	43
1690	12	36	35
1700	12	40	27

Anni Christi	Motus par[...] Circuli on which the 8 heaven [...]			
	Sig	gr	m	2a
1300	2	1	46	29
1310	2	2	39	31
1320	2	3	32	32
1330	2	4	25	35
1340	2	5	18	38
1350	2	6	11	39
1360	2	7	4	42
1370	2	7	57	44
1380	2	8	50	49
1390	2	9	43	40
1400	2	10	36	42
1410	2	11	29	48
1420	2	11	23	30
1450	2	12	16	33
1460	2	13	9	36
1470	2	14	2	39
1480	2	14	55	42
1490	2	15	28	45
1500	2	16	41	48
1510	2	17	34	51
1520	2	18	27	54
1530	2	19	20	57
1540	2	20	14	0
1550	2	21	7	3
1560	2	22	0	6
1570	2	22	53	9
1580	2	23	46	12
1590	2	24	39	16
1600	2	25	32	19
1610	2	26	26	23
1620	2	27	19	26

The small circle on which the 8 heaven doth move is in breadth from side to side 16. 8 gr. 37 and 26 seconde.

2.2. 'A table of the motion of the 8 heaven that I found in an old parchment bocke', Ashm. 244, fo. 54v. By permission of the Bodleian Library, University of Oxford.

microcosm and macrocosm and outlined how to make magical amulets. Almost all of Forman's extant writings were produced in the years between the dates of these two documents. That Forman wrote about subjects in 1606 that he had promised his readers in 1591 shows some continuity in his studies. It also highlights the gaps in the extant papers: if Forman wrote about cosmology prior to 1591, these notes are missing save the traces of them in his later papers. Another piece of evidence links *Longitude* and the 'Heavens', confirming that these two texts were part of the same project. Towards the beginning of *Longitude* Forman argued that God, as the creator of all things and source of all wisdom, had distributed knowledge across the ages just as he distributed skills and arts amongst the men of any generation. As St Paul said, God made many vessels to fill with different things, giving one man the knowledge of one thing, and another the knowledge of something else. Forman elaborated, drawing on a different Pauline epistle, 'to some the gifte of prophecie, to some the gift of healing, to some of doing wonders and miracle, to some the interpretation of thinges, and finding of hidden misteries, yet al is the administration of one spirit, and power of the holy Ghost'.[48] The 'Heavens' included a similar list in a discussion of 'howe the 8 heaven is assigned to the holly ghoste': 'For Paull saith, To som he gives the gifte of preachinge, to some of teatchinge, to som of healinge the sick and diseasede, to som of prophesinge and telling of things to com, to som of on thing, to som of a nother'. Forman concluded this passage 'yet all is the administration of on sprite and power of the holly ghoste', word for word repeating the phrase used in *Longitude*.[49] Elsewhere Forman added an astrological component to this argument,[50] but the similarities between the passages in *Longitude* and in the 'Heavens' probably indicates a kinship between these texts, perhaps in a parent set of notes. The passage in *Longitude* was predicated on the ideas articulated in the 'Heavens'. In *Longitude* Forman used this passage awkwardly to justify why he had the secret knowledge of how to find longitude; in the 'Heavens' the Pauline proverbs were integral to Forman's account of the analogy between the eighth heaven, the Holy Ghost, and man's body.

Across time Forman's writings became more sophisticated, better informed, and perhaps more deliberately arcane. As he constantly wrote, he often read, sprinkling the names of authors throughout his pages, though seldom including detail of the pages, titles, or editions of his sources. Stacked end to end these works would have filled several shelves in Forman's study in

[48] *Longitude*, sig. A3. The first half is from Romans 9: 21, the second from 1 Corinthians 12: 7–11.

[49] Ashm. 244, fo. 46.

[50] Ashm. 1436, fo. 139; 403, fo. 97ᵛ.

1606.[51] In *Longitude* Forman listed twenty-two authors from whom God withheld the secrets of longitude, beginning with Claudius Ptolemy, the great Alexandrian astronomer and ending with Cyprian Leowitz, a sixteenth-century German known for his prognostications, a treatise on the great conjunctions, and a defence of astrology. Forman also drew maxims from the standard medieval astronomical texts, Sacrobosco's 'De Spaera' ('Spheres'), the widely circulated account of Ptolemaic geometry, and the Alphonsine Tables, tabulations of the positions and movements of the planets. He cited two fifteenth-century authors, Georg Peurbach and Johann Müller (known as Regiomontanus), both reputed for their astrological as well as astronomical expertise and writings, and two sixteenth-century authors in addition to Leowitz, Pedro de Medina, author of the well-known treatise on navigation and Georg Stadius, best known for his astronomical tables.[52] In the 'Heavens' Forman's citations were more extensive, including, for instance, the ancient astronomers Hipparchus and Julius Africanus, perhaps drawing on references to them in Ptolemy's *Almagest* and Sacrobosco's 'Spheres'. He drew heavily on the teachings of Thabit b. Qurra (Thebit), the ninth-century Arabic astronomer, on the motions of the planets. And he cited books large and small by his near-contemporaries: the ephemerides of Michael Maestlin and Origanus (David Tost), and astronomical and astrological works by Girolamo Cardano, Hieronymus Wolf, Jean Taisner, Luca Gaurico, Giovanni Paolo Gallucci, Albert Pigghe, Peter Apian, Johannes Schöner, and others.[53] He cited manuscripts that he owned, such as 'an old parchment bocke writen by one Petrus Adamarus out of the bockes of Marsilius', which was actually a fourteenth-century text of Profatius Judaeus' 'New quadrant'.[54]

Forman's collection, or at least his reading, included the staple works of astronomy and astrology in the sixteenth century, though he did not mention English books. He departed from the canon in combining his study of these books with his study of magic, and over the years, despite the losses of his books, he had also built up a solid collection of magical texts. For instance, sometime in the 1580s he bought a copy of the 1567 edition of Cornelius Agrippa's *De occulta philosophia* and in 1592 he transcribed an old manuscript

[51] On identifying Forman's books, see pp. 28–30 above.

[52] *Longitude*, sig. A3^{v}.

[53] Ashm. 244, fos. 34–118 *passim.*

[54] This is Ashm. 360, fos. 49–61d. The text had a commentary by G. Machio (sometimes listed as Judeo Marciliensis), and was corrected and perfected by Petro de Sancto Adamaro—hence Forman's identifying it by the scribe and commentator. Cf. Ashm. 1796, fos. 55–76^{v} and see Lynn Thorndike and Pearl Kibre, *A Catalogue of Incipits of Mediaeval Scientific Writings in Latin* (Cambridge, Mass., 1963) for other variants of this text.

of the 'Picatrix', an Arabic magical compendium probably dating from the twelfth century.[55] The astrological and astronomical books occasionally touch on magic; and the magical books assume a basic knowledge of cosmography.

I have not located a model for Forman's blending of astronomy, astrology, and magic in any of his readings. He did articulate, however, the relationships between astronomy, astrology, and magic that underpinned 'Heavens' in some notes that date from either around 1590 or 1611. Probably borrowing from another author, Forman defined astronomy as the greatest science and divided it into five parts: astronomy, astrology, astromagic, geomancy, and alchemy. Astronomy, as one of the subdivisions, was the knowledge of the heavens, meaning the motions and properties of the stars and planets. Astrology was the reading of the significance of the stars and planets by judging their motions, places, natures, beings, and aspects. The operative part of astronomy was astromagic, the power of the stars to influence things, according to the knowledge of astronomy and the judgements of astrology. This was done by making rings, sigils, images, and characters at significant moments in order to enclose in them or stamp them with the virtues of the stars and planets. As astrology was the reading of the stars, geomancy was the reading of marks which were pricked in earth or sand, or written on parchment or paper: 'By the arte of geomancie youe may knowe sodainly all thinges paste present and to com.' The fifth art was alchemy, or 'alchemagic', the science of transmuting metals and making the philosophers' stone. In the science of astronomy as a whole, both the heavens and the earth had to be understood: for instance, the art of geomancy required the help of celestial astronomy.[56] Other taxonomies of the occult sciences stressed the dependence of the astrologer, geomancer, alchemist, and magician on astronomy.[57] Occult practitioners needed knowledge of the stars and they might in turn contribute to astronomical knowledge. For instance, one of the medieval traditions of commentaries on Sacrobosco's 'Spheres' was

[55] I have deduced Forman's ownership of a copy of Agrippa's work printed in Paris in 1567 from his notes to look further in the work and references to book, chapter, and folio numbers. For a discussion of the English reception of the Picatrix, including copies owned by Forman, Napier, Lilly, and Ashmole, see David Pingree (ed.), *Picatrix: The Latin Versions of the Ghayat al-hakim*, Studies of the Warburg Institute, 39 (1986), pp. xix, liii–lv; Sloane 3679 seems to be in Napier's hand. For the earlier reception of the 'Picatrix' see esp. Eugenio Garin, *Astrology in the Renaissance: The Zodiac of Life*, tr. Carolyn Jackson and June Allen (1983), esp. chs. 2 and 3. Although his copy has not yet been located, Forman recorded information from it throughout his notes: e.g. Ashm. 244, fos. 45, 97; 431, fo. 146^{r-v}; 1491, p. 1128. For Forman's notes on demon genitures from Marsilio Ficino, *De vita coeleitus comparanda*, see Ashm. 244, fos. 106–8; 206, fo. 22.

[56] Ashm. 392, fo. 46; cf. 1433, ii. 21–2^{v}, Forman's *c.*1606? notes on the philosophers' stone.

[57] Cf. Bodleian, Jones MS 1, fo. 49, a seven-part scheme ('astrologia, magia, divinatio, nigromantia, signatum, artes incertae, artes materiales') that Forman attributed to Paracelsus; John Dee's 'Preface' to Euclid, *Elements of geometrie*, tr. Henry Billingsley (1570); Paola Zambelli, *The Speculum astronomiae and its Enigma: Astronomy, Theology and Science in Albertus Magnus and his Contemporaries* (1982).

magical, culminating with the writings of Cecco d'Ascoli in the fourteenth century, and although the textual trail here runs dry Forman was probably an heir to this tradition.[58]

In 'Heavens' Forman touched on most of the subjects that he singled out as forthcoming at the end of *Longitude*. Fifteen years divided the publication of *Longitude* and the datable elements in 'Heavens', and I have been cautious not to ascribe Forman's later ideas to his earlier work. By 1591 his interest in the motions of the eighth sphere, the three sorts of hours, and the various methods of setting astrological figures had been kindled. These interests were explicitly astrological and magical. This is why Forman invoked the authority of hermetic knowledge in his engagement with the mathematical practitioners. While both the seaman and the astrologer were dependent on longitude, one to navigate the seas and the other to traverse an astrological chart, Forman's method for finding longitude remained a mystery. He thought that his understanding of the motions of the spheres contained the answer, and I suspect that his method included some form of astral divination.[59] Just before going to stay at Molyneux's house in the spring of 1591, Forman 'put the longitude in question'.[60] Perhaps he tested his method; or, since for him a 'question' was a type of astrological figure, he probably calculated the position of the stars at that moment and therein read his secret. Briefly Forman interloped in the activities of the mathematical practitioners, broadcasting his power to solve one of the great mysteries of nature. Thereafter he protested his authority and expertise together.

[58] Lynn Thorndike, *The Sphere of Sacrobosco and its Commentators* (Chicago, 1949); Thorndike, 'Robertus Anglicus and the Introduction of Demons and Magic into Commentaries upon the Sphere of Sacrobosco', *Speculum*, 21 (1946), 241–3; Thorndike, *History of Magic and Experimental Sciences*, pp. ii, v, vi, and *passim*. See also the tradition of talismanic magic attributed to Thebit and Ptolemy in Arabic texts tr. into Latin in the 12th cent., as discussed in Charles Burnett, 'Talismans: Magic as Science? Necromancy among the Seven Liberal Arts', in Burnett, *Magic and Divination in the Middle Ages: Texts and Technicians in the Islamic and Christian Worlds* (Aldershot, 1996), 1–15.

[59] See e.g. Ashm. 244, fo. 36^{v}, where Forman proposes a method to solve the mathematicians' problems of calculating the trepidation (an adjustment to account for the differences between the motions of the ninth and tenth heavens due to precession), concluding that they are the same because the ninth heaven has no natural motion at all; cf. Grant, *Planets, Stars, and Orbs*, 315.

[60] Ashm. 208, fo. 47^{v}. Forman used the phrase 'in question' to mean to conduct a trial or to assess, e.g. authors of medical treatises 'bring the science of physick in question wher it be a true science or no'; in 1593 the barber surgeons called Forman 'in question for my practice', Ashm. 208, fo. 49; 1491, p. 1276.

3
How to Write Like a Magus

Hood's book attacking Forman was published on 22 November 1591. The following evening as the sun was setting Forman read Hermes Trismegistus' *Poimandres*, an account of the creation of the world much like Genesis. Hermes, in a sleep-like state, has a series of delightful and frightening visions, through which Poimandres, 'mind of sovereignty', reveals the wisdom of creation.[1] The next morning Forman had the following dream:

> I sawe appearing in the clouds of heaven a man 10 tyms bigger and greter then any other man, with a marvailouse great face and his berd was not very longe but of a chestnut colloure, and a very high forhed. And he sate as in his magesty clothed downe to the feete in a purple gowne. And he loked very devoutly and held up his hands somwhat, and round aboute him shined a mervaylouse greate lighte & brightnes, moch brighter then the sonn. And when I sawe him me thought that yt was christe him selfe.

Forman identified with Hermes, like him a bedazzled initiate in the mysteries of God and nature. In the dream Forman put his face to the ground and cried for mercy. Everyone else was scared and ran away, but he continued to grovel and cry; 'the very power of the sprite of god' did not frighten him. He tried to hear what the man in the vision would say and could not. In the dream Forman 'thought with my selfe nowe shall I find mercy with the lord and obtein that which I have long desyred'. Then he woke up and sobbed.[2] Hood might have dismissed Forman as ignorant and perhaps even demonic, but Forman saw visions of Christ in his dreams and knew that his fortunes would improve.

The proximity of the publication of Hood's pamphlet and Forman's dream might be circumstantial, but it illustrates that throughout the year in which Forman published *Longitude*, he studied hermetic and alchemical texts. These writings promoted a definition of knowledge as arcane and divinely imparted. I have charted Forman's access to occult studies through the 1580s, read his gestures towards revealed knowledge in *Longitude*, and previewed his pursuit of astral magic in the 1600s. I now want to step back from these texts and to explore Forman's definitions of knowledge and his portrayal of his own authority throughout his writings. Then I will turn to the forms and genres in which

[1] Copenhaver (ed.), *Hermetica*, 1–7.

[2] Ashm. 1472, pp. 810–[11] (24 Nov. 1591).

Forman wrote, through him reflecting on how the form in which a text was published, in print or in manuscript, related to the subject matter and to the status, social, intellectual, and divinely sanctioned, of its author.

Hermes Trismegistus was the ancient Egyptian sage whose alleged writings prompted the doctrines and cosmology known as hermeticism. I will begin with Forman's debt to these traditions. Since the thirteenth century alchemical texts attributed to Hermes had circulated in Europe, and alchemy was often described as the hermetic art. In the late fifteenth century, following the fall of Constantinople, further texts attributed to Hermes were recovered, though these were more philosophical and had a distinct provenance from the alchemical texts. The texts were brought to Florence, translated from Greek to Latin by Marsilio Ficino, the humanist at work for Cosmo de'Medici, and printed as the *Corpus Hermeticum* (1463). Equipped with these and other Neoplatonic texts Ficino positioned man as an intermediary between the divine and the natural, the macrocosm and microcosm, and he presented natural magic as a theologically legitimate vehicle for man to achieve divine enlightenment and to become a magus.[3] Like Hermes, a magus literally permeated the mundane, celestial, and supercelestial spheres.[4] Hermes embodied inspired knowledge of the secrets of nature and hermeticism was more than the ideas expressed in the writings bearing his name.[5]

Forman never defined his own commitment to Hermes. He occasionally located the occult practitioner at the hub of the cosmos, defining, for instance, the astronomer as master of the greatest science, able to divine things past, present, and future and to influence them.[6] Practical knowledge, not natural or occult philosophy, was the subject of Forman's writings. But occult knowledge required wisdom and judgement and it was difficult to learn and complicated to write about. It was ancient and divinely inspired; it might be conveyed through texts, through experience, and through dreams and revelations. Hermes, Forman reminded the reader in *Longitude*, found the seven gold tablets and talked with the Holy Ghost (whom Forman equated with

[3] Yates, *Bruno*; Walker, *Spiritual and Demonic Magic*.

[4] Clark, *Thinking with Demons*; Webster, *Paracelsus to Newton*, 49, 57–8; Yates, *Bruno*, 22.

[5] For discussion of hermeticism and hermetism, see esp. Clulee, *Dee's Natural Philosophy*, ch. 1; Copenhaver, 'Astrology and Magic', esp. 283–4; Copenhaver, 'Natural Magic, Hermetism, and Occultism', esp. 272–5; Allen Debus and Ingrid Merkel (eds.), *Hermeticism and the Renaissance* (Washington, DC, 1998); Vickers (ed.), *Occult and Scientific Mentalities*, introduction; Webster, *Paracelsus to Newton*; and Robert Westman and J. E. McGuire, *Hermeticism and the Scientific Revolution* (Los Angeles, 1977). For ancient and medieval definitions of hermeticism, see Charles Burnett, 'The Establishment of Medieval Hermeticism', in Peter Linehan and Janet Nelson (eds.), *The Medieval World* (2001), 111–30; Copenhaver (ed.), *Hermetica*.

[6] Ashm. 392, fo. 46.

Poimandres), evidence that the 'creatures of God manifest his power and glory'.[7] A magus's authority was in his credentials as heir to divine and ancient knowledge, credentials that Forman articulated through his experience of true judgements, marrying a language of hermeticism with practical expertise.[8]

Forman most clearly declared the divine imperative of his knowledge in his alchemical writings. Around 1606 at the outset of an unfinished tract on the philosophers' stone, he addressed the reader:

And first to make the matter and way more plaine unto the reader of this my bocke the which I nowe here write not for any love I beare unto the wordle or people lyvinge: because both the wordle and people ar all Enimies unto me, and hate me and ever did. For I was born under such a constellation that the wordle people & hell should ever be my Enimies and againste me. And therfor I have noe love to them because they malign me without juste cause, and alwaies render me Evill for good & hatred for my good will. Neither doe I write this bocke for any profit or commodity I hope to have for my Laboure, nor for feare of any: But because arte shall not be buryed in oblivion and because knowledge shall not decay in the future tyme in the generations that shall com hear after & ar yet unborn. And because both those that ar nowe lyvinge and those that ar yet unborn shall knowe that god is almighty and giveth his giftes unto every man accordingly as he will and according to the capacity of the man (that because also the generation that is yet to com shalbe more righteouse than those that nowe live yet shall they swerve moch from god and true understanding) I have compiled by the grace and gifte of god this bocke, wherin they shall see the course of natur and facility of things done in tyme with discretion.[9]

Things done in time and with discretion meant according to astrological calculations. In 1609, in notes on the affordability of alchemical materials, Forman again digressed, this time reflecting back on three decades of study and work as an alchemist and astrologer-physician. He noted that knowledge could not be found in texts, nor by the traditional means of passing alchemical secrets from master to pupil:

For ther is a waie that goeth by tradition, that never came in bocks, which is easyly and spedily with small coste to be done as Experience hath showed to many. But this wai is hard to be found amonge men or of men, except a man have a greet and depe Judgment and be wise in workinge and a god among men.

[7] Forman, *Longitude*, sig. A3. Forman cited works attributed to Hermes throughout his notes and writings on astrology and alchemy.

[8] Cf. William Eamon, *Science and the Secrets of Nature: Books of Secrets in Medieval and Early Modern Culture* (Princeton, 1994); Pamela O. Long, *Openness, Secrecy, Authorship: Technical Arts and the Culture of Knowledge from Antiquity to the Renaissance* (Baltimore, Md., 2001); William F. Ryan and Charles B. Schmitt (eds.), *Pseudo-Aristotle: The Secret of Secrets: Sources and Influences* (1982).

[9] Ashm. 1433, ii, fo. 23^{r-v}. For more on this treatise, see p. 171 below.

He continued, for the first and only time acknowledging even a modicum of debt to the learning of someone he knew personally: 'Yet for my selfe I never lerned anythinge of any man, neither could I say that ever I was behoulding to any man for Art but to on simple fellowe, but to god and nature. For I was borne to find out arte and to make yt perfecte.'[10]

As St Paul had said, on the divine assembly line each man was fitted with different skills and virtues, and Forman was equipped as an astrologer-physician supreme.[11] The stars determined this, and his enmity with the College of Physicians verified it. In his 1607 plague tract Forman explained:

> because I knowe that in the course of heaven by the decre of god yt is set downe that the heavens by naturall course & influence shall bringe forth all manner of people, good and bad, and professores of all artes misteries craftes and sciences, and such again as shall dispise all artes craftes misteries and sciences.[12]

For every person born with a certain art, someone lacking in that capacity would be born. Forman had an uncanny aptitude for the astronomical arts and his enemies confirmed this. Elsewhere Forman extended this principle, 'for every man is not borne one for anothers health, because some be enemyes and unfortunate one to another by nature'.[13] Forman and his persecutors enacted a divine dialectic.

In this drama Forman cast himself in the age-old part of the magus and traced his predecessors in a series of genealogies of knowledge, often including Hermes Trismegistus. For instance in his earliest guide to astrological physic he outlined the history of astronomy: Abraham, according to Josephus, taught it to the Egyptians; according to Berosus, the Babylonian priest (in Annius of Viterbo's fifteenth-century forgery), Noah, Jacob, and Joseph also excelled in this study. Forman elaborated on Noah's knowledge of astronomy, noting that King Boccus had asked King Tractabar for a copy of the book of Noah that was owned by his astronomer, Sydrake. Forman had found this final detail in an old book, *The hystory of Kyng Boccus and Sydrake*, a compendium of information about subjects ranging from sex to science.[14] In other cases, such as in *Longitude*, Forman compiled genealogies of astrologers that ranged from Ptolemy to Guido Bonatti, the famous thirteenth-century astrologer.[15] He often included his name alongside those of renowned astrologers and alchemists, proclaiming

[10] Ashm. 1491, p. 1248. Cf. the verse preface to Forman's *c.*1597 alchemical commonplace book, Ashm. 1472, fo. 6^{r-v}.

[11] *Longitude*, sig. A3; see p. 50 above.

[12] Ashm. 1436, fo. 139.

[13] Ashm. 403, fo. 97^{v}.

[14] Ashm. 1495, fo. 5; *The hystory of Kyng Boccus and Sydrake* (*c.*1537). Forman's copy is in the library of St. John's College, Oxford. See also T. L. Burton (ed.), *Sidrak and Bokkus*, 2 vols. (Oxford, 1998).

[15] *Longitude*, sig. $A3^{v}$. See also Ashm. 1490, fo. 222^{v}; 1494, p. 174.

himself an heir to divine wisdom and ancient knowledge and advertising his authority and expertise.[16]

With God on his side Forman acquired the secrets of alchemy and astrology through dreams and experience. Texts were more problematic. Although Forman cherished and studied hundreds of alchemical texts, he did not learn the secrets of alchemy from them; for these he was beholden to God, and the elusive 'simple fellowe'.[17] Likewise, he discounted the value of his many astrological books, though he never explained how he learnt to read an ephemeris, cast a figure, or make a judgement.[18] In decrying texts on matters of love, he noted: 'I have reade manie bockes in my daies which have entreated of love, and sene manie experments wryten howe to obteine the love of maids, wives and wyddowes, but I never found any of them true as they ar set downe, but fals and deceighetfulle.' Sometimes love magic worked and sometimes it did not; 'For I have knowen som man hath proved an expermente and hath found yt true. The same man hath proved yt at another tyme and hath found yt fals and they knowe not the reason herof.' Forman's method was proven: 'But I have found by Experience that all consisteth in the tyme of doinge yt, for yf the tyme accordinge to the revolution of the heavens, and aspects of the plannets agre not to his working, all his works shall be in vaine, for all things ar done in tyme and bound for tyme.'[19] As an astrologer Forman knew that all matters, including love, depended on the positions of the stars. He had learnt from experience what he could not learn from books.

Forman's dreams document a more complex pedagogy. Dreams were vehicles for prophetic visions and alchemical knowledge. Forman marked dreams in treatises that he read, and he noted details about 'the angelic stone', a form of the philosophers' stone that endowed men with knowledge in 'dreams & otherwise'.[20] He kept a dream book, now missing, and in his casebooks he recorded the times of his dreams, cast figures to know what they prophesied,

[16] He did this most often by including his propositions amongst those of other authors. See for instance Sloane 2550, fos. 5–7; Trinity MS o.9.7, fo. 28ᵛ; Ashm. 389, *passim*; 206, fos. 24–9; 384, fos. 9ᵛ, 10, 13ᵛ, 27, 33, 68; 392, fos. 20–1.

[17] Ashm. 1491, p. 1248; see p. 57 above.

[18] Cf. 'The erection of thy figure by the oblique ascention, after Jhon de Regio Montano [Regiomontanus] . . . Loke fo. 122': Ashm. 206, fos. 76–[81]. On Forman's use of the system of Regiomontanus to cast figures, see John North, *Horoscopes and History* (1986), 162.

[19] Ashm. 390, fo. 29. See also Ashm. 363, fo. 132ᵛ; 403, fo. 81.

[20] Ashm. 1494, p. 623. The growing literature on dreams is surveyed in Patricia Crawford, 'Women's Dreams in Early Modern England', *History Workshop Journal*, 49 (2000), 129–41. For the relationship between dreams and astrology, as articulated by Cardano, see Siraisi, *Cardano*, ch. 8 and Grafton, *Cardano's Cosmos*, 158. Forman was particularly interested in the prophetic dreams of the sibyls, noting them and their interpretations in the margins of his copy of a sibylline text: Ashm. 1490, fos. 102–6. See Ashm. 802, fo. 26 for a prophetic dream of the 'Queen of Saba'.

and noted the events that followed.[21] At several stages he copied notes on twenty-one of his dreams into a commonplace book under the heading 'Of certaine dremes and visions that I have sene totching the philosophers stone'.[22] Some of these were about the philosophers' stone but most foretold his fortune in finding a wife, discovering hidden treasure, or securing invitations to dine with important people.[23]

Sometimes God worked through books and dreams together, as in the cases of alchemical texts that could not be read or even acquired without divine intervention.[24] For instance, on the morning of 4 January 1594 Forman dreamt that he encountered two men reading a book about the philosophers' stone, began to talk to them, and 'toke the bock to expound yt unto ym'. The next day around noon 'a strange man that dwelte at the gren dragon at holborn conduit [came] and broughte me this bocke & another lyttle bock of notes of astronomy to sell. And I bought them.' Forman duly recorded this note and the details of the dream that foretold this purchase amongst the pages of the book, a manuscript collection of alchemical notes previously belonging to Thomas Digges (1546–95), the author of astronomical and astrological publications.[25] Forman would encounter the other side of this black market in books several years later when the Cambridge students robbed his study.[26]

In another dream Forman was the only one who could read a book that an old woman was trying to sell. This dream is dated 31 October 1595:

I dremt that I was in a place by a passage wai and ther cam an old woman with a parchment bock in folio writen with many pictures, and she offred the bocke to mani to sell, and none wold buy it, because they said they could not read yt. And when I sawe them all refuse it I called the woman unto me and asked what I should give for the bocke & she toke me the book and I loked in yt and could reed and understand yt well. And the old woman put her hand upon my head and prayed over me & blessed me sayinge blessed arte thou my sonne that delightest in wisdom and seekeste after knowledge. To the shall the gates of all goodnes be opened, goe one and prosper. And she stood on my

21 See esp. Ashm. 234, fos. 123–4, 156ᵛ-7; 226, fos. 44–5; 219, fo. 136.

22 Ashm. 1472, pp. 807–[13]. There seems to be no order to these dreams, and the pages may now be bound out of sequence.

23 On the philosophers' stone: Ashm. 1472, p. [811] (7 Nov. 1587); p. 812 (18 May 1591). The last dream also appears under the heading of 'Del visions vel somne' (Ashm. 390, fo. 132ᵛ). On other matters: Ashm. 1472, p. [807] (27 and 28 Dec. 1602, 22 Apr. 1607); p. 808 (9 Oct. 1596, 20 Dec. 1597, 6 Mar. 1599); p. [809] (12 Sept. 1588); p. 812 (16 Nov. 1593).

24 Cf. Lucius' dreams and initiation into the cults of Isis and Osiris in Apuleius, *Metamorphoses*, discussed in Long, *Openness, Secrecy, Authorship*, 53; on Nicholas Flamel, an alchemical persona invented in the 16th cent. based on a medieval Frenchman, who reputedly also dreamt of an angel that prefigured his acquisition of a book, see Robert Halleux, 'Le Mythe de Nicolas Flamel, ou les méchanisms de la pseudépigraphie alchimique', *Archives internationales d'histoire des science*, 33 (1983), 234–55.

25 Ashm. 1478, fo. 48ᵛ.

26 See pp. 29–30 above.

right hand and I sate on a thing and my face towards the south and the people pressed moch aboute me wonderfully to heare what was written in the bock. By reason wherof I lefte [off] to locke farder therin, but I closed the bocke and did put yt in my bosom. And the old woman closed my girkin on yt. And I said mother give me leave to peruse yt thorowe and then com to me again and sai what I shall pai for yt. Soe she set me noe price but departed leaving the bock with me. And soe I awaked.[27]

Unlike the myth of the Sibyls, in this dream Forman saw the book before its price was demanded. In this dream Forman sat amidst a group of people with an arcane book cradled in his lap and an old woman standing by his side. He alone could read the text, but instead of expounding its contents to the eager audience, he closed it and clutched it to his chest. If such scenes occurred, no records of them survive. The page was Forman's arena and he pontificated throughout his life-writings, astrological handbooks, plague tracts, and alchemical commonplace books. He projected himself above all as an authority on astrology, endowed by God with knowledge of the workings of the microcosm. But he did not expose his words on the printed page; the constant motion of his pen, endlessly perfecting his writings and protesting his expertise, did not propel his words into print.[28] A plan to print a guide to astrology illustrates the complexities of Forman's attitude to his audience.

On 19 September 1599 Forman wrote to Richard Napier, the rector of Great Linford, Buckinghamshire:

I thought yt not amisse to signifie unto youe howe far I have proceded in the bocke that I told youe I mente to put in presse. I have halfe done. Therfore I pray forget not your promise for the answeringe of all invectives againste our profession that youe may have yt redy with expedition in the English tongu for all the wordle to vewe.[29]

The 'profession' which Forman and Napier shared was astrological medicine. Napier had consulted Forman in January 1597, and thereafter Forman had tutored Napier in astrology. They met occasionally in London and in Buckinghamshire and Forman sent Napier advice about books, recipes, herbs, and difficult cases.[30] Napier, perhaps bound by an oath, reciprocated with packages of food and books. One January, on receiving a stale turkey pie from

27 Ashm. 1472, p. 809 (31 Oct. 1595).

28 In a list of 'things Againste a Common wealth', probably drawn from another author and mostly concerning the timber supply, he included 'Printing of books, because yt hindreth scollars and writing and mainteyneth vice': Ashm. 195, fo. 151.

29 Ashm. 240, fo. 103.

30 Napier first consulted Forman on 22 and 26 Jan. 1597, Ashm. 226, fos. 3, 6. See also Ashm. 226, fos. 89^{v}, 184^{v}, 206; 208, fos. 59^{v}, 61^{r}; 219, fo. 79; 1488, fo. 89; 236, fo. 252^{v}; 802, fo. 152^{r-v}; 338, fos. 95^{v}, 98, 114. Forman's letters to Napier are listed in the Bibliography; I have not located any of Napier's letters to Forman.

Napier, Forman reminded him that 'I have done that for thee scoller that I have done for no man the like', and that he thus should take better care with the dispatch of his gifts.[31]

The half-finished book that Forman described in his 1599 letter to Napier was probably a manual of astrological physic. Through the 1590s Forman had written and rewritten several guides to the subject. Around 1594 or 1595 he compiled astrological rules relating to medicine in 'The grounds of arte gathered out of diverse authors' (hereafter 'Grounds of arte'), between 1596 and 1599 he incorporated much of this material under the title 'The astrologicalle judgmentes of phisick and other questions' ('Astrologicalle judgmentes'), and in 1600 he wrote a related volume, 'Liber juditiorum morborum' ('The book of the judgments of diseases'; only the title is Latin).[32] In 1599 Forman was probably preparing 'Astrologicalle judgmentes' for the press and he continued revising it for many years. These works spell out the rules for astrological medicine at great length, running to hundreds of pages. Napier fulfilled his promise, albeit belatedly, in May 1602 when he sent Forman 'A treatise touching the defenc of astrologie' ('Defenc') along with the usual gammon of bacon.[33]

[31] Ashm. 240, fos. 104, 110^{v}. Forman did not specify the year, though he noted that he had received Napier's offering on Tues., 30 Jan., which would make the year either 1599 or 1610. In 1611 Napier sent Forman '2 cheases and a lyttell bock of Merline': Ashm. 240, fo. 106. Perhaps this was the same book that Forman described in 1601: 'Mr. Horner in Croked Lane at the corner house a victeling house he hath merlines profecies in parchemente': Ashm. 411, fo. 163^{v}.

[32] I have taken the title of 'Grounds of arte' (Ashm. 1495) from fo. 11, though it might designate a section rather than the entire work. 'Liber juditiorum morborum' is Ashm. 355. There are multiple extant copies of 'Astrologicalle judgmentes'. Ashm. 403 is in the hand of Richard Napier and dates from *c.*1599 though the preface is dated 1596. Ashm. 389 is the only one in Forman's hand, is dated 1606, and contains examples from 1607. The most extensive, and latest version is Ashm. 363, in two hands, perhaps those of Thomas Robson and Sir Richard Napier (the nephew of Richard Napier), and, though it is dated 1600 in the preface, it contains examples through 1608. A fourth manuscript, Sloane 99, consists of the Introduction and chs. 6 and 7 only, and for these the text is the same as that for Ashm. 363. Cf. Forman's 'The groundes of physique and chirurgerie' (Sloane 2550, fos. 1–117^{v}), an undated treatise on medicine containing expositions of positions drawn from twenty-nine authors, a discussion of the four humours and four virtues, and a number of remedies, all drawing on alchemical and astrological principles. This work probably dates from *c.*1589, as Forman used a couple of examples from that year (fo. 19^{r-v}), styled himself 'student in astronomy and physic' as he did in *Longitude* (fo. 5), and the hand is small, tidy, and ornate as in his dated works from this period; see also Ashm. 1495, fo. 11. Later notes were added to Sloane 2550, e.g. one in 1596 on fo. 17^{v}. See also the accompanying 'A treatise of purginge', Sloane 2550, fos. 118–127^{v}; and Napier's copy of this: Oxford, Corpus Christi College MS 169, fos. 1–67.

[33] For a holograph copy of Napier's 'Defenc' see Ashm. 204, fos. 50–63, with the final pages bound in Ashm. 240, fos. 137–8. A partial, more legible transcript in a different hand is Ashm. 242, fos. 189–96. Neither of these is bound with Forman's 'Astrologicalle judgements', nor with Forman's papers. In Napier's record of the dispatch of his 'Defenc', an astrological query, he referred to it as his 'apology of Astrology': Ashm. 221, fo. 66. Two days earlier Napier recorded that he 'sente to London to D Dee and Forman the books I promised and a gammon of bacon', but his carrier, one father John Rutland, was not going to London that week so his boy returned with the books and bacon: Ashm. 221, fo. 56. For Ashmole's interest in these notes see Ashm. 1790, fo. 64.

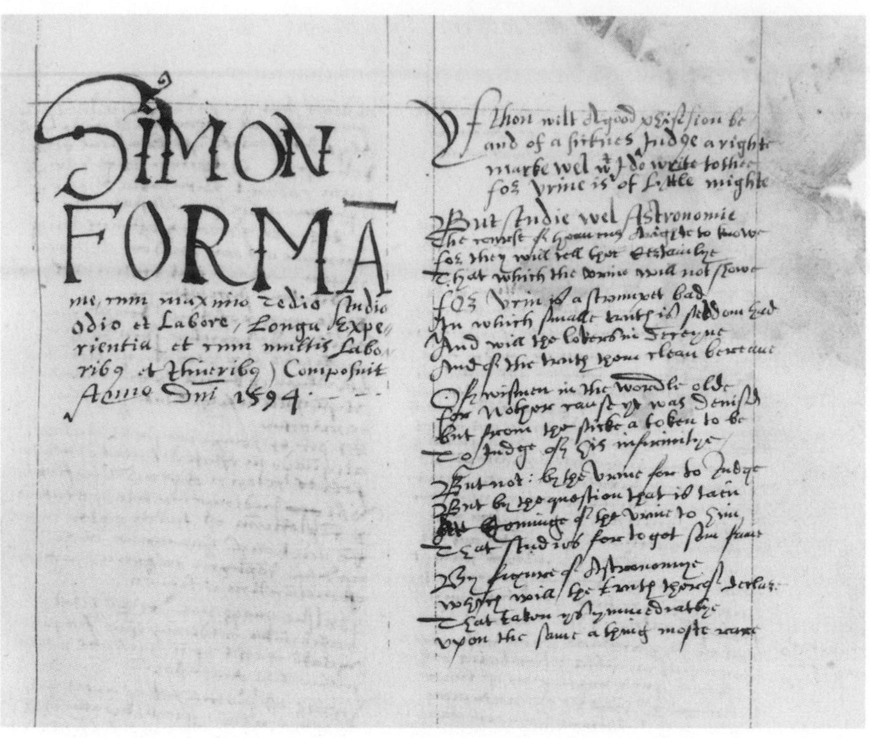
SIMON FORMAN
me, cum maximo tedio studio odio et Labore, Longu[m] Experientia et cum multis Laboribus et Itineribus) Composuit Anno Dni 1594

If thou wilt a good physicion be
and of a pisses judge aright
marke wel w[hat] I do write to thee
for urine is of little might

But studie wel Astronomie

3.1. Simon Forman, 'The grounds of arte', *c.*1594–5, Ashm. 1495, fo. 3. By permission of the Bodleian Library, University of Oxford.

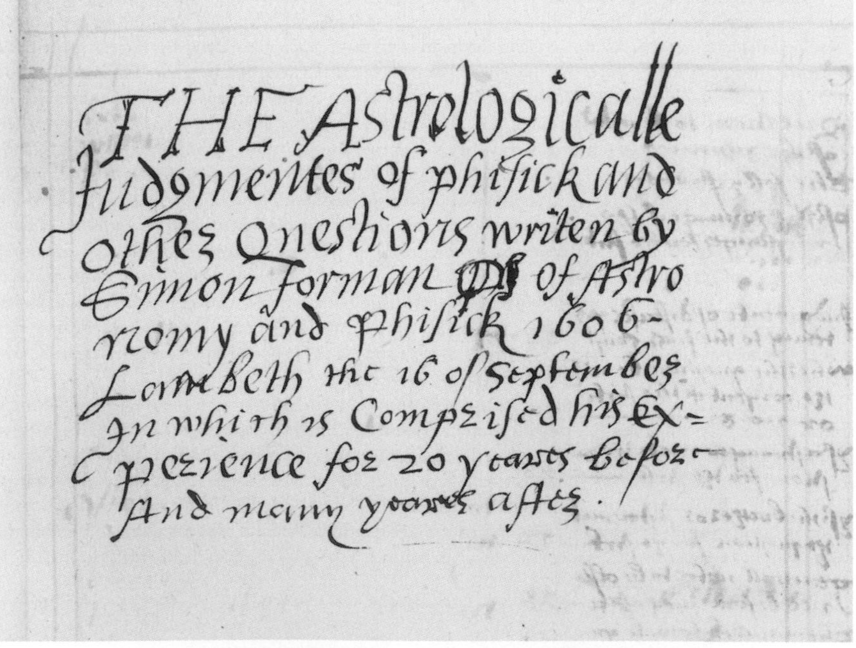
THE Astrologicalle
Judgmentes of phisick and
other Questions writen by
Simon Forman of Astro
nomy and Phisick 1606
Lambeth the 16 of September
In which is Compised his Ex=
perience for 20 yeares befor
And many yeares after.

3.2. Simon Forman, 'The astrologicalle judgmentes of phisick and other questions', 1596–9, with later revisions, Ashm. 389, fo. [6]. By permission of the Bodleian Library, University of Oxford.

3.3. Simon Forman, 'Liber juditiorum morborum', 1600, Ashm. 355, fo. 1. By permission of the Bodleian Library, University of Oxford.

50

A treatise touching the defenc of astrologie

3.4. Richard Napier, 'A treatise touching the defenc of astrologie', *c*.1599–1602, Ashm. 204, fo. 50. By permission of the Bodleian Library, University of Oxford.

Forman's project was never completed. He continued revising 'Astrologicalle judgmentes' at least through 1607, he seems not to have paired it with Napier's 'Defenc', and neither work was printed. Perhaps they never finished the project or decided it was not timely. Perhaps it was too expensive to print or too controversial a subject to be licensed for the press.[34] At the turn of the century Forman was thriving. He kept the doctors at bay, got married, bought a horse and new clothes, and had his picture drawn.[35] In 1601 John Chamber's *A treatise against judicial astrology* was printed, sparking old debates. Sir Christopher Heydon responded with *A defense of judicial astrology* in 1603, perhaps making the Forman–Napier venture redundant.[36] This debate and the accession of James VI and I in 1603 prompted strictures on printing astrological texts. For instance, Heydon's 1607 *An astrological discourse with mathematical demonstrations* was denied permission for printing and remained in manuscript until 1650.[37] Works like Forman's on astrological physic also remained in manuscript.[38] Nor were attacks on astrology destined (immediately) for print, such as Chamber's response to Heydon and a treatise by George Carleton which circulated in manuscript for twenty years before being printed as *Astrologomania* in 1624.[39]

When Forman wrote to Napier in September 1599, hundreds of astrological books and manuscripts could have been found in London. Astronomical primers often included astrological information.[40] Almanacs were printed annually, containing calendars of ecclesiastical holidays, the phases of the moon, dates of fairs or other local information, and prognostications about the weather, harvest, disease, and politics. They also advertised the services of their authors.[41] Extraordinary astronomical events, such as the conjunction of

34 F. S. Siebert, *Freedom of the Press in England 1476–1776: The Rise and Decline of Government Control* (Urbana, Ill., 1952), 59–85; Thomas, *Decline of Magic*, 344–5.

35 Ashm. 208, fo. 61 (doctors); 219, fos. 100^{r-v}, 106, 111, 135, 136^{v}; 208, fos. 61, 136, 226^{v} (wife, Jean Baker); 219, fos. 49, 62; 208, fo. 61^{v} (horse); 208, fo. 62^{v} (new clothes, picture).

36 For the slow printing of this book, see David McKitterick, *A History of Cambridge University Press*, i (Cambridge, 1992), 243.

37 Ashm. 242, fos. 1–13; Heydon, *An astrological discourse with mathematical demonstrations*, ed. Nicholas Fiske (1650). Heydon gave a fair copy of the text to Richard Forster, the physician, who gave it to Fiske. Fiske prepared it for publication, and Elias Ashmole subsidized the printing of the diagrams, *Ashmole*, ed. Josten, ii. 499–501.

38 For instance Mark Ridley (1560–1624), a physician and author of a treatise on the magnet, wrote a (previously unattributed) guide to astrology sometime between 1603 and his death: Ashm. 1501, i. For a guide to astrology devoted specifically to medicine written *c.*1620 and later owned and perhaps annotated by Thomas Harley, see Folger MS V.b.4. The date 1620 appears on p. 62. An exception is John Fage, *Speculum aegrotorum* (1606), on which see p. 68 below.

39 Bodleian, Saville MS 42; Allen, *Star-Crossed Renaissance*, 139–40.

40 Richard Dunn, 'The True Place of Astrology among the Mathematical Arts of Late Tudor England', *Annals of Science*, 51 (1994), 151–63.

41 Capp, *Astrology and the Popular Press*.

Saturn and Jupiter in 1583, spawned prognostications and these in turn kindled attacks against astrologers.[42] With the possible exception of his profitable activities in 1582, Forman seems to have been uninterested in the perennial activities of almanac-makers and oblivious to sensational prognostications, though he might have read and discarded these works, such as the mock-prognostication on which he jotted astrological rules and sent to Napier in 1597.[43] The 1590s were astronomically uneventful and astrologically quiet, though William Covell's *Polimanteia, or, the meanes lawfull and unlawfull, to judge of the fall of a common-wealth* (Cambridge, 1595) catalogued the arguments against divination and denounced astrologers, perhaps provoking Forman.[44]

The practice of astrology required a specialized array of books. Forman owned works on how to interpret the positions of the stars and ephemerides, tables of the heavenly bodies, such as the one that fell out of his saddlebag when he rode to Merley, Dorset, in 1601.[45] He bought these texts second-hand, such as the fifteenth-century manuscripts of Alcabitius' 'Introduction to astrology' and Geoffrey Chaucer's 'Treatise on the astrolabe'.[46] Persistent and eclectic in buying, borrowing, and copying books, his notebooks on nativities, for instance, began with the opening pages of an English translation of Johannes Schöner, *De judiciis nativitatum libri tres* (Nuremberg, 1545), a translation probably circulating in manuscript.[47] On the causes of comets, Forman did not hesitate to cite John Maplet's *The diall of destiny* (1581), a vernacular work summarizing scholarly accounts of the influences of the heavens on earthly events.[48]

Forman's astrological manual would have sat neatly on a shelf with the big Latin tomes on the subject, but next to English texts it was overgrown with detail.[49] When he drafted his first manual of astrological physic *c.*1594–5, he

[42] Allen, *Star-Crossed Renaissance*, 125.

[43] Forman's activities in 1582 are discussed in Ch. 1. John Cypriano, *A moste strange and wonderfull prophesie upon this troblesome worlde*, tr. Anthony Holloway (1595); Forman's copy is now bound in Ashm. 546.

[44] See also two mock-prognostications from 1591, Simon Smel-knauve [Anthony Munday?], *The fearefull and lamentable effects of two dangerous comets*; Adam Fouleweather, *A wonderfull, strange and miraculous, astrologicall prognostication.*

[45] Ashm. 208, fo. 64.

[46] Ashm. 360, iv, fos. 89–108b; v, fos. 116–28.

[47] Ashm. 206, fos. 8–18^v.

[48] Ashm. 384, fo. 78.

[49] For guides to astrology see Mary Bowden, 'The Astrological Revolution of the Seventeenth Century (1558–1686)', Ph.D. thesis, Yale University, 1974, 29, 36; Hugh G. Dick, 'Students of Physic and Astrology: A Survey of Astrological Medicine in the Age of Science', *Journal of the History of Medicine*, 1–2 (1946), 300–15, 419–33; Richard Dunn, 'The Status of Astrology in Elizabethan England 1558–1603', Ph.D. thesis, University of Cambridge, 1992, 30–41; Jacques E. Halbronn, 'The Revealing Process of Translation and Criticism in the History of Astrology', in Patrick Curry (ed.), *Astrology, Science and Society* (Woodbridge, 1987), 197–217, esp. 199; Thomas, *Decline of Magic*, 304–5. Some of the primary texts are surveyed by Allen, *Star-Crossed Renaissance*, 247–55. On the limited discussion of astrology in English

did not acknowledge astrological manuals printed in English. Perhaps he knew Andrew Boorde's outline of the principles of astrology or Fabian Wither's translations of the works by the well-known French astrologers Claude Dariot and John Indagine (or De Hayn).[50] The Indagine translation had been printed in 1558, and again in 1575, and Dariot in 1583. Perhaps Forman also knew Humphrey Baker's 1558 translation of an augmented version of Oronce Fine's more extensive and apparently less often reprinted work on judicial astrology.[51] Forman also neglected books on nativities, such as William Warde's translation in 1562 of a text attributed to Arcandam of Aleandri and Thomas Kelway's recently issued translation of Auger Ferrier's treatise on nativities (1593).[52] Even if Forman could not find these books second-hand, new editions were often available. Warde's translation of Arcandam was reprinted in 1592, Ferrier on nativities in 1593, and Dariot's and Indagine's works in 1598. Forman's astrological manuals had more in common with Francis Sparry's translation from the French of *The geomancie of maister Christopher Cattan gentleman* (1591) than these other books, though again he did not cite it. This work provided a thorough exposition of geomancy, modelled on Latin astrological works, and Sparry had corrected and added astrological information to the text.[53]

Most of these books were eclectic, describing astrology alongside other forms of divination such as physiognomy and chiromancy. Some were devoted to nativities or concentrated on the influences of the moon.[54] Medical astrology was represented throughout them. Indagine's book said little on the subject but the translator directed the reader to Dariot's work, which in turn contained a treatise on astrology and medicine, or mathematical physic by

medical books see Allan Chapman, 'Astrological Medicine', in Webster (ed.), *Health, Medicine, and Mortality*, 275–300. On Latin astrological texts available in England see for instance Roberts and Watson (eds.), *Dee's Library*, and the occasional Latin astrological book was printed in London, e.g. Cyprian Leowitz, *Brevis et perspicua ratio judicandi genituras* (1558), issued with Dee's *Propaedeumata aphoristica*: Clulee, *John Dee's Natural Philosophy*, 35.

50 Andrew Boorde, *The pryncyples of astronamye* (1547); Claude Dariot, *A breefe and most easie introduction to the astrologicall judgment of the starres* (1583); John Indagine, *Brief introductions* (1558). Forman included 'Dariotus' in a list of authors *c.*1589, probably indicating that he knew a work by Dariot in Latin or through citations in another source: Sloane 2550, fo. 1.

51 Fine, *The rules and righte ample documents, toutching the use and practise of the common almanackes, which are named ephemeredes.*

52 *The most excellent, profitable and pleasant book, of the famous doctor and expert astrologian Arcandam of Aleandri*, originally published by Richard Rowsat as *Canonicus Lingoniensis* (Paris, 1542); Ferrier, *A learned astronomical discourse.*

53 *The geomancie of maister Christopher Cattan*, sig. A3.

54 John Harvey, *An astrologicall addition* (1583); Richard Harvey, *An astrological discourse upon the great and notable conjunction of the two superiour planets, Saturne and Jupiter* (1583). See also *Key to unknowne knowledge*; Fage, *Speculum aegrotorum.*

G. C., perhaps one George Carey.[55] In 1583 John Harvey issued a translation of *Iatromathematica*, a brief treatise on decumbitures attributed to Hermes Trismegistus, along with an addition to his brother Richard's work on the conjunction of Saturn and Jupiter. In 1599 *The key to unknowne knowledge*, written by an unnamed surgeon, presented considerable medical instruction. Similarly, John Fage's *Speculum aegrotorum* (1606) contained the rudiments of astrological medicine.[56]

Forman's 'Astrologicalle judgmentes', like Sparry's translation of the book on geomancy, provided elaborate rules according to the twelve celestial houses; like Fine, Forman recounted Josephus' history of astronomy as an art taught by Adam to Seth. Yet, with the exception of Maplet's *Diall of destiny*, Forman showed no signs that he knew these or other English astrological books. Instead he drew heavily on Latin astrological texts, often denigrating their authors while flaunting his own learning. His silence about the English books suggests that he shunned the men who translated, augmented, and wrote them, though he might have obtained his supply of Latin books from the same sources as these men. Moreover, his terminology belies his engagement, whether in reading or in conversation, with English practitioners and proponents of astrology. For instance, he used the word 'querent' to describe a person posing a question to an astrologer, a word that probably became a part of English astrological parlance only in the 1580s.[57] Forman postured as a disciple of learned astrologers because he, with Napier's help, aspired to bring a new sort of astrological physic to London, complete with a defence of the art of judicial astrology, instructions for casting a figure, and the most perfect methods for judging the causes of a disease. Other English astrological books outlined the rudiments of astrology for any who could read the vernacular, leaving the debates about the validity and morality of astrology, expositions of different methods of calculation, and subtleties of interpretation to other books.[58] Forman was more ambitious. His expertise and authority, Napier's 'Defenc', and the legacy of the unprinted book that they hoped to produce illustrate the extent to which judicial astrolo-

[55] This identification is suggested by the references to 'Carey's mathematical physic' in Folger MS V.b.4, pp. 64–9, 84. Bowden, 'Astrological Revolution', 143 n., suggests that this is George Carew (1500–85), dean of Christ Church Oxford, though it might also have been George Carey, Second Lord Hundson (1547–1603), George Carew (d. 1612), George Carew (1555–1629), or another man of this name: *DNB*.

[56] Wither, G. C., and Fage promised further works, but none is recorded.

[57] Dariot, *Briefe and most easie introduction*. *OED*, 'querent' cites the 1598 edn., but it was first printed in 1583.

[58] For the complaint that astrologers obfuscated their art, see Thomas Brasbridge, *The poor mans jewel* (1592 [1578]), sig. A7^{r-v}. On the complexities of astrological expositions, see for instance Tamsyn Barton, *Power and Knowledge: Astrology, Physiognomics, and Medicine under the Roman Empire* (Ann Arbor, 1994); Ann Geneva, *Astrology and the Seventeenth Century Mind: William Lilly and the Language of the Stars* (Manchester, 1995).

gy, specifically astrological physic, could traverse conventions local and international, Latin and vernacular, scholarly and skilled.

Napier rehearsed the standard theological and historical justifications for judicial astrology, drawing particular attention to its importance in medicine. He included a long account of the history of astrology (which he noted was synonymous with astronomy), beginning with Seth or Abraham (depending on the source) engraving it on the twin pillars of knowledge, one of stone the other of brick, and thereby ensuring that it survived the Flood.[59] It was an ancient, legitimate, and divinely sanctioned art.[60] It had been 'pleasant & delightsome' for rulers, and was also 'commodious & fruitfull for it sheweth & teacheth us the wonderfulle vurse [verse] of the heavens'; it was beneficial or necessary for husbandry, navigation, medicine, law, and divinity.[61] This was the context in which Napier first mentioned medicine: without astrology to guide judgements about diet, the administration of medicines, and critical days, 'physicke is to be accounted utterly unperfect'.[62]

Napier challenged the standard objections to judicial astrology. These were, first, astrologers had not reached a consensus about the principles of their art. For instance, some cast nativities based on the moment of conception, others on the moment of birth. Secondly, prediction was incommensurate with Christianity. Even predictions that were correct, as by chance some would be, were of little value because there was no use in knowing what was inevitable. The debates hinged on this fulcrum, opponents stressing the supposed inevitability and rigidity of the things signified by the stars, and proponents stressing that the future could be altered. Thirdly, many philosophers, emperors, and divines throughout history had objected to astrology. Napier countered all of these objections. He catalogued the uses of astrology since antiquity, faced the theological objections, and addressed whether the stars carried any significance, especially 'whether a sound, & complete phisition can want the knowledge of Astronomie'.[63] For Napier and Forman, judicial astrology was legal, veracious, and essential to the art of physic.[64]

Forman had delegated the task of defending judicial astrology in general and defining its importance for medicine in particular to Napier. As Forman

59 Ashm. 204, fo. 50^{r-v}. 60 Ashm. 204, fos. 50–1, 52.

61 Although husbandry and physic often were associated with astrology, most commonly in almanacs, the other subjects are more unusual. He argued, for instance, that astrology was essential to divines because without it the Book of Job could not be understood properly.

62 Ashm. 204, fo. 53^{v}.

63 Ashm. 242, fo. 190.

64 There are marked similarities between Napier's arguments and those of Sir Christopher Heydon in the latter's response to Chamber, *A defense of judicial astrology* (1603). Compare for instance their discussions of the term 'mathematics': Ashm. 240, fos. 137–8; Heydon, *Defense*, 10.

reworked versions of his manuals he adjusted his definition of astrology and his persona as an astrologer. In 'Grounds of arte' Forman began with a biblical history of astrology, following Josephus and other sources. In the introduction to the 1599 draft of 'Astrologicalle judgmentes' Forman removed this transmission history, perhaps because Napier's preface would have made it redundant, and replaced it with an inspirational genealogy:

Never any man before my tyme that I could read or heare of did fynde this secret, nor the secrets of the judgments of diseases, nor shewe how to know the causes in his degrees of every disease and sicke person. But God that is the only giver of wisedome and knowledge hath given me the true knowledge thereof that all the world that heard me or sawe me have wondred at my judgments of the diseases of those that have bene sicke, when I have neither seene them nor their urine.[65]

In the *c.*1600 version of this text Forman replaced this passage with a more temperate one:

Manie notable and wise philosophers have written hereof some after one sorte and some after another, but diversely and uncertainly in manie things and very intricatly, but either thay lefte their bookes imperfect because thay did never attaine to the true knowledge thereof, and of the cause of the diseases, or ells if thay did know yet thay would not set it downe in their bookes, but did keep close the secrets thereof as thay do the philosophers stone.[66]

Some astrologers, Forman suggested, borrowed the code of secrecy of the alchemists, a code which he, in writing this book, was breaking. The history of astrological physic and the traditions to which Forman was heir could not be found in books.

As Forman drafted and redrafted his astrological manuals, he sought words to explain why he was writing them. Despite danger and suffering at the hands of his opponents, he explained in 'Grounds of arte', he had gained extensive experience as an astrologer-physician, and he wrote this tract in order to preserve his expertise for the benefit of posterity.[67] In the earliest version of 'Astrologicalle judgmentes' he noted that

Our ordinary practise and experience which we have obteyned of God by grace and by long experience and brought with many greefs sorowes calamityes imprisonments, hatred, disdaines and cares, and even with many hazards of our lyfe, from the yeere of our Lord God 1576 unto the yeere 1596, in which year I Simon Forman compiled this booke out of all my books of experience for the generations to come.[68]

[65] Ashm. 403, fo. 81. [66] Ashm. 363, fo. 132^{v}.
[67] Ashm. 1495, fo. 29. [68] Ashm. 403, fo. 81^{r-v}.

In the most extensive version of 'Astrologicalle judgmentes' Forman changed this passage again:

With much traville, many expences and many troubles hazards of my life and imprisonments, from the yeare of our lord god 1570, unto the yeare 1600, did I Simon F. the sonne of William the sonne of Richard laboure for experience to compell this booke of experience for the generation to come, that thay and their posterities may have a more briefer, truer, and more perfect waye for Judgmente of diseases and causes thereof then heretofor.[69]

Instead of denigrating the inadequacies of previous astrologers and their books, Forman stressed his experience, experience acquired through adversity and culminating in this book.[70]

Defending his reputation, vindicating his practices, preserving his expertise; this was why Forman wrote and planned to print 'Astrologicalle judgmentes'. His forum was England, his enemies the College of Physicians and opponents of judicial astrology. Though it was not printed, 'Astrologicalle judgmentes' circulated in manuscript in Forman's lifetime and beyond, apparently unlike Forman's other writings. Either by design or happenstance Napier acted as an agent for this text, probably having acquired a copy in 1599.[71] For instance, Matthias Evans, a Londoner known for his magical expertise, knew Forman's guide. Napier had lent him a 'booke written by Mr Forman of Astrology', but he was charged with being a conjuror and some of his books, including this one, were confiscated. Evans had recovered the book in 1621, and was writing to enquire whether Napier wanted it back.[72] Napier reputedly lent many people, including the young Kenelm Digby, whole cloak bags full of books to help with their astrological studies.[73] Perhaps Robert Burton borrowed a copy of this text from Napier or someone else, making note of seven lines of astrological rules attributed to Forman.[74] Later in the century a

69 Ashm. 363, fo. 132^{r-v}.

70 For a discussion of Forman's self-presentation in his plague tracts see Ch. 5.

71 'The Economy of Magic in Early Modern England', in Margaret Pelling and Scott Mandelbrote (eds.), The Practice of Reform in Health, Medicine, and Science, 1500–2000: Essays for Charles Webster (Aldershot: Ashgate, 2005), pp. 43–57.

72 Ashm. 421, fo. 170; see also fos. 168–9^{v} for a letter from Edmund Ferrers to Napier about these MSS. On Evans see Lilly, *Life*, 152–3; Lauren Kassell, 'The Economy of Magic in Early Modern England', in Scott Mandelbrote and Margaret Pelling (eds.), *Science, Medicine and Reform 1500–2000* (Ashgate, forthcoming); Michael MacDonald, 'The Career of Astrological Medicine in England', in Grell and Cunningham (eds.), *Religio Medici*, 62–90, esp. 85; Pelling, *Medical Conflicts*, 112; Thomas, *Decline of Magic*, 297, 413 n.

73 Lilly, *Life*, 79; Bowden, 'Astrological Revolution', 52. For a letter from the young Digby to Napier in 1624, see Ashm. 1730, fo. 166.

74 Robert Burton recorded seven lines of astrological rules attributed to Forman on pages interleaved with Ptolemy's *Quadripartum* (Paris, [1519]): Nicholas Kiessling, *The Library of Robert Burton* (Oxford, 1988), 246–7; J. B. Bamborough, 'Robert Burton's Astrological Notebooks', *Review of English Studies*, NS 32 (1981),

copy of 'Astrologicalle judgmentes' made by Sir Richard Napier passed through the hands of Richard Laford (b. 1620), a physician, and one Henry Gouldesburg, before being acquired by Ashmole in 1671.[75]

In early modern England astrology was taught through example and studied in manuscripts and printed books in English and Latin, some new, some second-hand. William Lilly was heir to this tradition, and his *Christian astrology* (1647), a massive guide to judicial astrology, transformed it.[76] This, like 'Astrologicalle judgmentes', was a huge compendium of rules for reading planetary positions, prefaced by rudimentary instructions for calculating an astrological figure. Lilly advertised it as the first such text printed in English, informed by the books and manuscripts of respectable astrologers not the quacks of present-day London.[77] Several decades later he specified that the instructions for setting a figure in the first part of the book were entirely his own work; but for the copious rules that filled the second part he had relied on the numerous manuscripts that he had collected and the rules that he had exchanged with 'the most able professors I had acquaintance with', only to find them defective.[78] Lilly's and Forman's astrological manuals perfected and promoted judicial astrology. Lilly consolidated his expertise as an astrological journalist of the 1640s, tutoring a nation in crisis in the language of the stars.[79] Forman was the astrologer-physician of Lambeth, renowned for his judgements in matters of love and disease, writing to preserve his art, establish his credentials, and vanquish his enemies.

267–85. For the possibility that as a young man Burton consulted Forman, see Rowse, *Forman*, 145–50; Barbara Traister, 'New Evidence about Burton's Melancholy', *Renaissance Quarterly*, 24 (1976), 66–70. Bowden cites references to Forman in Folger MS V.b.4 that I have not been able to locate: 'Astrological Revolution', 143.

[75] *Ashmole*, ed. Josten, iii. 1208.

[76] Geneva, *Astrology and the Seventeenth Century Mind*, 61–71.

[77] Lilly, *Christian Astrology*, sig. B2^{v}.

[78] Lilly, *Life*, 82. On the similarities between the systems for calculating figures of Forman, Napier, and Lilly see North, *Horoscopes and History*, 162.

[79] Lilly, *Life*, 80–1.

II

PLAGUE AND THE COLLEGE OF PHYSICIANS OF LONDON

In the summer of 1592 plague arrived in London and many people, including most of the members of the College of Physicians, fled the city. Simon Forman stayed behind. According to his account he had a divine prerogative to 'cuer the sicke and sore | But not the ritch and mighti ones | But the destressed poore'. Forman had performed occasional cures over the previous decade and in the summer of 1592 he, as he saw it, was chosen by God to learn about the plague. In June he had begun to have a swelling in his groin, and in July he took to his bed. When the unnamed people looking after him declared that he would die and abandoned him, Forman lanced his own sores and fainted. His servant, without realizing what he was doing, gave him 'A prentiouse water that I had | Whose vertue was from god above | To kill the plague and venome'.[1] Presently he revived and recovered. He had been ill for twenty-one weeks. As he had cured himself, by the grace of God, he then began to cure others. First he would lance their sores, then administer his vitalizing drink. When the plague abated and the physicians returned, they began a campaign against the irregular medical practitioners who had flourished in their absence, including Forman. The physicians pursued Forman for the rest of his life, and in spite of their efforts he established a thriving and lucrative medical practice.

Forman's recovery from plague is the opening episode in the psalm that chronicled his troubles with the College of Physicians.[2] In it he imitated the surgeons who stressed their personal triumphs at the outset of tracts on plague and other subjects.[3] However artful, Forman's medical writings were never

[1] Ashm. 240, fo. 25. The servant was probably Steven Mitchel, the son of Forman's step-sister. He had been apprenticed to Forman in 1588 and acted as a scryer, and, though periodically venturing to sea, was annually bound to Forman each spring through to at least 1593: Ashm. 208, fos. 43^{v}, 45^{v}, 46^{v}, 48, 49; 390, fo. 102^{v}. See also Ch. 1 and Traister, *Forman*, esp. 159, 229 n.

[2] Ashm. 240, fos. 25–7^{v}; 802, fos. 131–3^{v}.

[3] See for instance the opening of Guy de Chauliac's *Great surgery*, as discussed in Anna M. Campbell, *The Black Death and Men of Learning* (New York, 1966 [1931]), 3, 28–9. Personal experience as a practitioner if not as a patient was also prominent in new writings on medicine in the 16th cent., e.g. Leonardo Fioravanti, *A joyfull jewell*, tr. John Hester (1580), 10–12.

printed; he never became a respected medical authority, and has been remembered as he was portrayed by the College, as an ignorant and dangerous quack. The College Annals and Forman's extensive notes together allow us to reconsider their conflicts. Detailed records of such cases are scarce, and the physicians' and Forman's manœuvres reveal the complexities of establishing, maintaining, and challenging authority in Elizabethan London.[4] Plague frames these encounters. Through his medical tracts, particularly his plague tracts, Forman defined what amounts to a philosophy of medicine that was fundamentally astrological. He was a medical martyr, working against the corrupt methods of traditional physicians. God had chosen him to heal the sick and poor and taught him the methods to do so; physicians, he thought, killed by authority.

[4] For the definitive study of relations between irregular practitioners and the College of Physicians, see Pelling, *Medical Conflicts*. Forman's case provides a further illustration for many of her findings, but I have kept references to a minimum.

4

The College of Physicians and Irregular Medicine in London, *c.*1580–1640

When the noxious summer airs had cleared, the physicians returned to the city. The College met in November 1592 and they discussed 'the insolent and illicit practice of the quacks' and unanimously decided 'to summon them all'.[1] Forman was one of the many irregular medical practitioners (often referred to as 'empirics') who thrived in the periodic absences of the physicians, and he appears in histories of medicine as a typical example of the insolent, irrational, uneducated medical practitioner.[2] He was named in the College Annals ten times between 1594 and 1610, and in the late seventeenth century these records formed the basis of a history of the College in which Forman epitomized quackery, the ignorant, dangerous, and opportunistic practice of medicine.[3] Forman documented his encounters with the College in his psalm, diary, other life-writings, and astrological queries. With fanatical intensity, he paradoxically recognized the College's authority to regulate medicine and challenged the medical principles that they upheld. The plague of 1592–3 initiated Forman's success as a medical practitioner in London and occasioned him to write a treatise on the plague, a treatise that was also his first work on astrological medicine, and the plague of 1603 coincided with his final strategy against the physicians and inspired him to rewrite his plague tract.

On 8 March 1594 the Censors of the College of Physicians first examined Forman, eighteen months after the plague abated. They followed the standard procedure of assessing Forman's medical experience, methods, and learning, and they probably conducted the interview in Latin.[4] He confessed that he had

[1] Annals, 6 Nov. 1592, p. 77.

[2] For an account of physicians fleeing the city and 'empirics' usurping their position, see Thomas Dekker, *The wonderfull yeare* (1603), sigs. D3–4^{v}. See also Pelling, *Medical Conflicts*, 45–56; F. P. Wilson, *The Plague in Shakespeare's London* (Oxford, 1963 [1927]), 102–3.

[3] Charles Goodall, *The Royal College of Physicians of London, and an historical account of the College proceedings against empiricks and unlicensed practicers* (1684), 337–9. On Goodall's book, see Cook, *Decline of the Old Medical Regime, passim.*

[4] Margaret Pelling, 'Knowledge Common and Acquired: The Education of Unlicensed Medical Practitioners in Early Modern London', in Vivian Nutton and Roy Porter (eds.), *The History of Medical Education in Britain* (Amsterdam, 1995), 250–79, esp. 251; Pelling, *Medical Conflicts*, 30–1, 287.

'practised medicine in England for these sixteen years and here in London for only two years'. He said that he had cured twenty-three people of fevers with an electuary of roses and wormwood water. To a question about 'what authors he followed and what medical books he had read', he replied 'that he had read through one called Corkes and another called Wainefleet'. Forman then 'boasted that he made use of no other help in diagnosing diseases than his Ephemerides and that by heavenly signs aspects and constellations of the planets he could instantly recognise any one disease'. Forman did no better with questions about astrology, a central component of learned medicine but requiring a distinct level of expertise: 'his answers were so inadequate and absurd that it caused much laughter among those listening'.[5] Forman lacked deference and learning, flaunting his unschooled and unauthorized medical activities; his bold ignorance, not his astrology, was opprobrious. The report concluded, 'He was forbidden to practise and for his wicked and illegal practice he was fined £5 to be paid within 16 days. This he readily and faithfully promised to do'.[6] On 30 March 1594 Forman duly delivered the fine to the house of William Gilbert, then Treasurer to the College, later author of the treatise on the magnet.[7]

Forman's diary and other notes confirm that by 1594 he had occasionally practised medicine in London for at least two years and in England for at least sixteen, at times moving frequently and making many enemies.[8] In summer 1591 he had moved to London, published *Longitude*, and begun practising medicine there, though it was a hard year and he had very little money.[9] In the summer of 1592 he caught the plague and his recovery marked a change in his fortunes. Later he reflected that 'This yere I did mani notable cuers and began to be knowen and cam to credit.'[10] In February 1593 he noted that he was called before the Company of Barber Surgeons for his 'practice', but neither his nor their papers recorded what happened.[11] In April he changed rooms within the Stone House on Philpot Lane, moving from a small one at the top of the house that stank of the privy to a larger, more accessible and amenable one in order to

[5] On astrology and learned medicine see Chapman, 'Astrological Medicine', 283–6; Dunn, 'Status of Astrology', 37–41, 45; S. J. Tester, *A History of Western Astrology* (Woodbridge, 1987), 242.

[6] Annals, 8 Mar. 1593/4, pp. 84–5. Forman had informal contact with the physicians prior to his formal interview. He listed being warned on 14 Feb. 1594, called before them on 16 Feb. 1594, then warned on 6 Mar. 1594, and before them on 8 Mar. 1594, the date when his name first appears in the Annals: Ashm. 195, fo. 195.

[7] Ashm. 195, fo. 195. Gilbert was Treasurer from 1587–94 inclusive, and he was also present at the interview of Forman: William Munk, *The roll of the Royal College of Physicians of London*, i (1878), 78.

[8] Ashm. 208, fo. 45v; see also Ch. 1 n. 43.

[9] Ashm. 208, fos. 47v, 48; 1494, fo. 309v.

[10] Ashm. 208, fo. 48.

[11] Ashm. 208, fo. 49. I have not been able to locate Forman in the Company records.

4.1. Simon Forman's list of conflicts with the physicians on the end pages of a 1598 casebook, Ashm. 195, fo. 195. By permission of the Bodleian Library, University of Oxford.

accommodate his increasing number of clients.[12] In his diary Forman summarized his successes in 1593, though noting the malevolent effects of Mars.

This yere I loste moch money that I should have had for divers cuers that I did, & was besids that slenderly paid for many cuers that I did because I did not bargain with them first.

But my credit encreased & I got moch & this yere I cured A. Allen.[13]

But this yere yf I did entend to doe any thing what soever, yf I did tell any body of yt, I was prevented & did not doe yt or could have noe power to procead in yt.

Alsoe yf I did take any on hin hand to cuer and did bargain with him first then eyther I did not cuer him or ells I was not paid for yt when yt was done.

My knowledg in phisique and in astronomy did encrease and I began to com to credit and to get som thing about me.

Finally Forman noted, 'This yer I stilled my strong water by the which I got motch mony'.[14] Word of Forman's practices brought him to the attention of

12 Ashm. 390, fo. 60^{v}. This was probably a garderobe privy.

13 This was Avis Allen, Forman's mistress 1593–7.

14 Ashm. 208, fo. 49^{r-v}. He also distilled a strong water for the stone in May 1590: Ashm. 208, fo. 46^{v}.

the physicians, but his manner not his methods determined his conflicts with them.

Forman's papers also confirm that he lied to the physicians about his lack of learning. The Censors examined him a second time on 7 November 1595 and again found him 'completely ignorant'. Forman repeated 'that he had never read any writer in medicine except one of a certain Cockis', and he boasted 'that he practised medicine only by astrology'. The Censors described Cockis (previously Corkes) as 'an English writer, a very obscure man, absolutely unknown and certainly of no merit' and deemed Forman's knowledge of astrology inadequate. Forman, however, had been studying and practising physic, astrology, alchemy, and magic for decades and his notes are peppered with eclectic references to his extensive reading in these subjects. Robert Wainflete and John Cokkys (spelt variously with cs and ys) were both physicians in fifteenth-century England, though Cokkys has often been misidentified as Francis Coxe (fl. 1560), an astrologer, magician, and 'chymist' who authored three insubstantial publications.[15] On 2 February 1574 Forman bought a manuscript in Oxford, and duly wrote his name and the date in the front.[16] The volume contains two fifteenth-century items, a compendium of medicinal simples, arranged alphabetically, and a compilation of medical lectures by Cokkys from around 1450, hence the inscription 'IO COKKIS' on the fore-edge.[17] Forman soon added notes to pages interleaved throughout the volume, and over the next three decades he wrote all over it. He recorded letting blood to a John Waller in 1579. To the descriptions of different remedies and diseases, he added his experiences and those of other medical practitioners. To the gloss on Galen's description of the four complexions, he inserted notes on the 'Regimen sanitatis Salerni', perhaps from a translation printed in 1575.[18] He copied out long passages from Andrew Boorde's *The breviary of helthe* (1547) and Philip Barrough's *The methode of physicke* (1583).[19] In the latter Forman would have

[15] Robert (fl. *c.*1470–80) is the only Wainflete I have identified, but little is known about him or the treatises that he might have written: C. H. Talbot and E. A. Hammond, *The Medical Practitioners in Medieval England: A Biographical Register* (1965), 305. Forman seldom cited him, e.g. under the heading 'imagination' in a commonplace book that he compiled late in his life he noted, 'Wainflete saith fantasy and ymagination lieth in the foerpart of the brain and is hote and drie that it may the better comprehend things': Ashm. 1494, p. 601; cf. King's MS 16, fo. 59. Cokkys was a clerical physician in Oxford: Talbot and Hammond, *Medical Practitioners*, 134–6. The idea that Forman was citing Coxe seems to have been suggested by Sydney Lee: 'Forman', *DNB*.

[16] King's MS 16; Mary Edmond, 'Simon Forman's Vade-Mecum', *Book Collector*, 26 (1977), 44–60.

[17] Peter Murray Jones suggests that the first item was written by the Franciscan William Holm. *c.*1415, 'Reading Medicine in Tudor Cambridge', in Vivian Nutton and Roy Porter (eds.), *The History of Medical Education in Britain* (Amsterdam, 1995), 153–83, esp. 154. Cf. Edmond, 'Forman's Vade-Mecum', 46.

[18] *Regimen sanitatis Salerni*, tr. Thomas Paynel (1575).

[19] Edmond, 'Forman's Vade-Mecum', 52, 54, 56. It is uncertain which edn. Forman used.

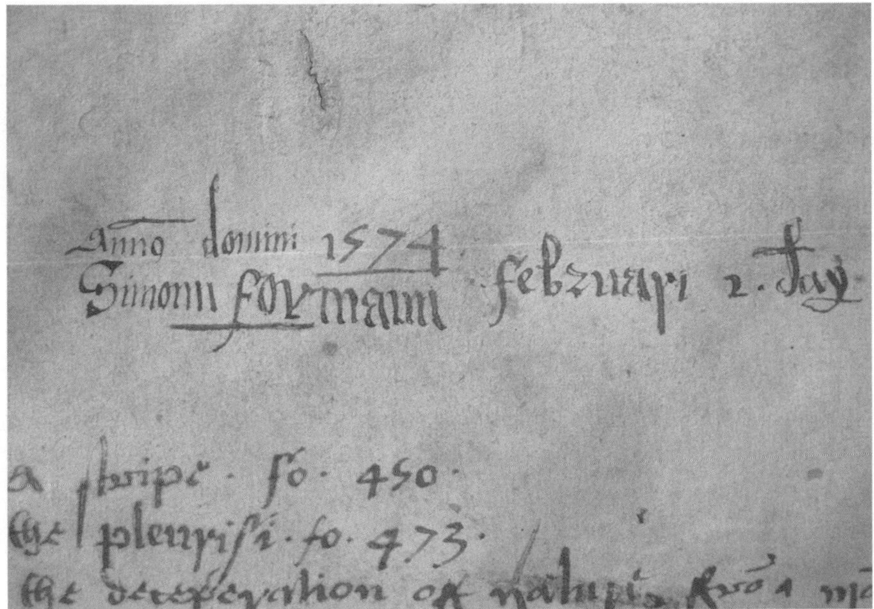

4.2. Simon Forman's note of the purchase of a book in Oxford on 2 Feb. 1574, King's MS 16, fo. 1^{v}. By permission of the Provost and Fellows of King's College, Cambridge.

found complaints that arrogant physicians did not heed experience but only studied books.[20] Perhaps Forman mentioned Cokkys and Wainflete to impress, and perhaps to appease the Censors; perhaps to mock them. Perhaps he cited them because their names were attached to orthodox, Galenic medical texts, though the physicians thought that they were out of date and obscure.[21] This text, and Forman's own writings from before 1595, document that he had studied much more than he admitted to the College.[22]

The Censors fined Forman £10 and committed him to prison.[23] Three weeks later, a Mr Willis presented a writ on Forman's behalf, and Sir John

[20] Barrough, *Methode of physicke*, sig. A5^{v}. Similarly, Sir Thomas Eliot defended his writings of vernacular medical treatises against the physicians who were opposed to him doing so: *The castelle of helth* (1572), sig. A3. See also Fioravanti, *Joyfull jewell*, sig. A3^{v}. Forman turned the rhetoric in favour of the physicians against them, such as inverting the meaning of the analogy to 'Blind Bayard', a mythic donkey, used by Boorde and Bullein: Ashm. 1436, fo. 142; 363, fo. 9; Andrew Boorde, *The breviary of healthe* (1557), sig. A2; William Bullein, *Bulwarke of defense against all sicknesse, sorenesse, and woundes* (1579 [1562]), fo. 10.

If I am correct in dating 'The groundes of physique and chirurgerie' (Sloane 2550, fos. 1–117^{v}) to *c.*1589, then the fifty-three authors that Forman listed as his sources would further illustrate the breadth of his reading prior to 1594.

[21] Jones, 'Reading Medicine', 154.

[22] 'A discourse of the plague' (1593), Ashm. 208, fos. 110–34; 'Grounds of arte' (*c.*1594–5), Ashm. 1495.

[23] Annals, 7 Nov. 1595, p. 97. Forman notes that he was released on 25 Nov. 1595: Ashm. 208, fo. 54^{v}. The Annals record the Censors' objection to this on 22 Dec. 1595: pp. 98–9.

Puckering, the Lord Keeper of the Great Seal, authorized his release.[24] When the Censors next met, on 22 December, they discussed Forman and protested against Puckering's decision.

Simon Forman, who a short time before had been put in prison on account of his illegal practice and remarkable audacity, was, on the authority of the Keeper of the Great Seal of England, freed from prison and set at liberty. It was therefore decided with regard to him, that four censors with Dr Smith, Oxon., should be sent to the Lord Keeper of the Great Seal of England to inform him why we had committed that impostor, Forman, to prison: and also to demand from his honour that the aforesaid Forman should be sent back to prison again, not by some new order but by the force and effect of our earlier command.[25]

They were not successful, though in January Edward Stampe, a lawyer, warned Forman about his medical practices and Mr Mosely, a physician, visited him to talk about a medicine that he had given to Elizabeth Watts at Billingsgate.[26] Despite the 'mani vexations by the doctors', Forman's busy medical practice continued unabated.[27]

The following autumn, on 3 September 1596, the Censors again interviewed Forman, now describing him as 'that bold impostor'. He 'confessed that he had given a compound water to Mr Sotherton in a burning fever and he had instantly died'.[28] Again the College asked 'in what grounds or for what reasons he practised medicine and how he could safely give medicine to the sick', and again he responded 'that he understood the nature of diseases and could prescribe only by astrology'. This time Richard Smith, physician to the queen, examined him in the rudiments of astrology, and he 'was found to be a mere impostor and ignorant in all that science, which confirmed the opinion of all present'.[29] Almost a fortnight later, on 15 September, at the request of the physicians, the lord mayor, Thomas Skinner, had Forman arrested.[30] Nine days later he was released from prison on terms which are not clear ('bailed by ye physicians'), only to be committed again on 30 September for another

[24] Ashm. 195, fo. 195; 208, fo. 54^{v}, where the date is given as 25 Nov. This might have been Timothy Willis, an alchemist who was himself called before the Censors in August 1596: Annals, 6 Aug. 1596, p. 102. See J. H. Appleby, 'Arthur Dee and Johannes Banfi Hunyades', *Ambix*, 24 (1977), 96–109, esp. 99.

[25] Annals, 22 Dec. 1595, pp. 98–9.

[26] Ashm. 208, fos. 56^{v}, 67. For cases in which Stampe summoned Forman on the request of his patients or their friends, see Ashm. 226, fo. 184^{v}; 219, fo. 42^{v}.

[27] Ashm. 390, fo. 60^{v}. Though he noted 'lyttle doing in physick' in the autumn of 1595: Ashm. 208, fo. 54.

[28] This might be the Timothy Sotherton who had consulted Forman on behalf of his sister a few months earlier, in July 1596: Ashm. 234, fos. 78^{v}, 79^{v}.

[29] Annals, 3 Sept. 1596, p. 103. This is the Richard Smith of Cambridge who died *c.*1599.

[30] Ashm. 208, fo. 57^{v}. The imprisonment by the College was entwined with the case of one Kate Whitfield, who had arrested Forman for beating her, and with whom much litigation followed: Ashm. 208, fo. 57^{v}; 234, fo. 102^{v}; 390, fo. 70.

fortnight.[31] On 7 October some officers of the College visited Forman in prison and asked whether he would give them a bond promising not to practise in London. He cast a figure to decide, and concluded 'the figure says do it not but stand to the law and trial therof. For they ar also weke and have as little power as my self; for I am determined fully to go to law with them; they will not go to law with thee, if they do they wil not continue it.'[32] The next day he cast another figure, decided to meet the demands of the College officials, was bound for £40 'not to meddle again in London after mai day next', and secured his release.[33]

From March 1596 six years of Forman's casebooks survive, clearly documenting the threat that he posed to the College.[34] He was consulted for medical services many times a day, and occasionally by members of the gentry such as Sir William Monson, an admiral. The Annals document the physicians' concern to protect their privileges, and accordingly their objection to practitioners who lacked appropriate credentials, prescribed remedies, and challenged their authority; they also document the limitations of their powers. Forman adopted the physicians' stress on authority and learning, turning their criteria against them. The difference between himself and the physicians was an ability to discern the causes of disease, he argued, not the credentials to prescribe remedies.

In 1604 Forman wrote the psalm of his troubles that began with his recovery from the plague and narrated his conflicts with the physicians. He conflated his first three formal encounters with the Censors into his 'first interview'. The Censors asked him where he learnt his skill and by what authority he impinged on their privilege, and they concluded that he learned his skill under a hedge. Forman replied aggressively:

> To this I answered them again
> I lerned it not of them
> Nor in great scolles, as they had done
> Nor yet amonge leud men
> Nor of those Emprickes which doe write
> Their bockes of fained lies
> As Gallin did: of paltrie pisse
> And pullse which they dyvise

He denounced their medical methods as 'toyes to mocke an ape | and physicks arte disgrace'. When again they demanded how he learned his skill, Forman replied:

31 Ashm. 208, fo. 57^{v}; 234, fo. 109^{v}.

32 Ashm. 234, fo. 111.

33 Ashm. 234, fo. 112; 195, fo. 195.

34 See Part III below.

Above from of the skies
Said I: wherin the course of nature
And hidden conninge lyes
For ther the truth of all is sene . . .

Forman justified his insolence. Regardless of what he might have said, he argued, the Censors had intended to commit him to prison from the start.[35] However much Forman might have asserted the authority of his art and his experience in his writings, he had no credibility with the College of Physicians. From Forman's point of view, the physicians were opposed to him because he did not have formal medical qualifications; from the College's perspective, as recorded in the formulaic Annals, Forman was ignorant of medicine and astrology and personally offensive.

These formal encounters between Forman and the physicians are only part of the story. He met their members and representatives informally, he defied their prohibitions, and he continued consulting the stars and prescribing remedies. These interactions document the plurality, volatility, and competition in medical care in Elizabethan and early Jacobean London. The physicians were not a monolithic body. Forman met them in the street and at the bedsides of his patients, though he seldom recorded whether these meetings were congenial or hostile. For instance, in December 1595 Forman met a Dr Wilkins (perhaps Ralph Wilkinson, a fellow of the College) at a patient's house in Chancery Lane; in January 1596 he went to speak to a Mr Katherine about leasing his garden, and there met John James, physician to the queen; and in October 1597 he bumped into Sir William Paddy, at the time a Censor, in Lombard Street.[36] In the 1590s he seems to have borrowed alchemical manuscripts from George Turner, periodically a Censor from 1591 to 1607 and perhaps also Thomas Moundeford, occasionally a Censor from 1595 and later President of the College.[37] Less ambiguously, Forman narrated several encounters between himself and physicians in his guide to astrology, 'Astrologicalle judgmentes', as examples of the superiority of his medical expertise over theirs. Two of these accounts involved one Dr Juthe Cittie, perhaps a foreigner, perhaps a pseudonym.

35 Ashm. 240, fos. 25–7^{v}; 802, fos. 131–3^{v}. As noted above, Forman was not imprisoned until his second examination: Annals, 7 Feb. 1595, p. 97.

36 Ashm. 208, fos. 55, 56^{v}; 226, fo. 234^{v}.

37 For a manuscript 'copied out of Dr Turners book' in 1593, see Ashm. 1490, fos. 57–61. Turner's wife, Anne, knew Forman and was implicated in the Overbury affair. Deborah Harkness has attributed a collection of alchemical manuscripts in the Ashmole collection to Moundeford, some of which include notes about lending texts to Forman: private correspondence 26 Feb. 2003. For Moundeford's copies of alchemical treatises later owned by Forman, see Ashm. 1423, i–iii. See also Ashm. 1459.

When Forman was out of town, a woman whom he had once treated had a relapse. Her husband summoned Cittie, who treated her for six weeks with no effect. When Forman returned, he was called to attend to the woman. He reported the following confrontation with Cittie:

I cam to her and met her doctor there, & had conference with him about her. And he demaunded of me this question, what is the reason Mr Forman that for these 6 weeks space I can not set this woman in her right wits, and you did once set her in her wits before when she was in this taking, and I have tryed all the wayes I can devise & can not do it. I answered him in this manner, the reason is because you do not know the cause of her frensy. And he answered again, I suppose the cause to be, by reason of melancholy humors in her matrix [womb] mixed with her menstrues. And I told him noe, quoth he let me try my skill once more. Do quoth I. He provided his medicine. Quoth I, when will you give it her. At such a tyme quoth he. Then quoth I, the tyme is evill for this diseaze, and again she will not take it. Why, quoth he? I know a reason to the contrarie quoth I.

As in *Longitude*, Forman protested his knowledge without revealing it:

When the tyme came he would have given her the medicin, but he could not make her to take it. When he saw that, Now, quoth he, let me see what you can doe. The next night following I layd a thing to her head, and the day following she was reasonably well come to her self but not well. Then I did so once more the night following again, and she was well thanks be to God, so that in two dayes we stopt the cause of her diseaze, which they could not do in 6 weekes because they did mistake the cause. Here you may see the skill of such Doctors as work without art.[38]

Another story about the same doctor followed, again illustrating the necessity of astrology to physic. This case concerned an ill gentlewoman who had been attended in her home, a house in the country. Her father had summoned Forman and played a prominent role in her case. When Forman arrived at the house he told the man that 'it was but a follie to bestow any cost on her: she would dy within 6 dayes following. And again I told him that he should give her no medicin, if they did she would be frantik within 6 howers after'.[39] Forman's advice was ignored, and the 'learned Doctor' (Dr Cittie) prescribed a glister. Within six hours, as Forman had predicted, the woman was frantic and it took four women to restrain her. The next day Forman again was summoned, and he found Dr Cittie at the house when he arrived. The following dialogue ensued:

[38] Ashm. 363, fo. 7.

[39] Ibid. In the second story Forman withheld the physician's name, though from the context it appears to be the same man. He noted that he did this because the man had shamed himself, and those who had licensed him to practise physic, the College of Physicians.

he demaunded of me, what I thought of her. Quoth I, she will dye within 3 dayes, except God give her longer life, as he did to Ezechiar the King. Why should you say so quoth he, and I see no signe of Death on her. Are not (quoth he) her eyes quick and her lips red, and a good colour in her face, and a reasonable good pulse . . .

Then in an aside, Forman reveals to the reader that the physician did not know that the woman was frantic, and that her colour came from striving. Forman had responded, 'what quoth I doest thou tell me of her eyes, of her lips, her nose or of her tayle, I tell thee she will dye, for art saith she will dye'. He had revealed his secret, to which Cittie responded, 'O quoth the Dr, you are one of them that is not free of our house, you stand much upon art, of which we have no skill.' Forman then launched a series of insults:

So it seemeth quote I, it were better for your credit, and also those whom ye deal with all, if you hath skill in art as you have not, but your owne talke, Quoth I, sheweth your ignorance. And such blind Drs as you are, quoth I, doe discredit art and your profession, and make mens bodies apothecaries shopps, & then to bestowe their monnyes idly to maintayne your follies and to kill themselves by your foolish doctrine.

The animosity was explicit, and the exchange continued, as Forman wagered his occupation on the young woman's life: 'This fellowe, quoth the Dr to the Gentlman, talkes he knowes not what. I will warrant your daughter, sir, quoth he. Do so quoth I, and if she overlive fryday next, I will never studie art, nor minister ani physick more'.[40] Forman left him to it. This was Wednesday; by Friday she was dead.

Throughout his notes and treatises Forman recorded medical gossip, reports of the cases of physicians, surgeons, and other medical practitioners gone wrong. Sometimes he noted that he would have provided a different therapy, such as bleeding and giving a syrup instead of purging, and occasionally he stressed the importance of astrological timing.[41] In 'Astrologicalle judgmentes' he reported that a lawyer, Mr Waldarne, had told him about a case in which ill-timed bathing proved fatal. Between 9 and 10 in the morning on Wednesday, 2 June 1602 a Mrs (Mary) Bret, aged 27, was persuaded by a woman in Chancery

[40] Ashm. 363, fo. 7^{v}.

[41] For the case of Dr Lane, 'an outlandish man', perhaps Roger Lane, who treated an 8-year-old boy who died, see King's MS 16, fo. 1^{v}. It is possible that this was not a first-hand account and that Forman copied it from another source, retaining the first person. Cf. Edmond, 'Forman's Vade-Mecum'. Further accounts appear under the heading 'Stories of certain sick folke trobled with strang dizeases': Ashm. 390, fo. 131. Around 1598 Forman noted that Elizabeth Norton, Mrs Pain's sister who lived by Rood Church Street, used to give glisters to men and women and set leeches: Ashm. 195, fo. 196. On 16 Nov. 1600 he noted that when a woman from Tower Street consulted him she told him about a case in 1596 or 1597 when a Dr Barnesby and a Dr Friar (perhaps William Baronsdale and Thomas Fryer, sen.) had treated a Mrs Scolles in Lothbury. She was suffering from a fever, they had let her blood, and she died the following day: Ashm. 236, fo. 246^{v}.

Lane (Susanna Gloriana) to take a bath. Bret, who had been married for six or seven years had not yet conceived a child, and the bath was supposed to facilitate a pregnancy. Instead, three hours later she was dead. An autopsy was performed, finding her sound in all parts except the womb, 'the which was very hard and shronke up like a purse, so that by noe meanes it could be opned'. Forman calculated the position of the moon at the time when Bret got into the bath to illustrate that certain therapies should be avoided when it was so situated.[42] Several other cautionary tales follow, one about a physician who almost killed a patient by administering a purge when the moon was eclipsed, and another about a man who fatally was let blood by a surgeon when the sun was eclipsed and died within a week. Forman did not name the surgeon, but he noted that he was acting under the counsel of the physician Ralph Wilkinson, perhaps the man that Forman noted meeting at a patient's house in 1595.[43] Elsewhere Forman noted that he saw one Merian Lerrat fail to remove a cataract because of the timing of the procedure, though he might have been reporting this case second-hand.[44] With all of these cases Forman demonstrated the dangers of medicine without astrology.

Forman saw himself as superior to other medical practitioners, whether learned physicians, trained surgeons, or others with medical expertise. The physicians saw Forman as typical of the ignorant, bold, and dangerous quack. He was one of the 714 irregular practitioners pursued by the College between 1553 and 1640. He was also amongst the twenty-one individuals named ten times or more in the Annals. The College's mechanisms for locating irregular practitioners and their procedures for summoning them were imperfect.[45] They asked questions and registered complaints, and like Forman they probably had their ears attuned to gossip about medical successes, failures, and wonders. Forman cultivated a reputation for his practice, and he annoyed the College with his defiance of their verdicts.

The College's dealings with other practitioners, especially the bold ones, informed their perennial encounters with Forman. The case of Thomas Hood, the mathematical practitioner who had dismissed Forman's method for finding the longitude, illustrates the procedure for licensing a university-educated physician. Hood had moved from Cambridge to London in the early 1590s,

[42] Ashm. 363, fo. [160ᵛ]. Forman only heard, or only noted, part of the story. On 14 June 1602 the Censors interviewed Susanna Gloriana regarding her prescription of a purgative and a bath for Mary Brett. Gloriana instructed Brett to wait until the end of the week before taking the bath, but Brett worried that her husband would object, so she went ahead with the bath on the Wednesday: Annals, 14 June 1602, p. 145, cited in Pelling, *Medical Conflicts*, 218.

[43] Ashm. 363, fo. 161.

[44] Ashm. 1495, fo. 501ᵛ; 403, fo. 176ᵛ.

[45] Pelling, *Medical Conflicts*, ch. 4.

bearing BA, MA, medical licence, and MD from the University of Cambridge. The Censors first examined him in October 1595 and he admitted to not having read Galen. He was sent away with a reading list, and because his behaviour was 'favourable and unassuming' he was not forbidden to practise. Just over a year later he was examined again, and announced that he had read two modern authors instead of Galen, 'because he [Galen] could not be greatly esteemed'. He was forbidden to practise. Perhaps a patron intervened, or perhaps Hood changed his tactics, and six months later he was again examined, this time succeeding in becoming a licentiate.[46] This is one of the many entries in the Annals in which there is almost no indication of the tone of the exchange.

The Censors expected the people that they interviewed to answer with deference and humility, and would accordingly respond leniently.[47] Forman was obnoxious and he annoyed the Censors; he also probably caused special offence to William Baronsdale, President from 1589 to 1600.[48] Throughout the 1580s other medical practitioners had persistently scorned the College and the Annals recorded their insolent and arrogant behaviour. They were 'shameless', 'bold', and generally ignorant or illiterate. For example, for almost four decades the Censors pursued David Ward, whom they described as a shameless, ignorant quack.[49] John Nott was similarly insolent, and despite interventions from his patrons, including Sir Francis Walsingham, Secretary of State, the Censors would not forgive his practice.[50]

The case of Paul Buck, a goldsmith by trade, had many similarities to Forman's. The Censors first examined him in June 1589, describing him as 'an ignorant fellow', 'renowned for his boldness':

> he confessed that he had neither received the benefit of a literary education nor had he occupied himself with any other form of learning: he boasted however that he knew very well how to cure everyone of diseases: he said he had practised medicine for six years in this City and had restored to health many by purgatives and correct diet.

[46] Annals, 17 Oct. 1595, p. 96; 25 Oct. 1596/7, p. 105; 5 August 1597, p. 106.

[47] See e.g. the case of a surgeon named Bewter: Annals, 25 June 1589, p. 58.

[48] Pelling, *Medical Conflicts*, 62. For the holders of the office of Censor see ibid. 27. For a list headed 'Doctor and Philosophicus', apparently listing people for and against Forman's case, see Sloane 2550, fo. 128ᵛ. The list beginning with 'Barbidel' (i.e. Baronsdale) included Atkins, Turner, Langton, Paddy, Nowell, Brown, Taylor, and Gilbert, all of whom served as Censors or were otherwise present during the period that the College pursued Forman. The opposite list included James and Johnson, who were Censors, and Pope, Hall, and Clarkson, who were present at interviews in 1595–6, and neither Wilkinson nor Moundeford was named. For a similar list by Napier of doctors dead and alive, see Ashm. 204, fo. 88.

[49] Annals, 2 May 1582, p. 11; 17 Sept. 1586, p. 43; 3 Nov. 1586, p. 45.

[50] Annals, 5 and 12 Feb. 1584, pp. 32, 33; 17 and 30 Sept. 1586, pp. 42, 43–4; 10 Nov. 1587, p. 48.

When they asked what medical books he had read, he replied Paracelsus and Erasmus.[51] They asked him to define 'inflammation' and the 'king's disease', and again his answers were inadequate. Buck was fined and imprisoned, only to be released by the lord mayor, Sir John Hart. Buck appeared again before the College Censors the following month and refused to assent to their order not to practise medicine; 'he declared that he intended to follow his profession on his own authority'. The Censors deemed such a response insolent and presumptuous, and again committed him to prison. Like Nott, Buck solicited a letter of support from Walsingham, and the Censors summoned him from prison to give him a further hearing; he refused to come. Buck defied the Censors' attempts to control his medical practices for the next two decades.[52]

Insolence and irreverence did not always spark an enduring animosity between the College and an irregular practitioner, a sign of the College's limited sources of information and its difficulties in exercising its authority. Many practitioners failed to honour a summons, either out of defiance or change in circumstance.[53] Some refused to heed further summonses, such as Edward Owen who was interviewed once in 1590, admitted administering purges at the instruction of a physician whose name he did not declare, and thereafter refused to appear.[54] Others, such as the Oxford-trained physician-surgeon John Banister, excused himself from not appearing in 1587 'because he had orders from the Queen to look after Lord Lidcot and restore him to health'; he was made a licentiate in 1593, though they had previously censured him for practising physic.[55] Some, such as John Gyle, made a rude appearance and then vanished. In June 1582 he 'confirmed and confessed' that he had prescribed a diet drink to three people, 'openly boasted of his skill in that part of medicine, flourishing his knowledge, and answering all questions with insolence'. Gyle's manner seems much like Forman's would be a decade later, though Gyle asserted that he could lawfully practise medicine without the permission of the College, something that Forman never explicitly stated. Gyle was committed to prison, but this was his only recorded encounter with the College.[56]

51 Perhaps he, the scribe, or the transcript of the Annals mistook Erasmus for Thomas Erastus, one of Paracelsus' great opponents.

52 Annals, 6 June, p. 58; 2 July, p. 59; 5 and 18 Dec. 1589, p. 61; 30 Jan., p. 65; 16 Feb. 1589/90, pp. 63–4; 8 May 1590, p. 78; 22 Dec. 1592, p. 81; 25 June 1593, p. 82; 25 Mar. 1594, p. 85; 3 July 1596, p. 101; 14 Oct. 1596, p. 103. He is last mentioned in the Annals in Feb. 1616/17.

53 For instance Annals, 1 Dec. 1587, p. 48.

54 Annals, 18 May, p. 66; 25 Sept., p. 70; 6 Nov. 1590, p. 71; 3 Dec. 1596, p. 104; 3 June 1597, p. 106.

55 Annals, 1 Dec. 1587, p. 48; Pelling, *Medical Conflicts*, 104–5. On Banister's support of alchemical and Paracelsian medicine, see Webster, 'Alchemical and Paracelsian Medicine', 327.

56 Annals, 25 June 1582, p. 12. See also the case of Robert Tanner, who was 'as distinguished for ignorance as for arrogance': Annals, 18 Dec. 1589, p. 61.

When Forman gave his bold answers before the Censors in 1594, they were familiar with this sort of behaviour and probably expected that if he did not disappear he would cause further trouble. Perhaps also Forman's reputation, from the longitude dispute or his earlier arrests, preceded him. Like many of these defiant practitioners Forman sought the support of a patron. This tactic had worked for Leonard Poe, a controversial figure whose many patrons secured him positions as a licentiate (with limitations) in 1598, then as royal physician and fellow of the College in 1609.[57] Forman noted the case of Poe, in October 1596 reminding himself to write to Sir John North, one of Poe's patrons, and others.[58] More mischievously, in the spring of 1598 Forman recorded details of two patients that Poe had killed with purges and another with ointments and fumigations.[59] Forman even aspired to the queen's patronage, again in early 1598, dreaming that 'the Quene did comend me moch for my skille & Judgment in phisicke & did chid with the doctors and railed on them more for trobling of me'.[60] A couple of weeks later he persuaded a man called Sellinger to speak to the queen on his behalf. Sellinger forced his way into her private garden, and was met by anger then calm, but there is no evidence that the queen intervened on Forman's behalf, as she had done for other irregular practitioners.[61] Undeterred, in January 1601 Forman cast a figure for the following question: 'Best to enterprise to obtain d. Jeames place physytion to the queen; whether I shall obtain it if I do'.[62] This was the recently deceased John James, a fellow of the College of Physicians since 1584 and a physician to the queen since 1595. Forman's less ambitious bids for patronage were more successful.[63]

Other irregular practitioners were perceived by the Censors to have poor manners and outrageous ambitions; some professed to have studied abroad, others to have learnt through experience, some to have practised at court, others to be expert in alchemy, but Forman alone asserted a singular expertise in astrology.[64] The case of the infamous John Lambe (d. 1628) provides a

[57] Annals, 18 Dec. 1589, p. 62; 30 June 1590, pp. 66–8; 22 Dec. 1590, p. 71; 5 Mar. 1590, p. 72; 7, 22 Dec. 1592, 20 Jan. 1592/3, pp. 78–9; 22 Apr. 1594, p. 85; 10 May 1594, pp. 86–7; 23 Dec. 1594, 10 Jan. 1594/5, p. 91; 22 Dec. 1595, p. 99.

[58] Ashm. 234, fo. 127ᵛ. [59] Ashm. 195, fo. 90ᵛ. [60] Ashm. 226, fo. 310.

[61] Ashm. 390, fo. 68ᵛ; e.g. Banister: Pelling, *Medical Conflicts*, 105.

[62] Ashm. 411, fo. 8ᵛ. Early in 1597 he dreamt about suggesting to the queen that he might help her to lift her skirts from the dirt in the street by causing her belly to swell with child: Ashm. 226, fo. 44.

[63] See for instance Thomas Blague's support for Forman, p. 94 below. Blague also supported other irregular practitioners: Pelling, *Medical Conflicts*, 219 n., 317.

[64] Pelling identifies six practitioners described in the Annals as astrologer, magician, wizard, witch, and sorcerer, and in all sources she finds six irregular practitioners described as astrologers and another six as magician, sorcerer, and wizard: Pelling, *Medical Conflicts*, 156–7.

useful contrast. In May 1619 Matthias Evans, the acquaintance of Napier's who had borrowed Forman's astrological manual, informed the Censors of seventeen cases in which Lambe had been paid large sums of money for providing physic. In three cases Lambe had conjured images in a crystal and in a fourth he had divined the identity of a future husband.[65] A decade later Lambe finally appeared before the Censors and presented them with a letter of support from the bishop of Durham. The Censors described Lambe as notorious for his knowledge of 'magic, astrology and of other mystic sciences', and renowned for the esteem in which a number of women of rank held him. They asked how he had learnt medicine, and, accommodating his lack of learning and intelligence, they questioned him on basic information about medicine, surgery, and astrology. He professed little expertise except the use of a few oils and purgatives, and said that the only astrology that he knew was what he had read in 'Caliman', by which he probably meant the tables or an astrological work by Georg Collimitius Tannstetter, an early sixteenth-century Austrian follower of Regiomontanus.[66] The Censors concluded that he was 'alien from all erudition, or rather completely stupid'.[67] Unlike Forman, Lambe was neither arrogant nor bold; throughout his examination he asserted, somewhat whimsically, his own ignorance. Like Forman, Lambe was notorious for his astrological, medical, and magical practices, and his popularity with women, but Lambe did not proclaim his astrological expertise nor fashion himself as a figure of opposition.

Forman's and Lambe's presumptions, not their astrology, offended the College. The Censors considered astrology to be a learned subject requiring specialized knowledge and expertise.[68] Respectable scholars practised astrology and physic, such as the Cambridge men Isaac Barrough, John Fletcher, John and Gabriel Harvey, Thomas Twyne, Richard Forster, and the Richard Smith who examined Forman.[69] Details of Forman's examinations would have been recorded in the book used for this purpose that is now missing, but the format of such an examination, adapted to allow for Lambe's apparent lack of ability, is documented in the letter that the Censors sent to the bishop of Durham reporting on Lambe's case. Their third question pertained to astrology: 'Being

65 Annals, 7 May 1619, p. 125.

66 Thorndike, *Magic and Experimental Science*, v. 348–9. See also Georg Collimitius Tannstetter, *Artificium de applicatione astrologie* (Argentorati, 1531).

67 Annals, 18 Dec. 1627, pp. 241–3. Lambe was murdered by a mob in London several months later: George N. Clark, *A History of the Royal College of Physicians of London*, i (Oxford, 1964), 259; *DNB*.

68 Chapman, 'Astrological Medicine', 283; Clark, *Royal College of Physicians*, 30.

69 Pelling and Webster, 'Medical Practitioners', 173, 204; Feingold, *Mathematicians' Apprenticeship*, 78, 79, and *passim*; Feingold, 'Occult Tradition', 81–4.

asked in Astrology what house he looketh into, to know a disease, or the event of it: and how the Lord Ascendant should stand therto.'[70] This was the point at which Lambe invoked Caliman, from whom he said he knew to look in the sixth house, but nothing more. To those members of the College who excelled in astrology, such as Robert Fludd, Arthur Dee, and Mark Ridley, such an answer was inadequate.

Not all astrologers were medical practitioners, nor all medical practitioners astrologers, and astrology was not the exclusive domain of learned physicians. Forman is invariably numbered among the notorious astrologers sometimes condemned as quacks, and sometimes lauded as the forefathers of the astrological boom of the Interregnum. These characters are as much mythological as real.[71] Glimpses of figures such as Sparry, Wither, and G.C. are visible in the handful of books that they 'Englished' and augmented. Almanac writers, many advertising medical credentials and services, provide a further measure of astrological expertise. But most of these men have left nothing to history but their names.[72] Forman was exceptionally visible, then and now, and, in part through his self-proclaimed and audacious defiance of authority, astrology and quackery have been conflated. He recorded the grounds of his opposition to the physicians and his resistance to their attempts to stop his practice. For Forman astrology was not an adjunct of medicine; medicine was an adjunct of astrology. In theory the members of the College accepted astrology as integral to, but only part of, medicine. The Annals record Forman's insistence that astrology was the singular means by which he practised medicine. He opposed the methods of university-educated physicians, objecting to the authority with which they practised and their lack of regard for the motions of the heavens. Astrology and authority were the meat of their struggle.

The first time that the Censors examined Forman they fined him £5; the second time they doubled the fine and imprisoned him; the third time he was again imprisoned. Forman fought back. The physicians never again succeeded in gaoling him, but their conflicts continued and the forum shifted from the College offices to the courts of law, and the evidence from the College Annals

[70] Annals, 18 Dec. 1627, pp. 241–3.

[71] Allen, *Star-Crossed Renaissance*, 50, 105, 137; C. Camden, 'Astrology in Shakespeare's Day', *Isis*, 55 (1933), 26–73, esp. 54; Dick, 'Students of Physic and Astrology'; Chapman, 'Astrological Medicine', 278; Thomas, *Decline of Magic*, 356–82; C. J. S. Thompson, *The Quacks of Old London* (New York, 1928), 31. For Forman's legacy in 17th-cent. accounts of astrology, see Lilly, *Life*, 17–23; John Melton, *Astrologaster or the figure caster* (1620), 21.

[72] E. F. Bosanquet, *English Printed Almanacks and Prognostications: A Bibliographical History to the Year 1600* (1917); Bosanquet, 'English Printed Almanacs and Prognostications: A Bibliographical History to the Year 1600, Corrigenda and Addenda', *The Library*, 4th ser. 8 (1928), 456–77; Bosanquet, 'Notes on Further Addenda to English Printed Almanacks to 1600', *The Library*, 4th ser. 18 (1938), 39–66; Capp, *Astrology and the Popular Press*, 293–386; Chapman, 'Astrological Medicine', 285; Thomas, *Decline of Magic*, 347–56. See 'Almanacs' in *STC*.

to Forman's notes.[73] As plaintiff and defendant, Forman was often involved in legal cases.[74] On 20 December 1597 the Censors attempted to arrest Forman on the bond that he had given the previous year, and a suit followed in which the College wanted three sureties, and settled for two. Forman recorded 'In this question I had the better and they ceased their suet for their own ease.'[75] In early January 1598 the physicians again took Forman to court for this bond and later that month Forman countered, serving Baronsdale with a subpoena.[76] On 7 and 11 October 1598 Forman cast astrological figures for the question 'howe the suet shall pass this Term between the doctors and myself & whether I shall overcom them or noe & what troble I shall have this term'.[77] Later that year 'the doctors arested me & I them & went to lawe together'.[78] Then the dispute was mutually resolved to Forman's advantage: 'I had the better for I cessed to call on the suet and they were glad and ceased also.'[79] In his 1604 psalm Forman summarized these encounters:

> And then they went to Lawe: and leste
> I should condem them all
> protracting out the tyme long space
> they lett the matter falle.[80]

This was not the end of the feud. In October 1599 Forman again sought an astrological answer to the questions of whether the physicians would do anything against him that term, and whether they could do him any harm.[81] In December his question was more specific: 'Whether ther be any troble towards me or by my drams of water & fling [?]'.[82] Retrospectively, Forman noted of 1599, 'This yere I was quiete from the doctors from imprisonment but I condemned them in lawe, & put them to silence for a whole yer after & a half.'[83] He had rented a house in Lambeth, beyond the College's jurisdiction, in

73 Although the Annals record imprisoning Forman on three occasions, he noted that they did so four times: 'And had moche troble amonge the docters for his practice for that he was not fre amonge them nor a graduat in the university, and was by them 4 tymes imprissoned and once fined, yet at the laste did overthrowe them all both in the common lawe and alsoe in the chancerie to their great sham[e].' Ashm. 208, fo. 225v.

74 See for instance the cases that he recorded in examples of astrological rules 'Of lawe and controversie' (Ashm. 392, fos. 172–80) and his litigious feud with Peter Sefton from 1596–1601, detailed throughout the casebooks and narrated by Rowse: *Forman*, 141–5. For court records involving Forman, see e.g. a bill of complaint brought by Audrey Sweyland: Public Record Office, Stac 5 s. 79/33, 12/34 and n. 124 below.

75 Ashm. 195, fo. 195; 392, fo. 172; 226, fo. 275v. 76 Ashm. 226, fos. 285, 292v.

77 Ashm. 392, fo. 172; 195, fo. 171. 78 Ashm. 208, fo. 59v. 79 Ashm. 392, fo. 172.

80 Ashm. 802, fo. 132. 81 Ashm. 219, fo. 170.

82 Ashm. 219, fo. 208. This has been crossed through and is difficult to read. If it reads 'fling', it could refer to his casting of astrological figures, though Forman does not elsewhere use this terminology. In Chamber's *Against judicial astrology* astrologers are referred to pejoratively as 'figure-flingers', 84. Perhaps it is a contraction of 'purging' or 'ring'.

83 Ashm. 208, fo. 61.

December 1597.[84] His neighbours conspired against him, and in June 1598 he moved back to the city.[85] His records are unclear about how long he stayed in London, and he may have maintained more than one household during this time. Throughout 1598 he looked for another house in Lambeth and he found one in February 1599.[86]

At some point around the turn of the century Forman had directly questioned the College's authority, an audacity signified by his purchase of a purple gown and a velvet cap, the dress code adopted by the College fellows a few years before.[87] According to Forman's account, though unconfirmed by the College, he challenged them to a debate.

From Cambridge and from Oxford both
I bid them chuse the beste
And through out Europe to dispute
To set us all at reste
Yf he in arte did vanquishe me
My selfe wold then give place
And leave their cytty and pryviledge
And they should have the grace

But yf my selfe did vanquishe him
Then I to beare the sway
Them selves to leese their pryviledge
Or ells to learne my waie
And course of physicke that I use
And leave their falls practice
Their pispots seges [siege, meaning stool] and their pulse
And learne late to be wise

This did I offer them ofte tymes
before the arch bishope
And in their Colledge before them
but none wold take me up
But this they said and did confes
my Judgment was moch better
then theirs because they had noe arte
And soe refused my proffer.[88]

84 Ashm. 226, fo. 268. 85 Ashm. 195, fo. 97^{v}; 208, fo. 59^{v}.

86 Ashm. 195, fos. 98, 111; 219, fo. 135; 411, fos. 32^{v}, 50^{v}, 103^{v}; 208, fo. 63^{v}; 392, fo. 142. On his return to Lambeth he seems to have held the parish offices of collector for the poor and sidesman, though his note is ambiguous: Ashm. 219, fo. 135.

87 Ashm. 208, fo. 62^{v} (1600); Pelling, *Medical Conflicts*, 281. In the same note Forman recorded that he grew his hair and beard. 88 Ashm. 802, fos. 132^{v}–3.

The physicians probably had another explanation for declining Forman's invitation to a debate.

Forman, according to the College's records, had not been formally summoned since 1596, when in November 1600 they tried again.[89] He refused to appear and sent a letter instead.[90] In January 1601, as already noted, Forman hoped to replace Dr James as physician to the queen, and that June the College had located Forman in Lambeth, beyond their jurisdiction. The following report was recorded in the Annals:

> Among the many unlearned and unlawful practitioners, lurking in many corners of this City, who were protected form the ordinary course of our laws partly by the very obscurity of the place and partly by the privileges of that see where they shelter, was one impostor by name, Forman who now was in the precincts of Lambeth. Here, just as if he were in a harbour, he sailed with great joy, pleasure and complete safety so that none of our officials could arrest him.

This was the territory of the archbishop of Canterbury, John Whitgift, and the Censors wrote to him 'to obtain his approval in order that by these plans all taking cover in the shadows might be routed from their hiding places'.[91]

In their letter, dated 28 June 1601, the Censors first stressed that Forman, 'an Intruder into the profession of Phisick', was dangerous to common people: 'Making a deceitful shew, and colour to the Ignorant people, that his skill is more then Ordinary, depending upon the speculation and insight of Nativities, and Astrology. Thereby miserably deceaving, the Innocency of such simple mynded people as resort unto him for councell.' The College had done everything within its power to stop him:

> We have heertofore convented him in our College assemblees and having made good and sufficient Tryall of his skill, as well in the one [medicine] as in the other [astrology]: have found him exceeding weak and ignorant in the very principles of them both, as appeereth by his most absurd answers, yet extant in our College book of Ordinary Examinations.[92] And thereupon, according to the Statutes of the Realme, We have heretofore utterly forbidden him to deale any further in practyse of that scyence, Wherein he hath so lyttle skill.

But he had ignored their injunctions and continued to infringe on their privileges.

> All which notwithstanding, the said Forman as we are infourmid, hath now placed him self in Lambheath beeing a Towne under your graces Jurisdiction. Mynding therby as

[89] Annals, 7 Nov. 1600, p. 130.

[90] Ashm. 208, fo. 62^{v}. The letter is not extant.

[91] Annals, 25 June 1601, p. 133.

[92] This book is missing.

yt shoold appeare, to abuse your honorable protection, touching the premises. In consideration wherof, we most humbly beseech your Grace that as well in Regard of the insufficiency of the man: as also for the better maintenaunce of our auncient privileges, he may be frustrated of his expectation in that behalf: and that by your graces favour, we may be ayded, and permitted, without any let or Impediment to use such lawfull and ordinary coorse as both holsom lawes and our privileges have provided for the supressing of him, and the lyke Offendors.[93]

Forman might have known about the College's approach to Whitgift, as the next month he noted that Alice Blague, his friend and client, had warned him to beware of the physicians. Alice was married to Thomas Blague, dean of Rochester, who also often consulted Forman. Blague had written a letter to Whitgift on Forman's behalf, and on 6 July 1601 Forman cast a figure to decide whether he should send it.[94] Two days later Forman cast another figure to decide whether he should have Blague appeal on his behalf to the Lord Keeper, now Sir Thomas Egerton.[95]

Meanwhile, at 11.30 a.m. on the day that the Censors had written to Whitgift, Whitgift was consulting Forman about his health.[96] On 4 July the archbishop had responded to the College:

Forman nether is, nor shalbe countenaunced by me: nether doth he deserve yt any way at my handes. I have hard very ill of him: in so much as I had a meaning to call him by vertue of the Commission Ecclesiasticall for divers misdeamaners if any man woold have taken upon him, the prosecution of the cause against him, in which mynd I remaine still. And therfore use your aucthorytie in the name of god. My Officers shall geve their assistaunce, or else they shalbe no Officers of myne.[97]

Whitgift assented to the Censors' request to act within his jurisdiction, placating them with a version of the truth. Whatever suspicious rumours he had heard about Forman, he had nonetheless resorted to the doctor himself.

What happened next can be partially reconstructed from Forman's notes, his psalm, and a letter that he wrote to Richard Napier in March 1603 complaining about his recent conflicts with the College, describing them as 'the furnace & trialle of adversyty'.[98] In September 1601 Forman had been introduced to Edward Seymour, first earl of Hertford (1539?–62), through Seymour's new

[93] Annals, 25 June 1601, pp. 133–4.

[94] For Forman's friendship with the Blagues, see Rowse, *Forman*, ch. 7.

[95] Ashm. 411, fo. 114.

[96] Ashm. 411, fo. 110^{v}.

[97] Annals, 25 June 1601, p. 134. The account in John Strype, *The life and acts of John Whitgift*, ii (Oxford, 1822), 457–8 seems to be drawn directly from the Annals.

[98] Ashm. 240, fo. 105. Cf. Isa. 48: 10, Dan. 3: 6–17.

wife, Frances, the daughter of Thomas, Viscount Howard of Bindon and widow of Henry Pranell. She had been a client of Forman's since at least 1597.[99] They both wrote to the archbishop on Forman's behalf, requesting that he grant Forman a licence to practise physic. The archbishop did not honour these requests, as Forman wrote to Napier: 'But he gives me fair words and soe dryves me of[f] with delayes sayinge the docters have written unto him, desiring him moste instantlye not to take parte with nor to graunt me any lycence for yf he should yt wold be much prejudiciall to them, to their privilege and alsoe to their proceadings . . .' Forman's disappointment with Whitgift was perhaps not unreasonable; this refusal of help 'makes his Gr. cold in that he absolutely of his owne clemency promised me at firste'.[100] Unfortunately Forman did not record what he and Whitgift talked about when they had dinner together on 28 December 1602.[101]

Forman appealed to Lady Hertford further, this time asking her to write to Sir John Popham, the Lord Chief Justice, and his son, Sir Francis Popham. As he told Napier:

> Again I caused my Ladi to write in my behalfe to my L. chife Justice, and to Sr Franncis Popham his sonne that his L. should not take parte with the Docters againste me, and he [Sir John Popham] retorned an aunsware, that he knewe me not, neither did he graunt any warrante that he knewe of againste me, but the docters cam to him in deed to have his hand to a generalle warrante & ther to he set his hand, but henceforth he wold be better advised.[102]

Though the Annals record cases of practitioners eliciting letters of support addressed to the College, here Forman used a patron to stay the hand of the legal authorities through which the College was obliged to enforce their judgements.[103] By March 1603, when Forman wrote to Napier, he was convinced that the physicians had been acting beyond legal means. His diary for 1600 records 'many sclanderouse speaches wer by the doctors and others used secretly against me'.[104] His psalm recounted that when they could not prevail in the courts, 'They rose fals sclanders then | One me without juste cause to make | Me be dispised of men'.[105] Law and slander had failed, Forman continued, so the doctors plotted to murder him:

99 *DNB*, Edward Seymour. Forman cast her nativity for the date 27 July 1578: Ashm. 423, fo. 59; see also 236, fo. 236; 208, fo. 64 (2 Nov. 1601); 411, fo. 161^{v} (24 Nov. 1601). She is not the Frances Howard, countess of Essex, who was involved in the Overbury affair.

100 Ashm. 240, fo. 105. 101 Ashm. 1472, p. [807]. 102 Ashm. 240, fo. 105^{r-v}.

103 Popham however had used up his credit with the College in his support of Thomas Rawlins: Pelling, *Medical Conflicts*, 239–40.

104 Ashm. 208, fo. 62^{v}. 105 Ashm. 802, fo. 131.

They soughte to have me slaine
Or poisoned by som stratagem
And therto ofte did fain
That certain men should com to me
To rid forth to the sicke
That by the way I might be kild
By som Inventyve tricke.[106]

In 1603, they almost succeeded:

And in the yeare of syxtie thre [1603]
Twise was I like bin kild
By their falls officers and knaves
That thoughte my blod have spild.[107]

Forman's fear of the physicians was nothing new, and on previous occasions he had planned to flee London and even England to escape them. On 30 October 1596 he cast a figure to determine whether 'To goe beyond sea and goe free' or not; the next month he asked three further questions about voyages.[108] Two years later, on 18 October 1598, he asked Sir William Monson for a ship, but Monson could not help him.[109] Forman seems to have been serious: on the reverse of the catalogue of the College's actions against him, he listed the things necessary to victual a ship.[110] A year later, now married, Forman considered moving to Essex. He decided against it, as a figure showed that, although the move would allow him to escape evil and imprisonment, 'in thend great suspision will grow on me . . . for some lerned cause'. The figure also showed that he would prosper by practising physic.[111] Discouraged from his plans to move, Forman never went further away from the City than Lambeth.

When he wrote to Napier on 16 March 1603 Forman's fears were immediate. He had returned to his house ten days previously, and 'used his practice', which seems to have meant that he saw his patients. The physicians' attorney had called on him, and Forman told him everything, though he did not record what this entailed. Fearing that the attorney would inform the physicians that Forman could be found at home, and that they would attempt to arrest him, he sent them a threat: 'I wish them to be better advised then they have bine. For yf they or any for them com and enter my house again as they have done, they shall never goe backe again to carry them newes howe they speed, yf they take not the better heed.'[112] Then he wrote to Napier for help, beginning his letter,

[106] Ashm. 802, fo. 132.
[107] Ashm. 802, fo. 132^{v}.
[108] Ashm. 234, fos. 120, 122^{v}.
[109] Ashm. 195, fo. 177.
[110] Ashm. 195, fo. 195; 392, fo. 172.
[111] Ashm. 219, fo. 124.
[112] Ashm. 240, fo. 105^{v}.

I knowe deare frind (since my laste beinge with youe) youe longemoch to heare of me, and of my estate, and howe I have hetherto passed, the mightie stormes, of soe greate a tempeste, the bellowinge of such a Company of Basan Bulles,[113] and the raginge waves of soe mighti a sea which in their fury have risine above their bankes and lifted them selves even up againste the heavens . . .

Thus he referred to the College. Forman continued, portraying himself as a martyr whose many and diverse strategies to appease the College had failed. The physicians,

whose furie non could tame, and whose displeasure non coulde quallifie, noe not any humble entreaty of my frinds, no offers of peace, noe giftes nor rewards, noe conditions, noe submission, nor yet any sacrifice offred to such a leude company of infernall gods, no nor yet the combate yt selfe could end their furie, nor in any wise asswage the inextinguible mallice of such fierce tygres, nor satisfie the gready pauches of such a sorte of devowringe wolves: finally ther is noe inferior die [?] to be found, nor noe hope of peace to be loked for at their hands, but they all cry out with on voice, Crucifie him, Crucifie him, Let him die and let his blod be upon us and on our children as those wicked Jewes did on Christe.[114]

Forman's life was at stake and he trusted in God to protect him against his enemies, even if He let them rage a while.

National events overtook the feud between Forman and the physicians. The queen died on 24 March, six days after Forman wrote to Napier. Perhaps this explains Forman's escape from imminent doom, though his notes do not contain comments on the death of the queen or the accession of the new king. Within a few months Forman had formulated a plan to secure his freedom and security. In late June 1603 he went to the University of Cambridge and obtained a licence to practise physic and astronomy, under the sponsorship of William Ward and Thomas Grimston.[115] This is probably the William Ward who became the regius professor of physic while at King's College Cambridge *c.*1591 and who is sometimes described as physician to the queen; perhaps he is also

[113] Psalms 22: 12.

[114] Ashm. 240, fo. 105; cf. 1436, fo. 139, Forman's 1607 plague tract where he portrayed himself as persecuted by 'som Carpinge momos [Momus] that will deprave me my sayinge and my doinge as they have depraved others more wiser and lerned then my selfe that have writen much truth and good herof. But thoughe they doe yt is not materiall I will suffer them as many of my predicessors in this science have done.' In 1619 another irregular medical practitioner, William Blanke, used similar imagery to describe his relationship with the College: Pelling, 'Knowledge', 267.

[115] Ashm. 208, fo. 225v; 802, fo. 133. The licence is Ashm. 1301, in poor condition, and 1763, fo. 44 is Ashmole's copy. *DNB*; John Venn and J. A. Venn, *Alumni Cantabrigienses, Pt 1. From the Earliest Times to 1751*, 4 vols. (Cambridge, 1922–7), ii. 269; iv. 335. Wood recorded that Forman stayed at Jesus College, Cambridge: Wood, *Athenae Oxonienses*, ii. 100. I am indebted to Frances Willmoth for confirming that the college records do not corroborate this: personal correspondence, 29 Nov. 2001.

the Cambridge man by this name who translated the work of astrology and astronomy attributed to Arcandam in 1562. Very little is known about Grimston except that he was a fellow of Gonville and Caius College. Cambridge was not lacking in scholars sympathetic to astrology and throughout the second half of the sixteenth century there had been an increase in the numbers of medical licences issued by the universities, occasionally, as with Forman, despite the disapproval of the College of Physicians.[116]

While Forman was away, plague had arrived in London, the physicians had fled, and Forman returned to cure the sick:

> Then cam the plague in sixtie thre
> whence all thes Docters fled
> I staid, to save the lyves of many
> That otherwise had bin ded.[117]

Now licensed to practise medicine and again spared from the plague, Forman was almost vindicated. He never again appeared before the College Censors, nor met them in the courts, and his fears seem to have diminished. He had become the astrologer-physician of Lambeth, renowned and notorious for his astrology and his defiance of the physicians. Yet his defence of his reputation and his liberty continued. In 1607 Sir William Paddy, a Censor from 1595 to 1601, reflected on Forman in a verse satire on medical practice, mocking his ignorance and aspirations:

> And doctor fforeman in art a poore man
> Although you know heavens privities
> By an Almanack out of date to tell a fooles fate
> And calculate nativities
>
> Though to your expence you did comence
> I th' universitye
> An also for such hap may wear a velvet cap
> And yt is the true diversity[118]

Paddy portrays Forman as a velvet-capped fool, absurd in his ignorance and posturing, yet Forman remained a threat to the privilege and status of the physicians and they continued to pursue him in his final years. They summoned him on 9 January 1607 and he sent a Mr Whitfield in his place: 'Mr Whitfield, who

[116] Pelling and Webster, 'Medical Practitioners', 192; R. S. Roberts, 'The London Apothecaries and Medical Practice in Tudor and Stuart England', Ph.D. thesis, University of London, 1964, 58–9.

[117] Ashm. 802, fo. 133.

[118] 'Let closestoole and chamberpot choose out Doctor', Bodleian, Rawlinson MS poet *160, fos. 183^{v}-5, stanzas 19, 20.

informed us that owing to more important business he [Forman] could not come then: nor would he come at any other time, unless a public pledge were given regarding his return.'[119] On 30 March of the same year two of Forman's patients presented evidence against him.[120] On 7 July 1609 the Annals record: 'The impostor Forman was to be summoned on the charge of Doctor Rawlins.' This was Thomas Rawlins, a physician-surgeon with an alchemical bent, himself only licensed in 1600 with the support of Sir John Popham.[121] In the summer of 1610, a year before Forman's death, the Annals recorded a final note about him: 'Recently indicted were three, namely Forman, Forester, and Tenant: against these the Fellows were asked to collect all the evidence they could regarding illicit and ill practice.'[122] On 25 June 1611 Forman cast a figure to know 'whether I shall have the better of this term of the doctors or noe and where they will proceed any farder against me or noe'. His conclusion was correct: 'They let the matter cease and proceded no further in it'.[123]

When the physicians summoned Forman in 1594 neither they nor he could have foreseen that their feud would last almost two decades; that Forman would audaciously challenge the College's privilege and status; and that the College would become the foil against which Forman defined his credentials and promoted his reputation as an astrologer-physician. In 1610 Edmund Dawson slandered Forman by impugning his authority in words that parody Forman's self-regard. Dawson, a woodmonger, and Forman were disputing a £72 fee for a property in Crooked Lane, and Dawson alleged that Forman had failed to take a degree in physic in England or abroad, was not permitted to practise physic by the College of Physicians or any English university, was unable to understand Latin, and practised a trade based on the self-proclaimed pretence that he had a special skill.[124] Forman had spent two decades building a reputation as a successful healer and asserting his expertise as an astrologer-physician. He had enlisted the authority of patrons, government officials, and the university of Cambridge to bolster his credentials as an astrologer-physician, credentials forged, he insisted, by his expertise in judging the influences of the stars.

119 Annals, 9 Jan. 1607, p. 191.

120 Annals, 30 Mar. 1607, p. 192. See p. 123 below. Forman recorded that the Censors summoned him on 31 Aug. 1607, and that he chose not to go: Ashm. 392, fo. 130ᵛ. This was not recorded in the Annals.

121 Annals, 7 July 1609, p. 11; Pelling, *Medical Conflicts*, 239–40 and *passim*.

122 Annals, the morrow of St John the Baptist's Day (24 June), 1610, p. 22.

123 Ashm. 392, fo. 175.

124 Corporation of London Record Office, City of London Sheriffs' Court Rolls, Box 4, 1610 bundle, dated 8 July. I am indebted to Martin Ingram for this reference. Forman's records of his disputes with Dawson are Ashm. 392, fo. 172.

5
Plague and Paracelsianism

An ignorant, audacious, illegal, bold, and wicked impostor; a quack. This is how the physicians described Forman during the two decades in which they failed to curtail his medical practice. They laughed at him, fined him, imprisoned him, sued him, and he thought they tried to murder him. What were they fighting about? He infringed on their privilege, challenged their authority, promoted his astrological methods, denounced their learned medicine, and administered remedies to thousands of people. I have charted Forman's conflicts with the College of Physicians, from his perspective and theirs. Here I will complete this story with an account of Forman's medical ideas, comparing them with those of his contemporaries and measuring how they changed during the two decades that he worked in London and defied the physicians, decades punctuated with outbreaks of plague in 1592–3 and 1603.

In 1592 God afflicted Forman with plague and spared him from it, appointing him to heal others as he had healed himself. But the physicians did not discern the stamp of God's authority on Forman's activities. Before his first interview with the Censors in 1594 he wrote a plague tract. In the summer of 1603 plague again arrived in London, Forman obtained a licence in astronomy and physic from the University of Cambridge, and later that year he rewrote his plague tract. To Forman plague signified the weaknesses of physicians and surgeons and the strengths of the astrologer. Outbreaks of plague disrupted the structure of medical provision in urban centres and provided an occasion for physicians, surgeons, and irregular practitioners to enact their rivalries. Plague was also an opportunity for physicians and clerics to dispute the contested boundaries between prayer and prescription.[1] In Forman's papers plague recurs

[1] The standard work on plague in early modern England is Paul Slack, *The Impact of Plague in Tudor and Stuart England* (Oxford, 1985). See also Andrew Wear, *Knowledge and Practice in English Medicine, 1550–1680* (Cambridge, 2000), chs. 6, 7; Pelling, *Common Lot*, ch. 2 and *passim*; Patrick Wallis, 'Plagues, Morality and the Place of Medicine in Early Modern England', *English Historical Review*, 71 (2006), 1–24; David Gentilcore, *Healers and Healing in Early Modern Italy* (Manchester, 1998), chs. 2, 5; Laurence Brockliss and Colin Jones, *The Medical World of Early Modern France* (Oxford, 1997), chs. 1, 6; Colin Jones, 'Plague and its Metaphors in Early Modern France', *Representations*, 53 (1996), 97–127. On the impact of the Black Death on medicine see Park, *Doctors and Medicine*, and McVaugh, *Medicine before the Plague*. On the historiography of plague,

as a theme binding his notions of expertise, authority, and medical knowledge. For him a body afflicted with plague was a stage on which God and the devil, the stars and planets, life and death, and physicians, astrologers, and quacks periodically rehearsed their contests.

Plague was a boon for Forman. His recovery from it in 1592 propelled him into success as a medical practitioner in London. In 1593 his practice grew, he began to clear his debts and to reclaim his pawned possessions, moved into a better room in the house where he lived, re-engaged Steven Mitchel, his step-nephew, as a servant, and bought a velvet gown.[2] He also wrote 'A discourse of the plague', one of his earliest medical writings, styling himself 'gent. practizar in physic and astrology'.[3] Forman met the College censors in the spring of the following year, 1594, and in his writings on plague he is already outspoken about his knowledge of astrological physic, and, more quietly, dismissive of formally educated physicians and surgeons. Over the next decade Forman rewrote this treatise at least twice and also compiled several general, lengthy treatises on astrological medicine. Forman's manuals of astrological physic provide copious lists of rules, occasionally prefaced with a history of those chosen to practise the art, culminating with himself, and interrupted with an account of one of his successful cases. His writings on plague are briefer, less compendious, and more polemical; they display his philosophy of medicine and the grounds of his opposition to the physicians and surgeons more explicitly than his other writings, and they do so across two decades.

Guides to astrology were scarce in Elizabethan England; plague tracts were common and formulaic and since the Black Death in the mid-fourteenth century hundreds had circulated throughout Europe.[4] Forman was engaging with an established, though heterogeneous genre. Some plague tracts were brief and anonymous, others sophisticated and signed by famous surgeons or physicians; some were theological, others medical, others melding physic for body and soul. Most began with definitions of plague, following Hippocrates, Galen,

see Faye Getz, 'Black Death and the Silver Lining: Meaning, Continuity, and Revolutionary Change in Histories of Medieval Plague', *Journal of the History of Biology*, 24 (1991), 265–89.

2 Ashm. 208, fo. 49; see also 390, fo. 60ᵛ. On subsequent clothing purchases, see Ashm. 208, fos. 57 (1596), 62ᵛ (1600).

3 Ashm. 208, fos. 110–34. This fills a full quire, which could have stood on its own. The title is on the front; there is nothing on the back of the final leaf. The title, some of the annotations, and the final page are written with a darker ink and were probably added at a later sitting. With the possible exception of Sloane 2550, fos. 1–117ᵛ (*c*.1589?), 'A discourse of the plague' is Forman's earliest known medical tract.

4 Slack, 'Mirrors of Health'. Cf. Colin Jones, 'Plague and its Metaphors'; Brockliss and Jones, *Medical World*, 38–42, 67–71. From the Black Death of the mid-14th cent. until 1500, 281 extant plague tracts were written: Campbell, *Black Death*; Pagel, *Paracelsus*, 172–87; Nancy Siraisi, *Medieval and Early Renaissance Medicine: An Introduction to Knowledge and Practice* (Chicago, 1990), 128, 189.

Avicenna, and the Bible. Air corrupted by evil vapours, dead bodies, stinking lakes, open caves, and the malign influences of planets, especially Saturn and Mars, caused plague; so too did an accumulation of foul humours through bad diet and large pores.[5] Information about how to predict a plague, how to prevent catching it, how to know what sort it was, how to cure it, and familial and civic responsibilities, might follow. Latin treatises contemplated the nature of fevers and cheap vernacular books advertised remedies from preventative amulets to palliative nostrums. Forman's writings on plague did almost none of these things. Instead they focused on the importance of knowing whether a plague had natural, demonic, or divine causes, and the astrological expertise necessary for making such judgements.

Astrology had become a point of contention in sixteenth-century plague tracts. The role of astrology in medicine was contested, astrology was increasingly theologically suspect, and it was becoming more specialized.[6] Most medieval plague tracts attributed plague to God's wrath, the malevolent influences of Saturn and Mars, and foul airs.[7] Sixteenth-century plague tracts reflected debates amongst physicians about the influences of the planets on the causes of disease.[8] For instance, Ficino suggested that plague was caused by the specific properties of the venomous air infecting the vital spirit, not its excess heat, moisture, or other qualities; Paracelsus stressed the interplay between man and the heavens and the creation of disease through imagined sin, describing plague as caused by God's retribution, shot from the firmament; and Jean Fernel postulated the notion of diseases of the total substance within a Galenic framework, attributing plague to the occult properties of the heavenly bodies.[9]

Forman's writings on plague, like most of his treatises, are incoherent, eclectic, and unusual. They are in English, and the earliest version is finished and copied and might have been destined for print: its subtitle is 'verie necessary for

[5] For a clear exposition in an Elizabethan plague tract see Thomas Lodge, *A treatise of the plague* (1603), sigs. B2^{v}–3.

[6] Grafton and Siraisi, 'Cardano and Medical Astrology', esp. 85; Siraisi, *Medieval and Renaissance Medicine*, 68–9, 111, 123; Brian Copenhaver, *Symphorien Champier and the Reception of the Occultist Tradition in Renaissance France* (The Hague, 1978), esp. ch. 1.

[7] Siraisi, *Medieval and Renaissance Medicine*, 128–9; Thorndike, *Magic and Experimental Science*, iii. 292–3, 289–91; see also 241, 242, 389, 520.

[8] For causation see Vivian Nutton, 'The Seeds of Disease: An Explanation of Contagion and Infection from the Greeks to the Renaissance', *Medical History*, 27 (1983), 1–34; Margaret Pelling, 'Contagion/Germ Theory/Specificity', in William Bynum and Roy Porter (eds.), *Companion Encyclopedia of the History of Medicine*, i (1993), 309–34, esp. 315.

[9] Thorndike, *Magic and Experimental Science*, v. 125, 297, 318, 330, 347, 439, 475, 542, 605–8; vi. 99–144, 158, 210–12. See also Brockliss and Jones, *Medical World*, 130–1; Pagel, *Paracelsus*, 174–80; Richardson, 'Generation of Disease', 184, 188–93; Siraisi, *Cardano*, ch. 7; Webster, *Paracelsus to Newton*, 56.

all men to reade and truely to remember'.[10] It remained in manuscript and seems not to have circulated. English, printed plague tracts abounded. Between 1486 and 1604 at least 153 medical books were printed in the vernacular in England. Twenty-three were devoted solely to plague, while many others had a chapter on it. In 1603–4 alone, twenty-eight books on plague were printed, though fifteen concentrated on the spiritual lessons of plague more than its physical causes or means of prevention.[11] Between 1592 and 1594, when Forman wrote his first plague treatise, one medical tract on plague, two medical tracts containing substantial sections on plague, three religious tracts on plague, and annual royal proclamations with rudimentary medical content were printed.[12] English vernacular medical works, with a few exceptions, contained standard expositions of humoral physiology and basic remedies, recycling material from earlier tracts without engaging with learned medical debates.[13] Innovations did appear in moral discussions about the uses of prayer and physic and the flight of physicians and clerics from the city.[14]

Few authors of Elizabethan plague tracts gave their opinions about astrology, and most of those who did were critical of it. The first vernacular plague treatise printed in England was a French work by Jehan Goeurot, translated as *The regiment of life* (1545). Goeurot explained that plague was caused by the will of God, as illustrated in the Bible; the heavenly constellations, particularly Saturn and Mars, following Ficino; the corruption of the air; and the abuse of things non-natural.[15] Throughout the century English plague tracts became more ambivalent about astrology. Thomas Cogan, in *The haven of health* (1584), attributed plague to God's anger, unclean living, unburied carrion, standing waters, and the influences of the stars, but he explained that, while the astronomers located its causes in the heavens, the physicians found them on earth.[16] In a 1583 translation of a work by Johannes Ewich, astrologers were

[10] Ashm. 208, fo. 110. In the 1607 version Forman wrote 'And marvaille not whie I write soe plain a waie but I doe yt to teach men to heal themselves': Ashm. 1436, fo. 142.

[11] Slack, *Plague*, 23–4.

[12] Anthony Anderson, *An approved medicine against the deserved plague* (1593); Brasbridge, *Poor mans jewel*; William Cupper, *Certain sermons concerning God's late visitation* (1592); Jean Goeurot, *The regiment of life, whereof is added a treatyse of the pestilence with the booke of children newly corrected and enlarged*, tr. Thomas Phayer (1560 [1545?]); Henry Holland, *Spiritual preservatives against the pestilence* (1593); Simon Kellwaye, *A defensative against the plague* (1593).

[13] Roberts, 'London Apothecaries', 64; Slack, 'Mirrors of Health', 252. Until the second half of the 17th cent. most tracts relied on material derived from the 14th and 15th cents., Slack, *Plague*, 24.

[14] Theodore Beza, *A short learned and pithie treatise of the plague*, tr. John Stockwood (1580), sigs. B8–C7ᵛ; Slack, *Plague*, 41–4.

[15] Goeurot, *Regiment of life*, sigs. K3–P5ᵛ. The plague treatise is an appendage to a larger medical work.

[16] Cogan, *Haven of health*, 262.

accused of falsely ascribing plague to a single cause.[17] Some plagues were caused by God; some by the putrefaction of air, water, and earth; and some, following Cardano, by infection.[18] Ewich underpinned his treatise with Protestant doctrines and stressed the importance of remedying the course of nature with good works, echoing the standard objection that judicial astrology was contrary to the doctrine of free will. From the 1570s, some English plague tracts dismissed the astrological causes of the plague outright. In a tract printed in 1578 Thomas Brasbridge outlined the usual four causes of the plague (the will of God, the influence of evil constellations, the corruption of the air, and the constitution of the body), only to note that there was no need for him to address the subject of evil constellations, 'espescially in such manner as the Astronomers do: who by their Ethnicall phrases, and kinds of speech in their Almanacks, and Prognostications, do seem, to favor or foster the idolatrie of the heathen'. Then he complained that he did not understand why astrologers wrote prognostications for unlearned readers and set down the rules of astrology, incomprehensible to all but themselves.[19]

In 1603 Thomas Lodge, the physician and poet, wrote *A treatise of the plague.* This was the most comprehensive English work on plague to that date, and it sidestepped the wrath of God, touched briefly on the malign influences of the planets, and dwelt on the natural causes of plague, a disease more secret and mysterious than any other.[20] Lodge, following Avicenna, described how malign planets corrupted the air and infected any who breathed it with evil vapours, thus corrupting the vital spirit. But Avicenna was an astrologer and astrologers, Lodge complained, wrongly asserted that 'any contagion or misfortune, incommoditie or sickness whatsoever may by reason of the starres befall man'.[21] The stars were perfect and therefore the stars could not cause plague:

> because contagion is no other thing but an infection proceeding from one unto another by communication of a pestilence and infected vapour, and by this meanes if the plague and contagion proceedeth from the starres, it should necessarily follow that by the definition of contagion, that the stares were primarily or formerly infected, if by their influence they should send a pernicious contagion among us.[22]

[17] Ewich, *Of the duetie of the faithful and wise magistrates*, tr. John Stockwood (1583), sig. ***2^{v}. Stockwood, a schoolmaster from Tunbridge, also translated Beza's plague tract.

[18] Ewich, *Duetie of magistrates*, sigs. ***3, ***4^{v}, ****5. Ewich gave Cardano's *De rerum varietate* as his source.

[19] Brasbridge, *Poor mans jewel*, sigs. A6–B1, esp. sig. A7^{r-v}.

[20] Lodge, *Plague*, sig. B3^{v}.

[21] Ibid., sig. B4^{v}.

[22] Ibid., sig. C1^{v}.

This was impossible. The celestial bodies were pure and divine and could not change their nature. Plague, he concluded, came not from the stars but from divine judgement and corrupt vapours.[23]

Lodge, Brasbridge, Cogan, and Stockwood had something to say about astrology, but the majority of English plague tracts did not.[24] When read alongside any of these works, Forman's texts are anomalous. They make more sense when set against the numerous alchemical and Paracelsian works that were printed in English in the 1570s and 1580s. During these decades John Hester (d. 1593), a distiller, and George Baker (1540–1600), a surgeon, and others translated several dozen works containing alchemical and Paracelsian remedies, and such remedies were also included in the works of other prominent surgeons such as John Banister (1540–1610) and William Clowes, Senior (1540?–1604). Elizabethan surgeons were especially receptive to the uses of alchemical remedies, though proponents of these methods and ideas could also be found amongst the physicians, most notably Thomas Mouffett (1553–1604). Historians have debated the extent to which the use of alchemical remedies was adopted without any concern for the theoretical teachings of Paracelsus. Most of the books translated and printed in Elizabethan England contained lists of remedies with little discussion of Paracelsian medical ideas; indeed some of the translators and compilers claimed, not wholly convincingly, that these ideas were so complicated that they did not really understand them.[25] These books document an interest in Paracelsianism beyond the recipes that they published. Forman gave them no credit, but communities of practitioners promoting alchemical and Paracelsian medicine and the tracts they published, along with the language of reform and opposition found in vernacular mathematical and medical works, informed his fashioning of himself as an astrologer-physician.

[23] Ibid., sig. C2. Also that year, two unidentified authors were less dismissive of celestial causes of plague, simply referring the subject to astronomers: S.H., *A new treatise of the pestilence* (1603); I.W., *A briefe treatise of the plague* (1603).

[24] Those that do not mention astrology at all are: Barrough, *Methode of physicke* (1583); William Bullein, *A dialogue bothe pleasaunt and pietifull, against the fever pestilence* (1573); Thomas Thayre, *A treatise of the pestilence* (1603). Pagel uses Thayre as a typical example of a traditional Galenic plague tract: *Paracelsus*, 173–4.

[25] The standard, though conflicting, works on Elizabethan alchemy and Paracelsianism are Debus, *English Paracelsians*; Kocher, 'Paracelsian Medicine'; Webster, 'Alchemical and Paracelsian Medicine'. On surgeons and alchemical and Paracelsian remedies, see esp. Kocher, 'Paracelsian Medicine', 466–73; Pelling and Webster, 'Medical Practitioners', 173–7. For contemporary complaints about not understanding Paracelsianism see Debus, *English Paracelsians*, 69; *The whole worke of the famous chirurgion Master John Vigo*, tr. George Baker (1586), Baker's preface to the reader, sig. ¶3. Baker says this amidst a denunciation of a recent book in which the author brags of his Paracelsian knowledge and expertise. This book is probably I.W., *A coppie of a letter sent by a learned physician* ([1586]).

Two plague tracts combined alchemical and Paracelsian medicine and provide a foil for Forman's writings and his oppositional persona. The first is a standard example in discussions of alchemical and Paracelsian medicine in Elizabethan England, the translation of a work by Leonardo Fioravanti as *A joyfull jewell, containing aswell such excellent orders, preservatives and precious practices for the plague*, begun by Thomas Hill, completed by John Hester, and printed in 1580. Hill, about whom little is known, wrote, compiled, translated, and prepared for the press works on astronomy, arithmetic, dreams, gardening, and other topics that were printed from the late 1550s through the seventeenth century.[26] Hester was a friend of Hill's who had set up shop in London as a distiller in the 1570s. From then until his death he translated and had printed numerous alchemical and Paracelsian treatises.[27] Fioravanti was an Italian irregular medical practitioner, originally from Bologna, who wrote numerous popular medical works recounting his miraculous cures.[28] Whether or not he was a Paracelsian depends on how the term is defined; he certainly promoted chemical and alchemical remedies and he, like Forman, portrayed himself as a force of opposition, wielding authority gleaned from experience not books.[29]

Most of Fioravanti's tracts, like other works translated by Hester, were collections of recipes. Fioravanti prefaced these with polemics on the merits of the new physic, borrowing the rhetoric of Paracelsianism and stressing the importance of experience and the inadequacies of the physicians.[30] In *A joyfull jewell* he outlined the standard causes of plague (God's vengeance, air corrupted through foul water, putrefied matter, or heat), he mentioned how a breakdown of the social fabric and fear exacerbated the disease, and he complained that physicians did not write about the pestilence because they did not encounter it in their everyday practice nor, as he had done, did they deign to travel in search of old men who had lived through it.[31] He began the substance of the book with seventeen cases from sixteenth-century Italy in which syrups, strong waters, electuaries, pills, and the occasional blood-letting or purge, prevented or cured the plague; then he recorded several dozen of his own recipes for quintessences, elixirs, balsams, oils, etc. His remedies to prevent and cure the plague

[26] For Hill's works see *STC*. Apparently Hill became ill in 1576 and entrusted the completion of this work to Hester, and Conrad Gesner's *The newe jewell of health* (1576) to George Baker. Hill however seems to have recovered and lived until 1599: *DNB*.

[27] *DNB*; Debus, *English Paracelsians*, 65–9; Webster, 'Alchemical and Paracelsian Medicine', 326–7.

[28] Eamon, *Science and the Secrets of Nature*, ch. 5.

[29] Ibid., 191. It would seem obvious for Forman to have modelled his persona on such a fellow medical maverick, though the only evidence that he knew of Fioravanti or read his works is a note about 'Mr Firovanto' and a secret for 'conjoining' mercury and copper: Ashm. 1494, p. 408^{v}.

[30] Fioravanti, *Joyfull jewell*, 3–8.

[31] Ibid. 7–8.

were learned through experience, his own and others', and he promoted the novelty of his methods and his knowledge. Forman's methods too were novel, but in his writings on plague he advertised neither the authority of accumulated expertise nor proven secrets, dwelling instead on the natural, unnatural, and supernatural causes of plague.

A second plague tract promoted alchemical and Paracelsian remedies and dwelt on the causes of plague, and unlike Fioravanti's, this work has no place in accounts of Elizabethan alchemy and medicine. This was a work by Pierre Drouet, translated by Thomas Twyne as *A new counsell against the plague* (1578). Half of Drouet's treatise concerned the causes of plague, and half its cure and prevention. He followed the convention of beginning with Hippocrates, Galen, and debates about the corruption of the air, whether from the influences of evil planets directly or from the more general putrefaction that followed their motions.[32] Echoing Paracelsus, he differentiated types of plague according to which organ (heart, brain, liver) was first afflicted. Unlike the other plague tracts printed in English, Drouet charted a particular course through the learned writings on the subject and across the medical practices of Europe. He liked to tell stories about himself, other physicians, and plagues. He recounted how the plague that the Paduan physician Montanus (Giovanni Battista de Monte, 1498–1552) reported in Lyons and Vienna in 1525 afflicted the substance of the heart, and the plague in Avernia in 1546 afflicted the brain.[33] He mentioned methods for drawing venom from the body that he had learnt in Paris in the 1550s studying with the famous physician Hollerius (Jacques Houllier, 1498–1562).[34] After that he had known a surgeon in Roan (Rouen?), an old man, who treated plague with blood-letting and vomits.[35] Around 1560 the physician to one Lord Vidam had taught him the merits of wearing a hazel nut filled with quicksilver around one's neck, a method, he noted, also endorsed by Ficino.[36] In 1564 he learnt how to make a plaster of red arsenic to place above the heart, though he noted that the merits of this method were debated by George Agricola and others.[37] Sometime in the late 1560s he travelled in England and Germany, both sites of plague in 1567, and everywhere he went he talked to people.[38] When passing through Antwerp an Italian surgeon taught him the powerful and convenient use of the Indian Nut (coconut) as an emetic; Leonard Fuchs, at his own house, told Drouet that electuary of either eggs or angelica was commonly used to cure and prevent the plague amongst the Germans.[39] Drouet wrote this book in

32 Pierre Drouet, *A new counsell against the plague*, tr. Thomas Twyne (London, 1578), sig. B3.

33 Ibid., sig. D4^{r-v}. 34 Ibid., sig. J2^{v}. 35 Ibid., sig. G4. 36 Ibid., sigs. E3^{v}–4.

37 Ibid., sig. E4. 38 Ibid., sig. H2^{v}. 39 Ibid., sig. G2.

Latin and it was printed in 1572, then again in 1576 before being translated into English in 1578.[40]

Having been in England in the late 1560s, Drouet probably knew the translator of his work, Thomas Twyne (1543–1613). Twyne translated half a dozen texts in the 1570s and was to become an astrologer, physician, and from *c.*1593 friend of John Dee.[41] Drouet claimed to have learnt nothing from the English, though he was impressed with the foreigners living and working there. For example, he met Giovanni Battista Agnello, an Italian who 'had spent all of his life in the art of Distilling', and who taught him how to make an opiate to purge evil humours and strengthen the heart and liver.[42] Agnello, Drouet reported, also practised medicine in England, noting the great success of his recipe for a purge containing two ounces of erysimum.[43] Drouet had also met one Jerome of Flanders, a surgeon working in London, who reported the effectiveness of salts in promoting sweat and combating the plague.[44] Drouet was worldly and well-educated, and he advertised these attributes in his book. Forman, in contrast, concealed the people with whom he spoke and, initially, the books he had read, promoting himself as an autodidactic not a man of letters.

When Forman arrived in London in 1591, other practitioners bearing few or foreign credentials had challenged orthodox medicine, promoted new ideas, and established themselves during outbreaks of plague. In the late 1560s Drouet had found plenty of knowledgeable foreigners and interested Englishmen in and around London, through the 1570s Twyne, Hill, and others translated various natural philosophical and occult works into English, and at the end of the decade they were joined by Hester in promoting alchemical and Paracelsian medicine. Through the 1580s the surgeons Clowes and Banister promoted alchemical remedies, and Mouffett engaged with the growing interest in Paracelsianism internationally. When Forman launched himself into the medical world of Elizabethan London in the early 1590s with his method for curing the plague and his treatise on the causes of the pestilence, if he had an informed audience, they would have known that, however idiosyncratic

[40] Pierre Drouet, *Consilium novum de pestilentia* (Paris, 1572; Argentorati, 1576).

[41] *DNB*. For Twyne's works see *STC*. For his friendship with Dee, see Roberts and Watson (eds.), *Dee's Library*, 15. When Drouet was in England, Twyne was probably either at Corpus Christi College in Oxford, where he was elected to a fellowship in 1564 and received his MA in 1568, or in Lewes, Sussex, where he subsequently settled as a medical practitioner.

[42] Drouet, *New counsell*, sig. F4^{r-v}. Giovanni Battista Agnello, or Agnelli, had published *Apocalypsis spiritus secreti* in London in 1566. This was printed in English as *The revelation of the secret spirit*, tr. R.N.E. (1623). His name was also anglicized to various forms of 'Lamb'. See Harkness, *Dee's Conversations with Angels* (Cambridge, 1999), 204; Harkness, '"Strange" Ideas', 152–4; Webster, 'Alchemical and Paracelsian Medicine', 305.

[43] Drouet, *New counsell*, sig. G3^{v}.

[44] Ibid., sig. H2^{v}.

Forman's ideas and practices, he was not as unusual as he thought.[45] He complained that the physicians had fled the city during the plague, but this was a commonplace.[46] Not everyone calling for a reform of medicine agreed with all or any of the teachings of Paracelsus; those who did follow Paracelsus drew distinctions between good Paracelsians and bad Paracelsians; and, as already noted, some promoted his methods though avowing not fully to understand his teachings.[47] Forman did not fashion himself as a follower of Paracelsus, though Paracelsus was one of the many authors on whom he drew, and he did not align himself with the English surgeons (Banister, Baker, Clowes) who promoted alchemical remedies, though he too distilled medicines. He ruminated on the divine and celestial causes of disease without ever clearly articulating a cosmology or natural philosophy. He traversed the terrain of scholarly and popular, ancient, medieval, and early modern writings on dozens of subjects, including natural philosophy, theology, history, and astronomy. In his writings on plague he blended medical and moral concerns, incidentally documenting his engagement with occult medicine.

'A discourse of the plague', though a fair copy, is rhetorically untutored and in what follows I have systematized Forman's arguments. He divided plague into three sorts, depending on whether it was caused by nature, the devil, or God, and devoted a section of his tract to each. The first part sketched the three types of natural plague caused by the revolutions of the heavens, motions of the planets, and influences of the stars, especially the malignant effects of Saturn and Mars. When Saturn was dominant, an abundance of melancholy mixed with phlegm caused the cold and black plague; when Mars was dominant, an abundance of choler caused the red and hot plague; when Saturn and Mars were both dominant, their combined influences caused a third sort of plague. Each of these diseases began with different signs and tokens, ran a different course, and required different remedies.[48] Forman would elaborate on these types in a later treatise.

The second part of the treatise considered how the devil, though constrained by God, caused plague. God commanded and compelled the devil to plague bad men, such as Ahab; He allowed the devil to plague good men whom he envied, such as Job; and sometimes the devil acted against God, such as when

[45] Harkness has identified 174 alchemical practitioners in London during the reign of Elizabeth: '"Strange" ideas', 151.

[46] Ashm. 208, fo. [126]; see also fo. 123^{r-v} and Ch. 4 n. 2 above.

[47] On reform with a distance from Paracelsus, see the works of Fioravanti, Drouet, and later Joseph Duchesne: *STC*. Banister, William Clowes, and others distinguished between good and bad Paracelsians: Debus, *English Paracelsians*, 69.

[48] Ashm. 208, fos. 110^{v}–14.

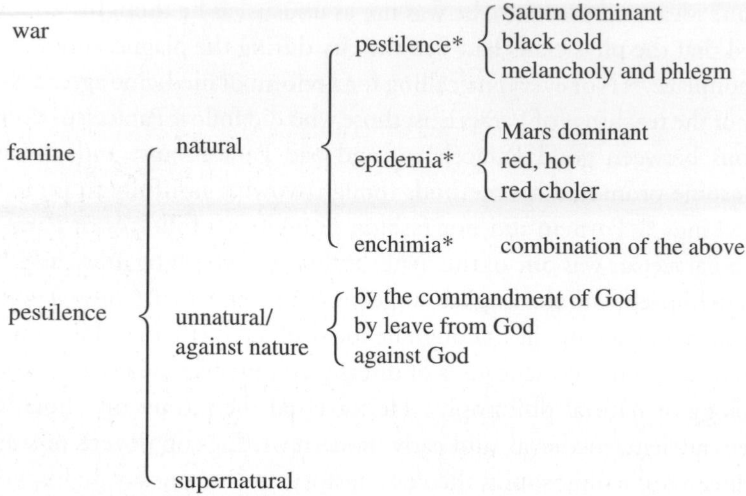

5.1. Simon Forman's typology of plague.
Note: This depiction is deduced from Forman's three plague treatises, though no such rigorous scheme was maintained throughout them. The terms marked with an asterisk are used only in the 1607 treatise, though the three types were described according to their characteristics in the earlier treatises.

he tempted Adam to eat the apple.[49] The third part of the tract, on the plagues of God, was less schematic, much longer than the first two parts, and progressed from an excursus on divine retribution for sin to the virtues and evils of the English. First Forman reflected:

But ther is noe Eva in England that dare eat an apple in paradice, for feare shee should be expelled from the joies of heaven and caste out into eternalle pain in hell fyer. Ther is noe wicked Caine in England, that darse to kill his brother Abell, because he is better thoughte of thene him selfe, for feare the Lord should curse him for hit and make him a vagabond.

There is noe Noah in England that will be dronken with wine . . .

Then he replaced the negative refrain (there are no such sinners in England) with the same in the affirmative (how many sinners there are in England), detailing the sins of the English from the oppression of the poor to the immorality of women.[50] Forman's haranguing concluded:

The lawes of England ar good, the countrie fertill and good, but the people verie bad, and never worse then nowe. For under the shadowe of religion and quarelle of god, they

[49] Ashm. 208, fos. 114–17. For possible echoes of Paracelsus, see Pagel, *Paracelsus*, 174–80; Webster, *Paracelsus to Newton*, 81.

[50] Ashm. 208, fos. 119, 121^{v}.

cover all kinds of sinne and villany that they commit against god, againste the church, againste their prince, against their countrie, againste their neighbours, yea and againste their owne soulles, selling them selves and their soules to the dyvell for lucre and gaine.[51]

Finally he noted that 'yt is no mervaille, thoughe the lord curse youe and your generacions and plague youe as he hath plagued them afore spoken of in tyme paste'.[52]

With a shift from moralizing to prophesying, Forman reflected on the importance of heeding the signs of God's displeasure. God had warned the English with an earthquake in 1576, famines in 1584–5, a comet in 1586, the Spanish Armada in 1588, and the plague of 1592–3, specifically a 'Saturnal' plague, beginning with pain in the head then 'tokens' on the body.[53] These events were the fodder of the many printed prognostications in England and throughout Europe, and in an unusual engagement with contemporary authors, Forman criticized Reginald Scot and John Harvey for belittling God's power in their books.[54] Chastizing the physicians, Forman concluded that penitence, not flight from the city, was the only way to escape the plague.[55] What began as an exposition of the astrological causes of the plague, ended with a peroration against the English who were too busy making money, drinking wine, and chasing women to repent, or too learned to recognize His signs. Forman thus turned from prognostication to history, righteously pronouncing on the causes of past plagues and declaring his version of Christian virtues.[56] As an astrologer, he had the authority and knowledge to discern the causes of plague, past and future.

All plague tracts mentioned the causes of the disease, usually distinguishing between God's wrath and the natural corruption of air. Depending on which cause the tract emphasized, plague treatises from early modern England are often classified as either medical or moral. Medical ones echoed Galen's precept that corrupt air and the corruption of the humours caused plague; moral ones were more concerned with sin and the wrath of God.[57] Occasionally a treatise addressed medicine for the body and soul in equal measures. For instance, Henry Holland's *Spiritual preservative against the plague* (1593) distinguished

[51] Ashm. 208, fos. 122ᵛ–3. [52] Ashm. 208, fo. 124ᵛ. [53] Ashm. 208, fo. 110ᵛ.

[54] Ashm. 208, fo. 131: Harvey, *A discoursive probleme concerning prophecies* (1588); Scot, *Discoverie of witchcraft* (1584). Forman kept notes on astronomical configurations during past plagues and rules for predicting future ones at least from 1592 to 1603: Ashm. 384, fos. 8, 30, 112, 169, 174ᵛ, 175ᵛ, 176ᵛ. For a discussion of prognostications relating to many of these events see Webster, *Paracelsus to Newton*, ch. 2. See also Ottavia Niccoli, *Prophecy and People in Renaissance Italy*, tr. Lydia Cochrane (Princeton, 1990); Laura Ackerman Smoller, *History, Prophecy and the Stars: The Christian Astrology of Pierre d'Ailly, 1350–1420* (Princeton, 1994). On providence see Thomas, *Decline of Magic*; Alexandra Walsham, *Providence in Early Modern England* (Oxford, 1999).

[55] Ashm. 208, fo. 131. [56] Ashm. 208, fos. 127ᵛ–9.

[57] See for instance Cupper, *Certain sermons*.

between supernatural and natural causes of plague and asserted the commonplace that a cure required repentance and physic, cleansing the soul then calling the physician. His contemporaries, he argued, were wrong to neglect physic in favour of prayer. As Luther had said, to neglect physic was like neglecting food, it was murder.[58] Like Holland, Forman was concerned about the natural and supernatural causes of plague but his emphasis was on the astrologer's ability to discern the causes of plague, not the conjunction of prayer and physic.

'A discourse of the plague' leaves arguments unfinished and meanders from one digression to the next. Forman needed more time in the library and a good editor. In 1603 there was another, more severe, outbreak of plague, and sometime between then and 1607 Forman radically revised his ideas on plague under the heading 'Forman's treatise on the plague'.[59] In 1607 he revised it again without giving it a title, Ashm. 1436.[60] Throughout these recensions Forman maintained the three types of plague (natural, unnatural, supernatural), but in the later versions he ranted less about God's punishments of the sins of the English and elaborated on the natural causes of plague, like many authors before him, dwelling on the corruption of air by standing water, foul winds, and dead carcasses, the malign influences of the planets, and the economy of the six non-naturals.[61] The third version omitted the section on demonic plague entirely, and limited the discussion of the divine causes of plague to the means of telling if a plague was supernatural or natural.[62] At the top of the pages of these sections in the *c.*1603 version Forman had noted 'I leve this

58 Holland, *Spiritual preservatives*, 178, 181–5.

59 Ashm. 1403. This contains a table of contents which does not reflect the organization of the MS, and in which sections were listed which are absent from the MS. In particular, it lacks the prefatory pages, which may account for why this text is undated. It seems that at some point Forman partially dismantled this treatise without discarding its remnants; it has multiple sets of pagination and foliation, and from these it appears that many pages have been excised.

60 Although Ashm. 1403 is not dated, that it preceded Ashm. 1436 is evident from the incorporation of marginal additions from Ashm. 1403 into the main text in Ashm. 1436. On fo. 1 Forman wrote, 'Of the plague generally and of his sortes. Of those things that moste commonly forshowe a plague.' This is the beginning of a list of contents, not the title of the work.

61 Ashm. 1436, fos. 38–42, 46–50, 55–6. The discussion of the six non-naturals seems to be missing and the text jumps to the internal causes of plague.

62 The 1607 tract is a complete, though not a fair copy, as its pages are of different inks and formats, and it has multiple pagination and foliation, all of which give it the quality of a composite like many of Forman's volumes. This volume begins with a dedication to the reader, a testimony of the author, and a preamble. The first two folios of the dedication to the reader were at some point damaged, and Ashmole has restored them. He transcribed the dedication to the reader and the author's testimony in full. William Black, while cataloguing the Ashmole MSS found these with Ashm. 1403, and they are now bound in Ashm. 1790, fo. 102. It is unclear whether Ashmole made these copies from Forman's damaged pages, or whether he had access to another version of this text. The dedication and testimony are both dated 1607, and this is in keeping with the contents of the MSS. There is a table of contents at the end, which in this case fits the text.

to devines', echoing the disclaimers in plague tracts by his contemporaries and restricting the concerns of the physician to diseases that were not caused by God.[63] Having excised the materials on demonic and divine causes of plague, Forman complicated its typology and elaborated its causes, thus replacing peroration with expositions of causality, especially astrological causality.[64] He also added information about signs of plague and death, significance of botches and carbuncles, symptoms of the disease, and a remedy and diet, stressing that he had cured many people with these methods.[65] In the new scheme, each of the natural plagues could have superior causes, inferior causes, or a combination of the two depending on the influences of the four imperial planets, Saturn, Jupiter, Mars, and the moon.[66] Astrological expertise could be used to predict a plague, its nature, and in particular cases whether it would result in death.[67] At every opportunity throughout the tract Forman complained that physicians and surgeons had neither the expertise nor the authority to deal with plague.

Forman's plague tracts were astrological tracts. Between completing 'A discourse of the plague' in 1593 and revising it in 1603 Forman wrote three manuals of astrological physic. He recycled passages from these guides into his plague tract; in particular he inserted in his 1607 plague treatise numerous passages from 'Grounds of arte', the guide to astrological physic that he compiled between 1594 and 1596.[68] This, like Forman's other manuals of astrological physic, listed thousands of rules for judging the astrological causes of a

63 Ashm. 1403, fos. 60–7, 70–93. These passages in Ashm. 1403 are slightly revised versions of the sections in Ashm. 208, fos. 114–17, 118–34. It seems that Forman did not complete the copy, and in Ashm. 1403 the description of the diseases of God leaves off after copying the first few lines from Ashm. 208, fo. 125ᵛ. On leaving things to divines, see Ambroise Paré's description of the divine causes of plague as 'fit to leave it to Divines': Ambroise Paré, *A treatise of the plague* (1630), 4. See also Paul Kocher, 'The Idea of God in Elizabethan Medicine', *Journal of the History of Ideas*, 11 (1950), 3–29, esp. 17; Kocher, *Science and Religion in Elizabethan London* (San Marino, Calif., 1953), 258–83.

64 In the 1607 plague treatise Forman added two further categories to the natural, unnatural, and supernatural causes of plague: plagues against nature were caused when a man or woman plagued another man or woman, and a fifth cause was when a man plagued himself: Ashm. 1436, fos. 5–8. Forman elaborated on this typology in the next section, again changing it slightly. The plagues of men were defined as coming from envy and malice, by which a man provoked the devil, the world, and the flesh. This resulted in the corruption of nature. This type of plague occurred within all parts of the social hierarchy: fathers plagued sons, mothers daughters, daughters mothers, and servants and masters plagued each other, all of which were supported with examples from the Bible: Ashm. 1436, fos. 11ᵛ–12ᵛ. He also elaborated on the different sorts of plague (plaga, pestis, pestilentia, epidemia) that are described in the Bible, noting that he was concerned with the latter two: Ashm. 1436, fos. 21–5ᵛ.

65 Ashm. 1436, fos. 59–68, 92–104, 107–13. There is a duplicate of fo. 68ᵛ on fos. 69ᵛ–70ᵛ; the cure for black plague is repeated, differently, fo. 78ʳ⁻ᵛ.

66 Ashm. 1436, fos. 13–15, 44–5. This section may be incomplete: the format shifts slightly and Forman's foliation jumps from 28 to 43.

67 Ashm. 1436, fos. 26–34.

68 Ashm. 1495. The latest dated addition to this text was in 1596, Ashm. 1495, fos. 484–7.

disease, generally organized according to the seven planets or twelve houses.[69] Forman's plague tracts followed this format, focusing specifically on the influences of Saturn and Mars. Moreover Forman saw the plague tracts as complements to the astrological tracts. He devoted separate chapters to Saturn and Mars in 'Grounds of arte' and 'Liber juditiorum morborum', and the influences of these planets and the varieties of plague that they caused figured periodically throughout 'Astrologicalle judgmentes'.[70] In 'Liber juditiorum morborum' he described the plague that resulted from the conjunction of Saturn and Mars, and referred to 'A discourse of the plague', concluding, 'Of this plague I have written a whole treatise of itself in Anno 1592 & 1593 the plague being in london, ♄ being in ♋'.[71] In the tenth chapter of 'Astrologicalle judgmentes' he again referred to his writings on the plague, this time in an explanation of how to judge whether a disease was caused by God or nature.[72] If it was natural, then the physician should get on with his job; if it was supernatural, then there was no medicine that could help and the physician should decline treatment. He digressed about disease as divine retribution for unrepented sins, began to give biblical examples, and cut himself short, noting 'but of this I have spoken more at large in a proper tratice that I made of the plague only', presumably meaning 'A discourse of the plague'.[73]

As Forman reused passages from one treatise or set of notes in another he left a slug's trail of information about his astrological studies. His conflicts with the physicians and his thriving medical practice were inscribed in these writings. Some of his ideas became more sophisticated, some more extreme, but he had arrived in London in 1591 with unorthodox ideas about the causes of disease and the authority of physicians and surgeons. They sought answers in flasks of urine where none could be found; he, by the grace of God, knew how to read the stars and to judge the causes of diseases. God had inscribed the past and the future in the motions of the heavens and gave men the knowledge of astrology so that they could appreciate His creation. This was how Forman began to explain the arts of the astrologer-physician and the importance of finding the causes of a disease in 'Grounds of arte'. As in the plague tracts, a disease might have natural, unnatural, or supernatural causes.[74] Natural things occurred in a natural course and order; things that were against nature were done by the devil, such as witchcraft; and supernatural events, such as the acts of God

[69] For details of Forman's astrological manuals, see pp. 61–5 above and Bibliography.

[70] Ashm. 1495, fos. 45–117ᵛ, 183–233ᵛ; 355, pp. 155–6, 161–3, 201–25, 253–76; 363, fos. 20, 21ᵛ, 132, 272, [330ʳ⁻ᵛ].

[71] Ashm. 355, p. 219. Ashm. 1411 is a copy of this. There may be an inconsistency here, as earlier Forman had said that this was the black plague.

[72] Ashm. 363, fos. 272–82. [73] Ashm. 363, fos. 272. [74] Ashm. 1495, fo. 4ᵛ.

recorded in the Bible, might defy these causes. Later in the tract he elaborated on the varieties of causes:

> Yf yt be naturalle yt is by influence of the heavens in his nativity, yf yt be supernaturall yt is the finger of god on a man or on his generations for som offence committed which remaineth on a man and somtimes on his posteritie throughe mani generations to com. And thei ar all sujecte to a certaine dizeas, as to some to die suddenly, som to have the kings eville, som the frenche pox, som the leprosye, and such like and all to die of one dizeas. And thes ar said to have such a dizeas by nature, but yt is supernaturall & naturalle alsoe.[75]

The categories of natural, unnatural (or preternatural), and supernatural were of growing concern for natural philosophers, and a variety of medical practitioners and clerics were increasingly consulted in cases of diseases attributed to demonic possession or witchcraft.[76] Most famously, in 1602 Edward Jorden and other physicians were consulted in the case of Mary Glover. Glover was suffering from hysteria, Elizabeth Jackson was accused of bewitching her, and the case hinged on whether the causes of Glover's illness were natural or demonic; if they were natural then medicine could heal her. A judgement of demonic possession prevailed, Jackson was imprisoned, fined, and pilloried, and Jorden published *A brief discourse of a disease called the suffocation of the mother* (1603), an explanation of the natural causes of hysteria and a discussion of the difficulties in treating it.[77] Jorden and Forman shared a concern for distinguishing between the natural and the preternatural, but Forman's plague tract singularly combined moral, medical, astrological, and preternatural philosophy, all in a vernacular tract on a specific disease.

I have already noted that Forman's concern for the demonic and divine causes of plague resonated with writings on the occult causes of disease. He dwelt on these topics in 'A discourse of the plague', pruned these sections back, then excised them in subsequent revisions. Throughout all of the

[75] Ashm. 1495, fo. 32.

[76] Stuart Clark, 'The Scientific Status of Demonology', in Vickers (ed.), *Occult and Scientific Mentalities*, 351–74; Clark, 'Demons and Disease'; Clark, *Thinking with Demons*, 233–50; Daston and Park, *Wonders and the Order of Nature*, esp. chs. 3, 4; MacDonald, *Mystical Bedlam*, 174; Michael MacDonald, *Witchcraft and Hysteria in Elizabethan London: Edward Jorden and the Mary Glover Case* (1991), p. xxxii; Erik Midelfort, *A History of Madness in Sixteenth-Century Germany* (Stanford, Calif., 1992), 153–7 and *passim*; Webster, *Paracelsus to Newton*.

[77] MacDonald, *Witchcraft and Hysteria*, contains facsimiles of the major tracts prompted by the case and a lengthy introduction. On debates surrounding other cases of witchcraft and possession in Elizabethan England and demonic explanations for diseases of the mind, see Clark, *Thinking with Demons*, chs. 26, 27; Kocher, 'Idea of God in Elizabethan Medicine', 20; James A. Sharpe, *Instruments of Darkness: Witchcraft in England, 1550–1750* (1996), ch. 8 and *passim*; Thomas, *Decline of Magic*, 482–91; D. P. Walker, *Unclean Spirits: Possession and Exorcism in France and England in the Late Sixteenth and Early Seventeenth Centuries* (1981).

versions, though most explicitly in his 1607 draft, Forman combined Galenic and Paracelsian definitions of disease. According to the former, plague was defined in terms of a humoral imbalance within the body; according to the latter, plague could be attributed to specific substances, whether astral or not, invading the body from without and disrupting or blocking the spirits specific to the brain, heart, or liver.[78] This dichotomy provides a useful framework for analysing Forman's rather muddled ideas on plague and should not be taken as representative of categories which he employed. Throughout his plague tracts he correlated the four humours, the effects of Saturn and Mars, and the three sorts of plague that they caused.[79] In his 1607 tract he digressed on the subject of infection, echoing Paracelsian notions. Air was the breath of God, source of blood and life, vitalizer of the soul. If fumes and vapours corrupted the air, it infected the blood, spreading to the heart and brain and disrupting the habitation of the three principal spirits of man and jeopardizing the residence of the soul. For as pure and sweet meats were the natural food of the body, pure air was the natural food of life.[80] Later in the treatise, next to a passage on the infection of the heart, Forman noted 'Paracelsus'; otherwise he was silent about his debt to Paracelsian ideas about the plague despite his intense reading of Paracelsian writings after 1600.[81]

The Bible was the only authority that Forman cited in his 1593 plague tract; in the later versions, as well as shifting the balance to the natural causes of plague and explicitly attacking the physicians, Forman adorned his arguments with references to other authors, probably drawn from a handful of texts. He cited ancient, medieval, and modern experts and he disagreed with all of them on specific points about the nature of plague and the state of the humours.[82] He copied passages directly from 'Grounds of arte', naming many authorities including the great astronomers Ptolemy and Albumazar and great physicians Hippocrates, Galen, and Avicenna in support of astrological medicine.[83] For

78 Clark, 'Demons and Disease', 42–4; Clark, *Thinking with Demons*, 226–7; Hutchison, 'Occult Qualities', 240–1; Pagel, *Paracelsus*, 174–82; Webster, *Great Instauration*, 287. I am not here accounting for the role of the occult in Galenic teachings, on which see for instance, Copenhaver, 'Scholastic Philosophy and Renaissance Magic', 525–30.

79 Ashm. 1436, fos. 90–104. For Forman's discussion of the humours see Ashm. 355, pp. 15–126; 1494, p. 542.

80 Ashm. 1436, fo. 54^{r-v}.

81 Ashm. 1436, fo. 133^{v}. On Forman's reading of Paracelsian texts see Chs. 8 and 9 below. As early as 1591 he had encountered Paracelsus' description of how plague proceeded from the opilation (blockage) of the spirit in English translations of 'De natura rerum' and 'De natura hominis': 'The 7 bookes . . . toching the nature of thinges' and 'Two bockes . . . concerninge the nature of man': Ashm. 1490, fos. 199–220; see Ch. 1 n. 32 above on this text.

82 See for instance references to Valasco de Taranta (fl. 1382–1418), presumably his tract on plague, *Tractus de epidemia et peste*, first printed in Basel in 1464: Ashm. 1403, fos. 44^{v}–45; 1436, fos. 55^{v}, 92, 97, 104.

83 Ashm. 1495, fo. 6^{r-v}; 1436, fos. 135^{v}–8, 144.

the most part Forman used these citations to establish received opinions, then to counter them. In the discussion of the word epidemia, he noted the definitions of the Parisian physician Hollerius (with whom Drouet studied) amongst others, only to conclude,

Thes and all such vain exposisions of Epidimia I let passe, which divers authors have set down according to their own minds and suppositions and accordinge to their owne Invention, not knowing the disease nor nature therof. Wherfore in fewe wordes and plainly, youe shall well understand what we mean by this word Epidemia in this our Booke.[84]

Similarly, under the definition of the word pestilence, Forman quoted the Arabic medical authorities Haly Abbas and Avicenna, and concluded 'But I saie the pestilence or plague of pestilence is an infectiouse disease and infecteth the blode of man by reason of the ayer or smell therof whereof ensueth the botch and the blain and the token'.[85] Again he supported his position with examples from the Bible.

Righteous and alone, in his writings on astrological physic and plague Forman promoted a Paracelsian and astrological philosophy of medicine. A denunciation of other medical practitioners was integral to his project. The prudent physician, Forman argued, judged whether the cause of a disease was natural, unnatural, or supernatural, and the only true way to know this was to read the stars, not to discern it from a patient's urine, pulse, or siege (stool). In 'Grounds of arte' Forman asserted that the physician must first be an astrologer:

For noe man auughte to studdie phisickus excepte he be well sene in astrologie. For yt is impossible to give a juste judgmente of the state of a dizeas only by seeinge the urine or by feeling the puls or sidge, by the sight of ani urine or seinge the sicke, for a man by astrologie wille saye more by a question demaunded for the state of the sicke, for his sicknes and diseas, and totchinge life and death, or cueringe of the party hurte or sicke, then ten phisisions that shall see the urine or speke with ye sicke bodye. For many ar sicke yt knowe not their owne dizeas nor the cause, nor depnes therof. & by astrologie yt is to be knowen and by noe means ells, because ye bodies of men ar subjecte to diseases accordinge to the influence of the heavens, for a superioribus regmitur inferiora. For yf a man marke well all diseas ar either naturalle supernaturalle or againste nature.[86]

More than a decade later, in his *c.*1607 plague tract, Forman concluded that astrology was neglected by his contemporaries: 'For men in thes dais ar ashamed to learne art which their predecessors used, and to be skillfulle in

84 Ashm. 1436, fo. 58^{r-v}; cf. Jacques Houllier, *De morbus internis libri II* (Frankfurt, 1589).

85 Ashm. 1436, fo. 87^{v}.

86 Ashm. 1495, fo. 32.

supernalle causes, but they thinke that the whole scope of physicke and state of the sicke for judgemente of the cause of the diseas of the sicke is tyed to a pispote a pulse or sedge.'[87] If God was the cause of a disease, then the only medicine was repentance. Physicians who disregarded astrology, potentially acted against God, and did as much harm as good.

Forman intertwined ideas about how to practise medicine and define a disease with a promotion of the arts of the astrologer-physician and condemnations of other medical practitioners. He did not articulate a Paracelsian philosophy of medicine, but he did denounce the methods of erudite physicians, positing an eclectic brand of astrological medicine instead. According to Forman, without astrology a physician could not know whether a disease was natural, supernatural, or unnatural, and if it was natural, which influences caused it. Without this knowledge, one could only treat the symptoms, not the causes, of a disease. As Forman noted in his 1607 plague tract: 'It is impossible for any man to be a perfecte phisision or chirurgion, be he never soe great a clarke, without astrology. For he that knoweth not the course and alterations of the stares and planets above can never know the state and alteration of mans body beneath.'[88] He struck at the core of learned medicine, challenging the methods of diagnosis and treatment.[89] Previous generations of physicians, he noted in 'Astrologicalle judgmentes', had not so wilfully neglected the place of astrology in physic:

> when they them selfes do verie well know, that their authors do forbid them to deale or medle in physick without astrologie. For that none can be cured, but by chaunce without the counsel of the starres and knowledge in Astrologia. And he that is Ignorant in astrologie, is so far from the true knowledge of medicin and physick that he is not worthie to be called a phisicion but an Impostor or an Intruder.[90]

Physicians, Forman insisted, were acting against their own traditions.

Forman was insistent about the importance of knowing the causes of a disease in order to cure it. In 'Astrologicalle judgmentes' he wrote that 'except thou knowe the cause of the disease, and take it away, there can be no effecte, it is not so much materiall to knowe the disease as to knowe the cause of the disease';[91] in the 1607 plague tract he concluded, 'And the ground of phisicke is thus. Take away the cause, and the effect will followe. He saith not: take awaie the pain or

87 Ashm. 1436, fo. 135^{r-v}.

88 Ashm. 1436, fo. 141^{v}; on his condemnation of surgeons see also 1436, fo. 142, and 363, fo. 9.

89 Roberts, 'London Apothecaries', 111–12. For Galenism see Nutton, 'Seeds of Disease'; Temkin, *Galenism*.

90 Ashm. 363, fo. 8^{r-v}.

91 Ashm. 363, fo. 132.

diseas but take a waie the cause of the paine or diseas.'[92] In 'Astrologicalle judgmentes' he gave a vivid example.

I take a threed or a string and tye it about my thomb or handwrest verie hard, and thereby my hand and arme doth swell much. I com to a physicion, putting a glove upon my hand that he can not see the string whereith my finger is bound which is the cause of the swelling of my arme. I showe myne arm to the physician. He administred many medicins to me, but all helpes not because he findeth not the cause. But when he seeth the string, he taketh it away, and when it is gone myne arme and hand waxe well of them selves or with verie few medicins.[93]

Forman's hypothetical physician found the thread, but in practice causes were more difficult to discern and physicians looked for the wrong signs. Urine, according to Forman, was deceitful: it varied according to what someone ate, how much he or she exercised and slept, and other factors.[94] The pulse, the siege, the complexion, and other non-astrological means of diagnosing the balance of the humours were equally misleading. Late in his life, in an alchemical commonplace book Forman condemned the practices of physicians outright:

For they wold mak the pisse & excrement of the bodi to be greter then the bodie yt cam from. Contrary to arte and the true principles of phisicke and philosophie. And they thrive therafter for wher they cuer on they hurte 20, and where they helpe on they kill 20. Therfore they ar but emprikes, conicatchers ^mountebanks^ quacksalvers and bobtailles. And when they were not able to attain to the trewe science of phisick, which is Astrologie, yt is so depe and tediouse, for that they were lasy and ydelle and not borne to be phisitions but Intruders. Then they began to write bocks of pisspotes and pulses, seges and other excrements, and so corrupted by tracte of tyme the true science of phisicke, and have filled the wordle with their vain bables and pispot doctrine. By which means they bringe the science of phisicke in question whether yt be a true science or noe. For yf physicke be a science it moste have true and infallible groundes. For yf the grounds of phisicke be false the science cannot stand but moste faill, and yt moste be accounted a cosseninge trade & crafte and no science. Then yf they will make a pispote a sidge a puls or a mans talle the ground of physick as toutching the cause of the discasc, thes ar all ſalse. Ergo their proffession & way of physicke is false like them selvs. And by this meanse phisick is noe science but a cossoning trade to conicatch and deciev men, &c as in my other bock of judgments.[95]

His 'other bock of judgments' probably referred to 'Astrologicalle judgmentes'.

Not only did a physician need astrology to judge the true cause of a disease, he needed it to know at what time a remedy would be effective. Astrologers knew the times of life and of death, of sickness and of health, according to

92 Ashm. 1436, fo. 145. 93 Ashm. 363, fo. 8^{v}. 94 Ashm. 363, fo. 5^{v}; 1495, fo. 3.
95 Ashm. 1491, pp. 1274–5; see also 1457, fos. 53–4^{v}, a fragment defining good medicine.

experience.[96] Timing was essential, and Forman frequently noted this in his writings after 1600. In 'Astrologicalle judgmentes' he wrote,

And for myne own part, I know this and the inhabitants of London and the countrys adjoining can wittnesse the same, and some learned men in this land that have seene the experience therof. That in one hower the course of heaven a man will give a medicin shall cure a diseaze, that missing such a tyme, a man may give a hundered medicins and not cure it.[97]

In his 1607 plague tract Forman was more specific, stating that if someone who had seen many physicians and taken much medicine came to him at the right time, he could heal that person within six days.[98] A practitioner who did not heed the stars 'gives the sicke many medisons and makes his bodie an appoticaries shope, and yf he healpe on sick yt is more by chanch then by any good judgmente'.[99] Often Forman argued that an ill-timed remedy would harm the patient:

so they try experience upon mens bodies, when they neither know the estate of mens bodies, nor the cause of their diseases. And then give them such medicins as worck so extremly, that nature not being able to beare the force therof, or because it worketh on a contrarie cause, that manie tymes through blind ignorance and follie they turne up their heales and bidd men good morrow at midnight.[100]

Forman used a similar argument in the psalm about his troubles with the physicians:

And he that knoweth not the cause
of sicknes doth but mar
what others make, and wold doe good
leud empricks all doe spille

by followinge of leud fansies such
As want righte physicks skill
For as the blind man hits the marke
by chanch and not by skille
Soe doe thes dotinge doctors ofte
Cuer one, and ten doe kille.[101]

Physicians who did not heed the timing of the stars could not know the causes of a disease, and thus ministered blindly. More perished in a year from ignorant physicians than would have perished if they had taken no physic.[102]

96 Ashm. 1436, fo. 135.
97 Ashm. 363, fo. 8.
98 Ashm. 1436, fo. 143.
99 Ashm. 1436, fo. 135.
100 Ashm. 363, fo. 3^{v}.
101 Ashm. 802, fo. 131^{v}.
102 Ashm. 1436, fo. 135.

Forman extended this theme. Physicians who prescribed without consulting the stars and thereby harmed people were acting as instruments of divine retribution. God sent unrepentant sinners to evil physicians. In his *c.*1607 tract he ranted,

> for thy hard harte, for thy uncharitablenes & unmercifulnes, for sinne and dissobedience, he [God] will deliver thee over into the handes of eville phisitions (but not of good phisisions) that they maye make experience on thy bodie, punish thy carkess and make an appoticaries shope in thy belly and consume thy wealth, and bringe thee to beggery and to a miserable estate alsoe of thy bodie.[103]

Physicians were morally reprehensible and in his writings Forman often threatened them with God's wrath. At one point he described the mouth of hell as opened wide ready to swallow them, and lawyers:

> it were no greate matter if the world were well ridde of all such caterpillers of the commonwealth, for the one makes rich men poore, but they never make poore men rich, and the other makes whole men sick, but they never macke sick men whole, the one consumeth a mans felicitie, & the other a mans libertie, and both a mans wealth . . .[104]

In another passage he was more direct: 'Of such fellowes we have to manie in England, butt their names of Doctourshipe doth cover their knaveries when plein experience showeth their ignorance. & yet they thinck they may kill men by authority, but yet I will them to remember this that they must all come to Judgment for it'.[105] And again, 'But remember this all yee ignorant phsicions and unskillfull surgeons, that you must all come to judgement, and give account for everie finger, for everie hand, and for everie arme, legg and member that you have cutt off, or causeth to be lost thorough your ignorance, and for everie one that hath dyed through your follie.'[106] In his *c.*1607 plague tract Forman likewise promised, 'But yf thou have done eville in thy profession to the hurte of many as thou haste, then what saith the judge: goe ye cursed quacksalvers into eternall paine to be punished your selves, as youe have punished many others throughe your negligence and folly. And youe shall not com thence untill youe have paid them the utter moste farthinge.'[107] As far as Forman was concerned, the physicians and surgeons who practised medicine without astrology were dangerous. They might not have been accountable to greater authorities in this world, but they would be in the next. He, in contrast, saw himself as acting according to the will and course of God.

[103] Ashm. 1436, fo. 73. [104] Ashm. 363, fo. 3^{v}. [105] Ashm. 363, fo. 4.
[106] Ashm. 363, fo. 9. [107] Ashm. 1436, fo. 144^{v}.

Avaricious and ignorant impostors, quacksalvers, and sinners. This is what Forman called the physicians. Throughout the 1590s and 1600s Forman fought with them, wrote and rewrote numerous astrological and medical treatises, and conducted thousands, if not tens of thousands of consultations. He fashioned himself as a medical martyr, preserving the true place of astrology in medicine in defiance of those falsely bearing the authority of physicians. His antagonism to the College was integral to his philosophy of medicine. But his thriving medical practice, as documented in the casebooks, threatened the College of Physicians as much, if not more, than his ideas.

III

THE CASEBOOKS

In January 1607, after a three year respite, the Censors of the College of Physicians again summoned Forman. He refused to appear without a public pledge that he would not be detained. By March the Censors had secured witnesses of Forman's malpractice. A Mr Pelham, 'professor of medicine', reported that Forman had used the following methods to gain money: 'Firstly he asks the name and place of habitation of the client: then (as he openly confesses) he makes an effigy [astrological figure]: thirdly just as if he were a prophet he foretells the disease and fate of the patient: finally he prescribes medicaments.' Pelham also reported that Forman had diagnosed one Humphrey Weld as dropsical when he was suffering from arthritis. The Censors also heard from Jacob Saterthayte, who brought further allegations against Forman:

> for when he had come to him [Forman] at his home, he [Forman] first asked him [Saterthayte] his name and then where he was staying: thirdly he fashioned an effigy and gave an opinion regarding the disease. He demanded ten pence from him for one medicament: for another five shillings and for two purgatives four shillings.

On this evidence, the College again summoned Forman, and he again refused to appear.[1]

The testimonies of Saterthayte and Pelham are the only extant accounts of Forman's medical practices by his contemporaries. In contrast, Forman's methods are vividly portrayed in his astrological and medical writings and meticulously recorded in his casebooks. The casebooks are not transparent, however, and the information they contain was inscribed within and refracted through the practical and intellectual processes through which it was recorded. The following chapters outline how to read Forman's casebooks and provide a picture of what exactly happened in his consulting room.

1 Annals, 9 Jan. 1607, p. 191; 30 Mar. 1607, p. 192.

6
How to Read the Casebooks

Before a Square Table, covered with a greene Carpet, on which lay a huge Booke in *Folio*, wide open, full of strange Characters, such as the *Ægyptians* and *Chaldaens* were never guiltie of; not farre from that, a silver Wand, a Surplus, a Watering Pot, with all the superstitious or rather fayned Instruments of his cousening Art. And to put a fairer colour on his black and foule Science, on his head hee had a four-cornered Cap, on his backe a faire Gowne (but made of a strange fashion) in his right hand he held an Astrobale, in his left a Mathematicall Glasse.[1]

This was John Melton's portrait of an astrologer.[2] To find him you followed a gaggle of women down the backstreets of London to his house, and once before him you could ask, for a price, the whereabouts of lost 'money, silver-spoones, rings, gowns, plate, or linnen', how many children you would have, how many husbands, and which would love you best. In exchange for your money you would get many words of little value.[3] Melton criticized the astrologer for professing 'an absolute and exquisite knowledge in philosophy, astronomy, physike, metaphysikes, the mathematikes, and astrology', while he was really a mountebank who deluded his clients, 'creatures so ignorantly obstinate' that they would not hear a word against him.[4] Despite the astrologer's dubious learning and empty results, he attracted a steady and devoted clientele.

The problem of explaining the credibility and popularity of astrologers has endured, and as Forman figures amongst the back-alley practitioners that Melton mentioned, so he has played a role throughout histories of astrology in early modern England. Sometimes he figures as a charlatan, sometimes as a womanizer, and sometimes as a testament to the popularity of astrology.[5] He

[1] Melton, *Astrologaster*, 8. Melton purports to be writing about a Dr P.C. in Moorefields, but also mentions 'Doctor *Fore-man* at *Lambeth*' to conclude the list of 'the cunning Man on the *Bank Side*, Mother *Broughton*, in Chicke-Lane, yong Master *Olive* in *Turnebolestreet*, the shag-hair'd Wizard in *Pepper-Alley*, the Chirurgion with the Bag-pipe Cheeke' (21). For a summary of this work see Allen, *Star-Crossed Renaissance*, 135–9.

[2] On Melton (d. 1640) see *DNB*. [3] Melton, *Astrologaster*, 4–5. [4] Ibid. 5, 7.

[5] Traister, *Forman*, is an exception. See also her 'Medicine and Astrology in Elizabethan England: The Case of Simon Forman', *Transactions and Studies of the College of Physicians of Philadelphia*, 11 (1989), 279–97; Traister (ed.), '"Matrix and the Pain Thereof": A Sixteenth-Century Gynaecological Essay', *Medical History*, 35 (1991), 436–51.

ASTROLOGASTER,

OR,

THE FIGVRE-CASTER.

Rather the Arraignment of Artlesse Astrologers, and Fortune-tellers, that cheat many ignorant people vnder the pretence of foretelling things to *come, of telling things that are past, finding out things that are lost, ex-* pounding Dreames, calculating Deaths and Natiuities, *once againe brought to the Barre.*

By Iohn Melton.

Cicero. *Stultorum plena sunt omnia.*

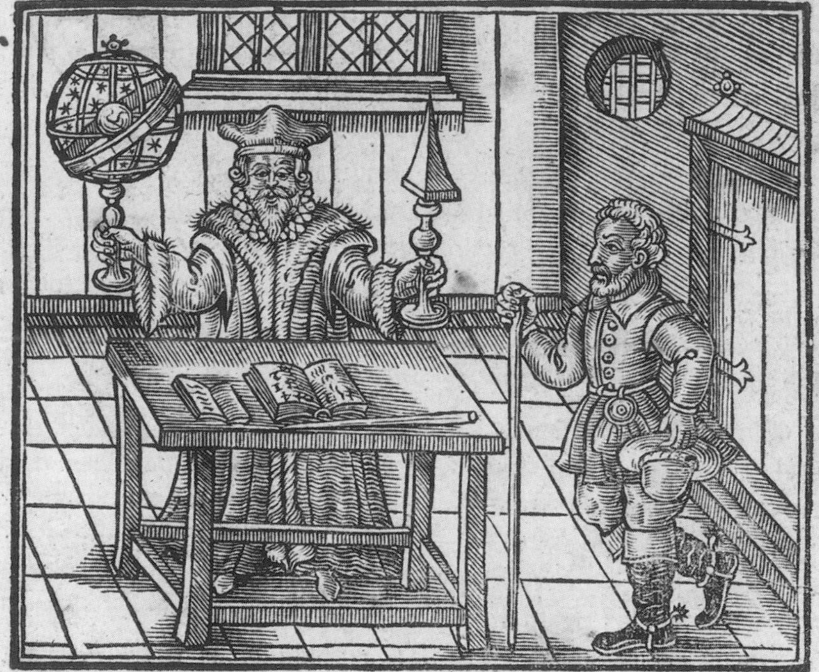

Imprinted at London by *Barnard Alsop*, for *Edward Blackmore*, and are to be sold in *Paules* Churchyard, at the Signe of the

6.1. John Melton, *Astrologaster* (1620), title-page. By permission of the Folger Shakespeare Library, Washington, DC. Shelfmark: STC 17804.

also features in histories of quackery which similarly attempt to explain the appeal of irrational remedies.[6] Some studies chart the popularity and decline of astrology in almanacs and other printed texts.[7] Others explore the solace that the astrologer's social and cosmological framework provided in a world where people experienced much anxiety and little medical efficacy.[8] However much Forman was a living stereotype, his papers, particularly his casebooks, meticulously document the popularity of an astrologer-physician and the dynamic between him and his patients and clients. Casebooks record the droves of people who consulted astrologers, and the astrological fodder for which they paid. The English records are remarkable. Forman, Napier, Lilly, and John Booker (1603–67) each recorded more than a thousand consultations a year. Their querents came from all levels of society and asked questions about lost property, missing persons, maritime adventures, business prospects, legal matters, preferment, politics, love, life expectancy, hidden treasure, the philosophers' stone, and pregnancy, disease, and death.[9] Keith Thomas mines these records to explain the belief in astrology, and he identifies two motives impelling people to consult an astrologer: the need for information which no other agency could provide, and the need for advice. The astrologer's function, Thomas concludes, was psychological: he helped to lessen anxiety. In addition, astrology provided an intellectual framework within which to make sense of personal, social, and political events.[10] People believed in astrology because it made sense and it made them feel better.

While Thomas's evidence is for the most part anecdotal, Michael MacDonald

[6] Porter, *Health for Sale*, 165; Thompson, *Quacks of Old London*, 31. Thompson draws most of his material from Goodall, *Royal College of Physicians*. On quackery see also Gentilcore, *Healers and Healing in Early Modern Italy*; Mark Jenner, 'Quackery and Enthusiasm, or Why Drinking Water Cured the Plague', in Grell and Cunningham (eds.), *Religio Medici*, 313–39.

[7] Allen, *Star-Crossed Renaissance*; Capp, *Astrology and the Popular Press*; Chapman, 'Astrological Medicine'; Patrick Curry, *Prophecy and Power: Astrology in Early Modern England* (Cambridge, 1989); Geneva, *Astrology and the Seventeenth Century Mind*.

[8] MacDonald, *Mystical Bedlam*; Ronald Sawyer, 'Patients, Healers and Disease in the Southeast Midlands, 1597–1634', Ph.D. thesis, University of Wisconsin, 1986; Thomas, *Decline of Magic*.

[9] Thomas, *Decline of Magic*, 362–82. This relies primarily on the manuscripts in the Ashmole collection in the Bodleian. For the numbers of people consulting Napier, see MacDonald, *Mystical Bedlam*, 26. For a survey of English casebooks 1500–1700 see Lauren Kassell, 'Simon Forman's Philosophy of Medicine: Medicine, Astrology and Alchemy in London *c*.1580–1611', D.Phil. thesis, University of Oxford, 1998, appendix 1. See also Beier, *Sufferers and Healers*, 51–96, 120–6; Duden, *Woman Beneath the Skin*; Brian Nance, *Turquet de Mayerne as Baroque Physician: The Art of Medical Portraiture* (Amsterdam, 2001); Sophie Page, 'Richard Trewythian and the Uses of Astrology in Late Medieval England', *Journal of the Warburg and Courtauld Institutes*, 64 (2001), 193–228; Katherine E. Williams, 'Hysteria in Seventeenth-Century Case Records and Unpublished Manuscripts', *History of Psychology*, 1 (1990), 383–401.

[10] Thomas, *Decline of Magic*, 378, 391–3. Cf. John Henry, 'Doctors and Healers: Popular Culture and the Medical Profession', in Stephen Pumfrey, Paolo Rossi, and Maurice Slawinski (eds.), *Science, Culture and Popular Belief in Renaissance Europe* (Manchester, 1991), 191–221.

armed himself with a computer and approached the wealth of data in Richard Napier's thirty-seven years of casebooks statistically.[11] He accounts for any social or ideological variables which would have skewed the group of people who were represented in Napier's casebooks before drawing conclusions about who consulted him and why, considering Napier's personality, prices, and beliefs, and the social variables of sex, age, marital status, and place of residence of Napier's patients.[12] Ultimately these statistics provide the basis for a broader discussion of attitudes to mental illness for which Napier's astrological casebooks are a unique source. Astrology is not the focus of MacDonald's study; he nonetheless stresses that astrological physic provided a holistic framework within which disease could be rationalized and treated.[13] This is particularly the case for the 5 per cent of Napier's cases that MacDonald classifies as mental disorders.

In a study of Napier's medical cases as a whole, Ronald Sawyer foregrounds the role of astrology, arguing that 'the astrological techniques helped doctors conduct a systematic consultation while seeming to place the clinical interview in a fruitful context for the patient by providing the symbolic, interpretive, therapeutic, and social dimensions necessary for the completion of a successful healing act'.[14] MacDonald has cogently argued this case in a further effort to move away from functional explanations of the belief in astrology. The historian's project, MacDonald suggests, is no longer to explain why people believed in astrology, but why its prestige declined as its popularity grew. His subject is an English astrological tradition, beginning with John Dee, through Forman and Napier, all of whom linked astrology and medicine. MacDonald concludes that the difference between the astrologer and other medical practitioners lay in the astrological figure: this was an opportunity for interaction and negotiation between the practitioner and his patient, thereby enhancing a practitioner's abilities to make clinical assessments. Furthermore, astrology added a cosmological and social dimension to the egocentric experiences of disease and healing, and 'At its best, astrological physic was regular medicine with a greater symbolic significance and probably a greater psychological impact.' Astrology was integral to Napier's and other astrologers' success not simply because of its powers as a system of explanation, but because once a diagnosis had been made a series of therapeutic procedures could then follow to correct any discrepancies between the physician's and the patient's understanding of the disease.[15]

[11] Thomas shies away from statistical analysis of questions asked, noting that 'the registers [casebooks] are too erratic to lend themselves to statistical summary', *Decline of Magic*, 364, 379. He does calculate figures for Lilly's and Booker's records, 379 n.

[12] MacDonald, *Mystical Bedlam*, 30.

[13] Ibid. 175, 183, 194.

[14] Sawyer, 'Patients, Healers and Disease', 293; see also Sawyer, '"Strangely Handled in All her Lyms": Witchcraft and Healing in Jacobean England', *Journal of Social History*, 22 (1988–9), 461–85.

[15] MacDonald, 'Career of Astrological Medicine', 13–14, 17.

Table 6.1. *Sex and type of all consultations, March 1596–February 1598*

Type of Consultation	Female	Male	Unrecorded	TOTAL	% female	% male	% unrecorded	% TOTAL	% of medical
Medical: direct[a]	1359	905	0	2265	60.00	39.96	0.00	82.07	89.60
Medical: vicarious[b]	160	48	55	263	60.84	18.25	20.91	9.53	10.40
TOTAL MEDICAL	1519	953	55	2528	60.09	37.70	2.18	91.59	n.a.
TOTAL NON-MEDICAL[c]	134	99	0	233	57.51	42.49	0.00	8.44	n.a.
TOTAL	1653	1052	55	2760	59.89	38.12	1.99	100.00	100.00

[a] Consultations in which a person consults Forman on their own behalf.

[b] Consultations in which a person consults Forman on behalf of someone else, with or without that person's knowledge or consent.

[c] For non-medical cases it is not useful to distinguish between vicarious and direct consultations.

MacDonald and Sawyer maintain Thomas's agenda for explaining the role of astrological medicine in easing the anxiety that vexed life in early modern England, while shifting the emphasis from the psychological to the social and therapeutic role of the astrologer. I have discussed these studies at length because they underpin the methodological groundwork for what follows. Forman taught Napier astrology, and their methods were for the most part similar, though their personalities and social positions were very different. My starting point is not to ask why people believed in astrology, but what information Forman's casebooks document about his clients and his ideas and practices.

Forman's casebooks survive from 17 March 1596 to 29 November 1601 and they record on average 1,200 consultations a year.[16] I have entered information from the first two years into a database, and I will draw on these data throughout the following chapters. Between March 1596 and February 1598 Forman recorded 2,760 consultations (see Table 6.1). Of these 92 per cent were for medical questions and 60 per cent were with women. Even if women consulted Forman more often than men because they suffered more illnesses, they were also more inclined to consult him for non-medical cases, on behalf of other people (vicariously), and in person.[17] It would seem that Forman's casebooks confirm Melton's impression that women favoured astrologers. The makeup of Forman's clientele differed little from those recorded by other medical practitioners. Physicians, astrologers, and surgeons were popular with women.[18] Various reasons for this disparity have been suggested, from a practitioner's sex appeal to the tendency for women to internalize tensions which men expressed, for instance, at riots.[19] As the Casanova of the astrological consulting rooms and the Elizabethan Pepys, Forman has a reputation for seducing his patients and writing about it.[20] Whatever Forman's therapeutic skills or personal

[16] Ashm. 234, 17 Mar. 1596–19 Feb. 1597; 226, 20 Feb. 1597–20 Feb. 1598; 195, 20 Feb. 1598–8 Feb. 1599; 219, 8 Feb. 1599–31 Dec. 1599; 236, 2 Jan. 1600–17 Dec. 1600; 411, 26 Dec. 1600–29 Nov. 1601. Copies of casebooks for 11 May–5 Sept. 1603 are Ashm. 411, fos. 164–79 and these are discussed p. 157 below. One peculiarity is that, while the majority of Forman's MSS seem to have survived, more than half of the volumes of casebooks seem to have gone missing.

[17] Full details of these data are in Lauren Kassell, 'Casting Figures for Disease: The Patients of an Astrological Medical Practitioner in London, 1596–1598', M.Sc. dissertation, University of Oxford, 1994.

[18] For the College of Physicians, the popularity of irregular medical practitioners with women was axiomatic: Margaret Pelling, 'Compromised by Gender: The Role of the Male Medical Practitioner in Early Modern England', in Hilary Marland and Margaret Pelling (eds.), *The Task of Healing: Medicine, Religion and Gender in England and the Netherlands, 1450–1800* (Rotterdam, 1996), 101–33, esp. 112.

[19] See for instance Beier, *Sufferers and Healers*, 217, 241; MacDonald, *Mystical Bedlam*, 39; Steve Rappaport, *Worlds within Worlds: Structures of Life in Sixteenth-Century London* (Cambridge, 1989), 11.

[20] The phrase is from MacDonald, *Mystical Bedlam*, 37. For references to Forman in the literature on women's health, see Patricia Crawford, 'Attitudes to Menstruation in Seventeenth-Century England', *Past and Present*, 91 (1981), 47–73, esp. 54; Anthony Fletcher, *Gender, Sex and Subordination in England 1500–1800* (New Haven, 1995), 63–5; King, *Hippocrates' Woman*, ch. 10; Anne Laurence, 'Women's Psychological Disorders in Seventeenth-Century Britain', in Arina Angerman *et al.* (eds.), *Current Issues in Women's History*

charms, it was not unusual that women consulted him more often than men.[21] While a woman's sex might have made her more prone to illness, gender was not only a factor influencing who consulted Forman in the first place; it was also an integral component in what happened in the consulting room.

The question of why so many people, particularly women, consulted Forman cannot finally be answered, but it is possible to reconstruct what happened between Forman and his patients. Two conclusions will emerge. First, astrology was integral to Forman's procedures. The casebooks embody this: as material objects they were present in the consultation and exposed the astrological component of Forman's expertise. This is not to say that the patient necessarily believed in astrology; indeed, the astrologer had to establish his authority and to negotiate a diagnosis and a therapy. Secondly, astrology was particularly necessary in dealing with women's diseases because women were perceived as duplicitous.[22] The astrologer, unlike other medical practitioners, could discern the often concealed sexual activities and emotional preoccupations of his patients, factors considered essential to a woman's health. Astrology and gender, from Forman's point of view, were inextricably bound together: his astrological skills entailed an ability to win the trust of women.

These conclusions could not be drawn from the casebooks alone. Fortunately, Forman provided a methodological complement to them: again I will draw on his manuals of astrological physic, particularly 'Astrologicalle judgmentes'. For the present purposes this work had two important features. The first was a long introduction that outlined how to hold an astrological consultation and make judgements.[23] The second was a series of stories interjected throughout the text illustrating the necessity of astrology to physic, and portraying Forman's successes. In the introduction, Forman told the reader that there were three questions which the astrologer should ask at the beginning of every consultation. The first question was the sick person's names. If a consultation occurred on behalf of another person, this revealed the sex of that

(1989), 203–19; Hilda Smith, 'Gynecology and Ideology in Seventeenth-Century England', in B. A. Carroll (ed.), *Liberating Women's History: Theoretical and Critical Essays* (Urbana, Ill., 1976), 99–101. Forman recorded fifty-six instances of sexual intercourse ('halek') with fourteen women, some of whom were his patients, between 1582 and 1607, most of these being with his wife in 1607. These records are concentrated in his diary, casebooks, and esp. a 'diary' for 1607, Ashm. 802, 152^{r-v}. In most cases these are astrological notes, kept to document the fate of his relationship with a woman and the moments at which his children might have been conceived.

21 MacDonald, *Mystical Bedlam*, 36–7; Sawyer, 'Patients, Healers and Disease', 469; Thomas, *Decline of Magic*, 365. An exception was the practice of Joseph Binns, a surgeon, who saw more men than women: Beier, *Sufferers and Healers*, 55–6.

22 Fletcher, *Gender, Sex and Subordination*, 73–4.

23 In this discussion I focus on the most extensive version, Ashm. 363, fos. 1–9^{v}. An early version of this introduction appears in Ashm. 1495, fos. 29–32.

person, and in all cases made it possible to locate previous records. The next question was the sick person's age, as close as could be known. This was because diseases were age specific, not because Forman planned to cast a nativity. The third question, in cases where the question was not asked by the sick person directly, was whether or not the person who had brought or asked the question had come at the request and with the consent of the patient.

Forman made it clear that these formulaic interviews were controversial. He defended these questions in the form of a refutation, or mock interview:

> These men and such like I know will sey unto me many tymes behind my back, as well as they have some tymes sayd unto my face. Why should this Phantasticall Fellow demaund such foolish Questions? Is it Materiall to know the Name of the sick, or is there any difference in Names, or is ther any thing to be knowen by once Name? Or in the Age of the Parties? Or is it to any purpose whether the sicke bodie doth send him selfe or no? Cometh not all to one end, or will not the Judgment be all one? To which I answere and say, No Sir, it is not one.

Forman also told of attempts to prove him wrong by changing the name of the patient from John to Joan, or the proverbial replacement of human urine with that of a horse. The astrologer's questions exposed such impostors.[24]

Based on the time that a patient had come to him, or, in the case of written requests, the time when the letter had arrived, Forman would construct an astrological figure. Astrology was by definition a written art. Whether making a prediction, casting a nativity, electing the best time to do something, or, as Forman mostly did, casting horary figures for the moment at which a question was posed, a figure needed to be drawn, and from it calculations made. The figure was a square divided into twelve sections, each representing a section of the celestial orb and called a house. The positions of the signs of the zodiac were located on the edges of the houses, and the five known planets, the moon, and the sun were likewise mapped.[25] Each house represented a set of categories: the first house represented the person who was ill, and was the house of life; the second represented the relationship between the patient and the physician, especially whether the physician would be paid well; the third represented the third party, in cases where the question had been asked on behalf of the sick person; the fourth represented the medicines and the ends of every cure; the fifth represented the four virtues (attractive, digestive, retentive, exclusive) and indicated which had been weakened; the sixth represented the infirmity; the

24 Ashm. 363, fos. 2^v–3.

25 These methods were described in numerous printed astrological handbooks of the 17th cent., in particular Lilly's *Christian astrology.* For other accounts of medical astrology see Dunn, 'Status of Astrology', 112–21; MacDonald, *Mystical Bedlam*, 26; Sawyer, 'Patients, Healers and Disease', 279–87.

seventh represented the sick person; the eighth, similar to the first, was the house of life and death; the ninth was the house of the physician; the tenth was the house of God, and showed whether the disease was supernatural; the eleventh, much like the fourth, represented the nature of the medicine, and how to begin and end a cure; and the twelfth represented whether a disease had natural or unnatural causes, such as witchcraft.[26] Obviously there was some overlap between these categories. Each house also represented a part of the body, a social relationship, and a deviant situation, though the scheme was not rigorous. The thousands of possible positions of the planets correlated to rules for interpreting them, ranging from the general ('party feareth to die and is aferd of death') to the specific ('the partie hath surfeited with muskadell and oysters' or 'the woman was frayted and toke her diseas with fear of som that come to serch her house for starch').[27] For medicine, the first, sixth, and eighth houses (virtues, infirmity, death, respectively) were the most important, and the presence of an evil planet, particularly Saturn and Mars, in them was ominous. In cases where the client would ask subsequent questions, Forman would again cast a figure according to the time of the question, though the initial figure retained a particular significance.[28]

Forman drafted instructions for holding an astrological interview in 1594, the year after he first was called before the College of Physicians. As he did not record how he learnt to cast a figure, so he likewise omitted to record how he established the procedure for his interviews. Little had changed in the way Forman conducted a consultation between this 1594 account and the reports of Pelham and Saterthayte thirteen years later.[29] The extant casebooks, however, do not span the full period that he was an active astrologer-physician, a period in which he repeatedly revised the manuals recording his methods.

Any systematic records that Forman might have kept in the 1580s have not survived, but his records of disputes about payments for his services in his diary throughout this decade partially document his medical practices.[30] Likewise, he used examples in his treatises and notes that date from the early 1580s

26 Ashm. 363. I have deduced these categories from Forman's chapter headings.

27 These are from Forman's judgements on the first house, Ashm. 363, fos. 30^{v}–44^{v}. For fear and disease see David Gentilcore, 'The Fear of Disease and the Disease of Fear', in William Naphy and Penny Roberts (eds.), *Fear in Early Modern Society* (Manchester, 1997), 184–208.

28 Ashm. 1495, fos. 494, 502, 505.

29 In 'The grounds of arte', composed at least a decade earlier, Forman gave slightly different criteria: (1) time; (2) name; (3) in the case of a woman, whether or not she was married; (4) who sent the urine: Ashm. 1495, fos. 29^{v}–30. In the accounts of Pelham and Saterthayte with which this part began, they mentioned only that Forman asked the name and place of habitation.

30 The case that Forman mentions the most frequently is that of Agnis Cole, whom he first treated on 27 Sept. 1584: Ashm. 208, fo. 39^{v}; 1495, fo. 501; 389, fo. 494.

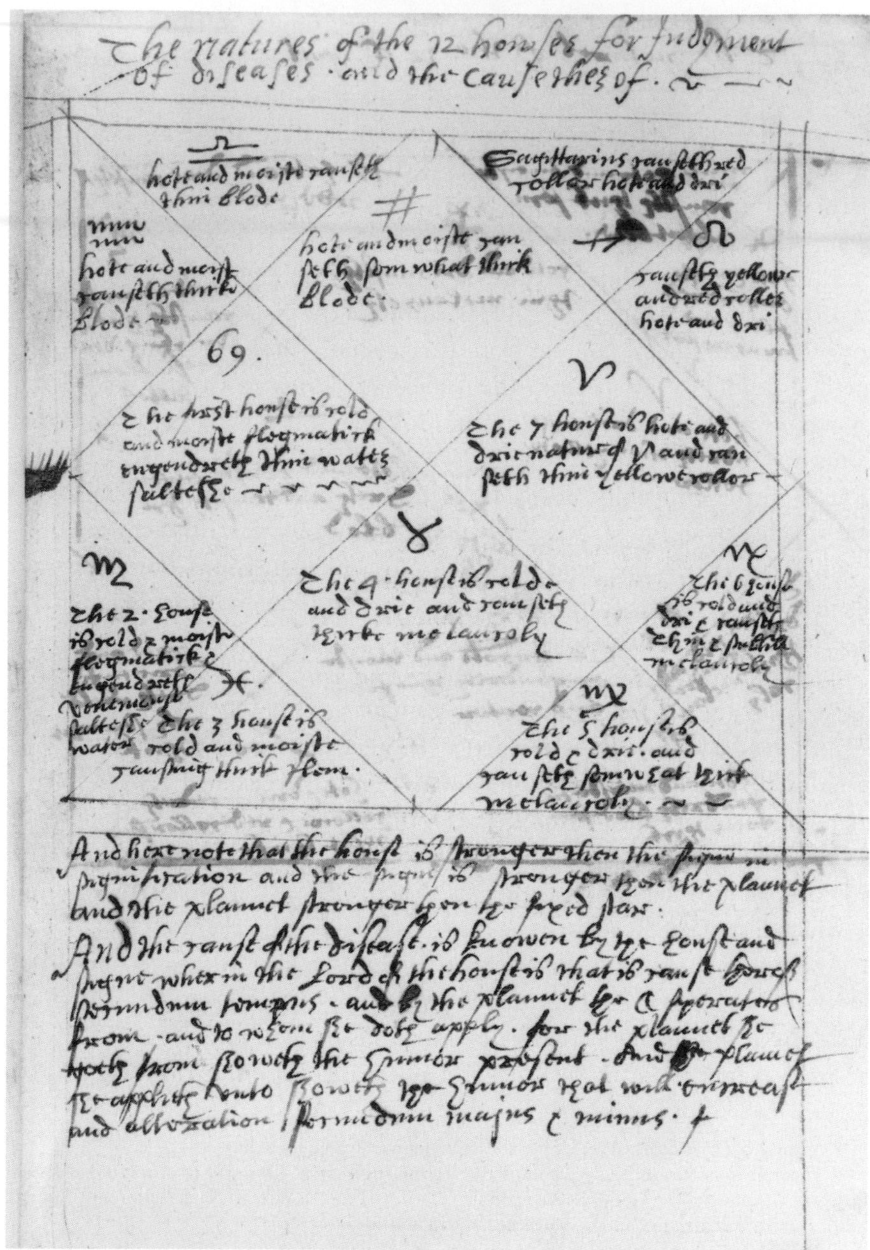

6.2. 'The natures of the 12 howses for judgment of diseases and the cause therof', Ashm. 389, fo. [11]. By permission of the Bodleian Library, University of Oxford.

To knowe in what place of the body every planet doth cause distempratur or diseases & what pt they rule 153

	♃	♂	☉	♀	☿	☽	♄
♈	hart bark	head face	thighs	feete	leggs	knes	stomak
♉	belli mawe	nek throte	knes	heade face	fete	lege	hart bark
♊	reins kidnis	Arms shoulders	Legs	nerk throte	head face	fete	belly mawe
♋	privie parte	stomak	fete	arms should=ers	nerk throte	heade & face. ey.	reins kidnis
♌	thighs	hart & bark	heade & face	stom=ake	Armse & shoulders	necke & throte	genitals & privie parte
♍	knees	belly & mawe	necke & throte	harte bark	stomak	arms shoulders	thighs
♎	Legs	reinse & kidneis	Arms sholders	belly & mawe	harte bark	stomak	knes
♏	feete	privi pte & stones	stomak	reines & kid=neis	belli & mawe	harte & bark	Legs
♐	heade & face	thighs	harte & bark	privie parte & stons.	reins & kidneis	belly & mawe	feete
♑	necke & throte	knes	belly and mawe	thighs	privi pte & stons & vulva	reins & kidneis	heade & face
♒	Arms shoulders	Legs	reins kidneis	knees	thighs	privie parte stones & vulva	nerk throte
♓	stomak	feete	privie parte stons & vulva	lege	knes	thighs	shoulders and Arms.

This table haue I set downe by experience 1603. formen. march 8

6.3. A table 'To knowe in what place of the body every plannet doth cause distempratur or disease & what part they rule'. Ashm. 355, p. 153. By permission of the Bodleian Library, University of Oxford. At the bottom is written, 'This table have I set downe by experience 1603, Forman, march 8'.

through 1607, and recycled them between the drafts of his guide to astrological physic.[31] Forman tended to use recent examples. For example, he wrote 'Grounds of arte' between 1594 and 1595 and most of the examples in it are from 1593–5. Forman's non-medical treatises are also rich with examples, particularly from the 1580s when little is known about him, and less about his medical activities.[32] There are several isolated pages throughout the volumes of Forman's papers which look like pages of casebooks, though they contain consultations at greater intervals. The earliest of these is from 1587, a year in which the only other records of Forman's involvement in medicine are a few examples scattered in his astrological and medical writings. Another example is from 1592, and three are from 1595.[33] Although Forman occasionally recorded that he earned much or little from practising physic in his diary, sometime after 1593 he began to be consulted with increasing frequency. It is quite likely that he kept casebooks from an early date, but little more can be said. It can also be presumed that he continued to keep casebooks, though perhaps in a different form, after 1603.[34] Separate notebooks were dedicated to maritime questions and nativities, and there was probably also a book of prescriptions and payments.[35]

The extant casebooks are now bound as annual volumes running from March through February. Forman kept them as unbound notebooks, filling one every few months and recording incidental notes about gossip and expenses, for instance, on the papers at the beginning and end. Some of these casebooks may have gone missing or been stolen during Forman's various losses of his books and papers. In November 1596, for instance, he cast a figure for a 'book of judgements of physic' to discover whether it was lost or stolen; this was probably a casebook.[36] Some sources described the destruction of the casebooks by Anne Turner or Jean, Forman's widow, during the Overbury affair, which would explain the loss of those after 1603, probably the date when Frances Howard first consulted Forman.[37]

31 Ashm. 1495, 389, 403, 363. They also appear in his notes on women, Ashm. 390, fos. 175–89.

32 See notes on missing and stolen property, Ashm. 205; 208, fos. 181–99; navigational questions, Ashm. 802, fos. 234–75; geomantical questions, Ashm. 354.

33 In chronological order: Ashm. 390, fo. 160; 208, fos. 37–8; 240, fos. 13^{v}, 14^{v}. There are several pages of Forman's notes on consultations bound with Napier's papers, which Forman might have sent to Napier, Ashm. 1488, fos. 23–8. The examples from 1587 are Ashm. 1495, fos. 495, 501; 390, fo. 195^{v}. The same examples are used in Ashm. 403, fo. 177^{v}.

34 Rowse states that Forman's medical practice got smaller as his clientele became more elite. His evidence for this is a notebook which he incorrectly identifies as Forman's 'pocket book' for 1609, Ashm. 338. This notebook is not Forman's, but Richard Napier's, and it records various details of his visit to London, including shopping for books, visiting friends, and casting their nativities, see esp. fos. 77^{v}, 96, 90, 120; Rowse, *Forman*, 246, 251–3.

35 Ashm. 802, fos. 244–75 (maritime); 206, fos. 226–436 (nativities).

36 Ashm. 205, fo. 23.

37 Rowse, *Forman*, 261; White, *Cast of Ravens*, 123.

Forman wrote according to the rules of astrology, spurred by his compulsion for detail. His records were systematic, designed so that he could consult them at a later date. If a patient returned for further consultations, or if he heard news about the outcome of a case, he looked up his earlier notes; often he noted the death of a person, even if it was contrary to his predictions. William Lilly commended him for this empiricism.[38] Forman also used his casebooks to test his system and to exemplify his guides to astrology.[39] He kept these records alongside others, of payments, therapies, his travels, dreams, aspirations, nativities, and more. As well as documenting the mundane details of Forman's astrological practice, they record his penchant for observation; they lack, however, the complex authority of his other notes and writings. Together the casebooks and these other writings allow me to recreate, then to begin to explain, the scene in the astrologer's study which Melton so vividly described.

The casebooks embody the difference between Forman and other physicians, surgeons, apothecaries, and irregular medical practitioners; he kept them because he was an astrologer. A patient could consult Forman at home, or send for him to come to his or her house. If he or she brought her urine, he would disregard it. Instead, he would enact the strange ritual of asking questions and writing the answers in his book. Then he drew a figure, and perhaps consulted several other books. What happened next is less clear because the casebooks become less systematic. Presumably Forman delivered a verdict, his judgement. In some cases this was accepted, medicines prescribed, and the consultation was concluded within a few minutes. In many cases it was not so simple. Forman and the patient would then negotiate the reading of the figure.

Urinoscopy was at the heart of Forman's objections to how humanist physicians diagnosed a disease. He dismissed the inspection of urine as a viable means of assessing the cause of a disease yet he acknowledged that most patients would expect the physician, whether an astrologer or not, to inspect their urine. In 'Grounds of arte' urine was a central feature of the consultation:

The first thinge to be noted is the instante tyme when the question is made or the urine broughte. For somtimes on bringeth a urine to a phisision, and he is not within, and the partie leaveth the urine with som of his servants, or with som frind or neighboure, or at his house put in at a windowe, or other wise wher he shall finde yt, or to be

[38] Lilly, *Life*, 17–18.

[39] Some of Forman's examples date from a period when his casebooks survive, but are not recorded in them. Many of these are for people with whom Forman was particularly friendly, suggesting that for these cases he kept supplementary sets of notes, as, for instance he seems to have done for nativities, maritime questions, and geomantical figures—e.g. the case of William Allen, 22 Mar. 1597, with direction to 'loke 1597 the 16 March pm at 15 p 1 fig per infirmata'. This is an example in 'The grounds of arte' though it is not recorded in the casebooks: Ashm. 1495, fo. 496.

delyvered unto him at his cominge home. Then in such a case he shall take the question when the water is delyvered unto hime, or when ye partie commeth to hime for his answere. But yf youe find the water by chaunch then shall youe take that question of that urine when the partie that brought it coms for his answere.[40]

A flask of urine, Forman argued, indicated nothing about a disease. Rather, it was a token of the patient's will to be healed. Again, in 'Grounds of arte' Forman wrote, 'For the urine, in my opinion, at firste time amonge the old philosophers was dyvised to be broughte to the phisision to knowe the dizeas. Not for that the dizease or life death can be perfectly decerned by a urine, but by bringinge the urine yt is a token from the sicke to knowe his diseas by makinge ye question for the sicke.'[41] Forman omitted his reflections on the token-value of urine from his later astrological manuals, but he returned to the subject in an entry on 'Urina' in an alchemical commonplace book. Urine 'was ordeined at first a monge phisitions to be broughte from the sicke person as a token that he was desirous to have his health, and not that they should loke into the urine to see his desease or the cause therof. For yt is not to be sene in an urin or pisspot.' He continued,

For yt is read in the Actes of the appostells howe many came to Peter, Paulle, Jeames, & Jhon and other of the Appostelles. And they brought with them the handkerchers, aprons, gloves, partlotes of the sicke (what to do) as a token from the sicke that they were willinge to have their health, and to knowe the cause of their sicknes, and whether they should lyve or die. Not that yt was seen in the handkercheifes, partlokes, or aprones of the sicke or any thing ells what they asked, but it was a token from them that they had a will & desier to have their health and that they did belive that through the power & grace which god had given them they could helpe them.

Soe the urine was firste dyvised amonge the docters to be broughte as a token from the sicke to showe that they wold knowe the cause of their diseas, and whether they might have healpe or noe. Not that yt was seen in the urin, but that they through their skill and arte should try them, and tell them and not truste to the urine.[42]

In practice, Forman's definition of urine as a token would have allowed him to fulfil the expectations of his patients without compromising the principles of astrological physic.

Talking to a patient, Forman insisted, was also a false means of assessing a disease. In one of his numerous perorations on the failures of physic without astrology in 'Grounds of arte', he noted,

for a man by astrologie wille saye more by a question demaunded for the state of the sicke, for his sicknes and diseas, and totchinge life and death, or cueringe of the party

[40] Ashm. 1495, fo. 29; see also 1457, fos. 53–4, and p. 119 above.
[41] Ashm. 1495, fos. 31^{v}–2.
[42] Ashm. 1491, p. 1274; e.g. Acts 19: 12.

hurte or sicke, then ten phisisions that shall see the urine or speke with ye sicke bodye. For many ar sicke yt knowe not their owne dizeas nor the cause, nor depnes therof & by astrologie yt is to be knowen and by no means ells.[43]

In the later version of this introduction Forman stated at the outset that if a sick person or his or her representative volunteered a diagnosis, this information should be disregarded; the astrologer should have asked the series of questions at the beginning of a consultation, and these would enable him to determine the causes of the affliction.[44] As Forman stated succinctly late in his life, 'ther is no true way to knowe a mans disease by his water, pulse, sedge or talk, but by arte Astronomicalle'.[45]

In 'Astrologicalle judgmentes' Forman implied that his method of questioning had led to the accusation that he relied on his patients to tell him the states of their bodies. He countered this:

Some again will say we talked with the sick party & he tells us the whole state of his bodie and disease. I graunt that it is good in dangerous diseazes to se the sick and to talcke with him, and to take all the Informations you can, or that he or these that be about him can give you. But what can he or she say unto you. They can say perhaps they have a burning fever, or they vomit much or sowre, or that they have much paine in their head, stomak and back, or that they have the stangerie, gowte or palsey or atche in their bonnes, or the pox, or that they cannot sleepe or eate their meate or such like, but what is all this to the purpose to a man of art. He can cure him never the sooner for all this, because he knoweth not the cause of this distemperature. For the sike although he can tell the physicion his diseaze and paine, yet he can not tell him the cause of his paine, which is the cheefest thing, and the ownly thing which a physicion must and ought to know . . .[46]

Information about the patient was important, but it was not the basis of the diagnosis; rather, it was the basis on which astrological rules were consulted and the stars read. Forman boasted that he could make an accurate diagnosis when he had seen neither the patient nor her urine. The particulars of the situation and the timing of the question were enough. He wrote that God

hath given me the true knowledge thereof that all the world that heard me or sawe me have wondred at my judgments of the diseases of those that have bene sicke, when I have neither seene them nor their urine. And sometymes they have bene 100 myles of[f] and more, yet have I told their diseases and whether they might be remedyed or no, so perfectly that many have said I did it by the divell or by nigromancy, or by some familiar spirit.[47]

43 Ashm. 1495, fo. 32.
44 Ashm. 363, fo. 2.
45 Ashm. 1491, p. 1274, dated *c.*1609.
46 Ashm. 363, fo. 6v; 'cause' is written in red ink.
47 Ashm. 403, fo. 81.

Likewise in the case of one Lady Hawkins, Forman noted that they 'suspected me to be a magician &c. because I told her disease and sawe not her water'.[48] In most cases Forman discerned the cause of a disease in an astrological figure, though occasionally he used other forms of divination. The time at which a question was posed or urine brought or sent was factored into these calculations. These methods were open to imputations of magic and trickery but also enabled Forman to have a minimum amount of contact with his patients, freeing him of the association of talk with women, and of physical operations with the manual craft of surgeons, two associations which might lessen a physician's prestige.[49]

Forman's clients were querents, posers of questions, and these questions carried a particular significance.[50] In 'Grounds of arte' he explained, 'youe shall marke specially his demand for sometimes the partie that cometh saith Sr I am com to you to have your councelle one [on] this urin of on[e] that is sicke and sayeth not I would know his disease, nor whether he will live or die'. Other times they asked what the disease was, whether the party would escape it or not, what was good for the party, could the physician help him, whether a woman was with child, or whether the party had the disease which was suspected or not. The question, like all else, was governed by the heavens:

> somtimes they aske one thinge, somtimes they aske another, for the minds of people are variable and divers even accordinge to the motions of ye heavens and aspects of the plannets and stars. And a man shall have noe power to goe to demaund a question of the state of the sicke, whether they determine neither to ask any thinge totchinge the sicke, but when his mind doth accord with the heavens, and when the hevens doe accord to the end of his entente to showe the juste end therof.[51]

In theory the content of the question was integral to the time at which it was asked.

In the casebooks, Forman did not record specific questions that he was asked, but reduced them into categories.[52] Eight per cent of his cases record no type of question at all, though most of these were probably for disease. Most of the cases recorded 'diz', an abbreviation for disease. Occasionally Forman recorded more specific questions, 'mend or pair' (worsen) or 'live or die'; in addition, 5 per cent of the women who consulted Forman asked if they were

48 Ashm. 1495, fo. 486 (28 Mar. 1595); 208, fo. 53ᵛ. This was probably Margaret, second wife of Sir John Hawkins (1532–95), *DNB.*

49 Pelling, 'Compromised by Gender', 107, 111.

50 Forman habitually used the word 'party' in the casebooks.

51 Ashm. 1495, fo. 31ᵛ.

52 Napier seems also to have done this, cf. MacDonald, *Mystical Bedlam*; Sawyer, 'Patients, Healers and Disease'.

pregnant, which he designated with various abbreviated forms of 'utrum mulier sit gravida'. He also noted whether a person was having a second or third consultation, for those who chose to ask a series of three questions, usually at weekly intervals. This was important because the position of the stars at the first consultation remained of utmost importance.[53] Although Forman's categories might have effaced his querents' words, they nonetheless represent an element of diversity. They also make it clear that a question was asked, and an answer was expected.[54]

The casebooks, however, are less illuminating about Forman's answers. Most of the entries (more than 90 per cent) contain secondary information: some combination of symptoms, causes, personal histories, and prescriptions. The records of symptoms were formulaic and included various internal pains, vomiting or nausea, swimming in the head, or fevers, and it is unclear whether these were articulated by the patient or whether Forman deduced them from the positions of the stars, or, as is most likely, from some combination of the two. Cases linked only by chronological succession suggest the extent to which Forman read the disease from the position of the stars. Figures were cast to the minute, but the planets did not move across the houses so quickly. For instance, on 4 May 1596 a 40-year-old woman asked Forman about disease and he recorded 'her water sprinkells she hath not her course'. Three hours later a 25-year-old woman again asked about disease. The entry began 'she is trobled with the toth ach much and arising in her stomake redy to vomit'. Two hours later a 30-year-old woman sent a question, or perhaps urine, and the entry began 'she is moch trobled with the toth ach her urine sprinkells moch'.[55] These were the only cases mentioning toothache in the second quarter of 1596, perhaps a coincidence, but probably the result of the positions of Saturn and Venus. These examples illustrate the necessity for caution in assuming that Forman's patients articulated the symptoms that he listed.

There is further evidence that Forman charted the stars and then mapped the disease onto the patient's body. On 6 May 1596 at 7 a.m. Forman recorded the following about a 17-year-old man: 'moch pain stom[ach] ready to vomit pa[i]nd head & harte & in the throte or neck of ♃ in ♈ ☾ sg a ♄ ap ☉ [Jupiter in Aries moon significator aspecting Saturn applying to the sun] pox or measles it seams'. Ten minutes later, without casting a figure, he recorded the following about a 21-year-old woman: 'much paind stom lik to vomit pand neck & head

53 Ashm. 1495, fos. 494, 502.

54 On patient–practitioner expectations and contracts see Pelling, *Medical Conflicts*, chs. 7, 8; Pomata, *Contracting a Cure*. Occasionally Forman recorded a contract in the casebooks, e.g. Ashm. 219, fo. 133ᵛ.

55 Ashm. 234, fos. 28ᵛ–29 (Keelle, Morley, Cooke).

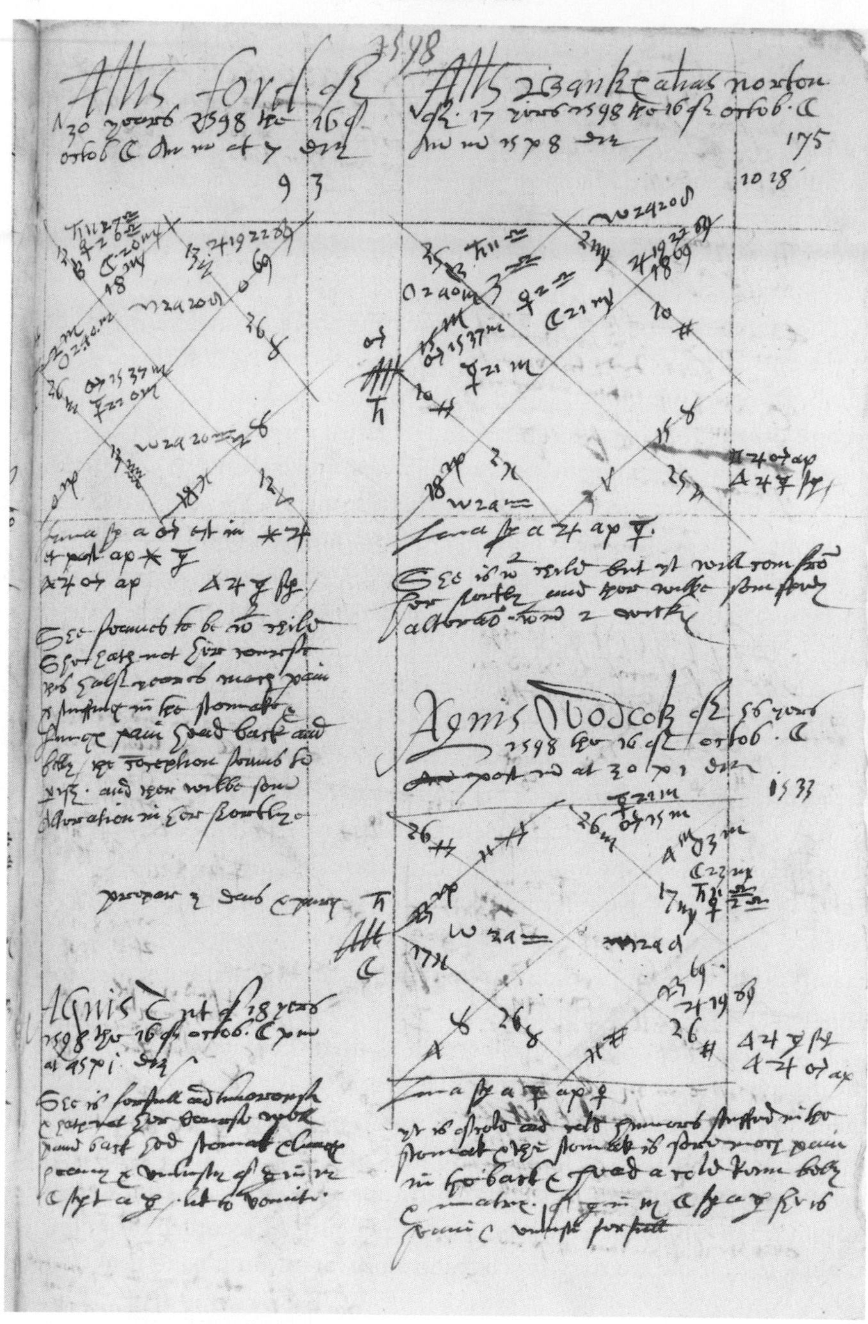

6.4. Entries in Simon Forman's casebooks for 16 October 1598, Ashm. 195, fo. 175. By permission of the Bodleian Library, University of Oxford.

she hath not her course paind harte fed & lims of ♃ in ♈ ☾ sg a ♄ ap ☉ [Jupiter in Aries moon significator aspecting Saturn applying to the sun] thought & grife & yt breds the pox or measell often this humor'.[56] In both cases the astrological notations were the same. The same causes of disease, however, did not necessarily mean that the symptoms were identical. On the morning of 14 May Forman recorded that a 50-year-old man, a 30-year-old woman, and a 15-year-old girl all had taken 'grief & cold'.[57] In each case this had resulted in a stoppage, the man's in his kidneys, and the woman's and the girl's in their wombs.

At the end of some of the entries Forman recorded information which either contradicted or corroborated the previous symptoms. In one case he recorded that a man had much pain in his side, stomach, and head, made a note to prepare, purge, and bleed him, attributed the cause to choler and phlegm in the belly, and then added that he suffered from diarrhoea, vomiting, and wind.[58] If indeed the descriptions of the diarrhoea, vomiting, and wind were the man's, then Forman had calculated the cause of the disease and decided a course of therapy before being told these symptoms; or perhaps he recorded them for good measure. In the case of a young woman Forman recorded 'yt is in her matrix impostume of grosse blod & collor stom belly hed reins [kidneys]', then added 'her right leg is swollen & hath an yssue menstruall'.[59] In a more complicated case in which a woman asked Forman if she was pregnant, he had trouble making a judgement. He recorded that she had a fever, was fretful, nauseous, did not menstruate, and had pain in her heart and kidneys. He predicted that she would have the green sickness and concluded that she was not pregnant, then added, 'but yet by the judgment of this figure she seems to be with child'. An uncertainty had prompted him to re-examine the astrological figure: 'this wentch was well ynough but she was supposed to be with child, she was very big'.[60] In all of these cases Forman's judgements were tempered with information that the patient volunteered or Forman elicited or observed.

Because of the ambiguity of the secondary information in the casebooks, aside from the prescriptions, it is difficult to quantify. A fuller picture of what happened in his consulting room can be recovered from individual cases, particularly those where a patient returned for frequent consultations. Forman's regular clients, however, were atypical. They consulted him more frequently

56 Ashm. 234, fo. 30ᵛ (Woods, Harrice).

57 Ashm. 234, fo. 37ʳ⁻ᵛ (Skinner, Barnard, Hillar).

58 Ashm. 234, fo. 14 (Dai, 10 Apr. 1596).

59 Ashm. 234, fo. 16ᵛ (Newman, 15 Apr. 1596).

60 Ashm. 234, fo. 34 (Painter, 11 May 1596).

Table 6.2. *Frequency of consultations, March 1596–February 1598*

Number of consultations	Cumulative	%	Non-cumulative	%
1	2183	77.27	1855	84.97
2	328	11.61	195	8.93
3	133	4.71	62	2.84
4	71	2.51	25	1.15
5	46	1.63	17	0.78
6	29	1.03	17	0.78
7	12	0.42	4	0.18
8	8	0.28	4	0.18
9	4	0.14	1	0.05
10	3	0.11	0	0.00
11	3	0.11	1	0.05
12	2	0.07	1	0.05
13	1	0.04	0	0.00
14	1	0.04	0	0.00
15	1	0.04	1	0.05
TOTAL	2825	100	2183	100.00

The column headed 'cumulative' counts the total numbers of consultations (e.g. a person who asked a second question also asked a first); the 'non-cumulative' figures count individuals according to the number of questions asked (e.g. only one person had nine consultations).

than the majority of his patients, and could afford to do so.[61] Accordingly the variables of friendship and wealth must be kept in mind. In 1596 and 1597, 15 per cent of Forman's patients returned to him at least once; in other words, of the 2,183 people who consulted Forman over these two years, he saw 311 of them twice or more and 133 at least three times (see Table 6.2). Most of the return consultations were within the same quarter. Forman's most regular client was Hugh Broughton, the scholar and divine with a passion for prophecy and chronology, who was worried about his career and posed fifteen questions within eighteen months.[62] Unlike Broughton, most of Forman's regular querents asked medical as well as non-medical questions. The cases of two women, one who consulted Forman eight times, the other seven, are particularly elaborate and instructive.

The first is Brigit Allen, who consulted Forman five times in May 1596. On the first consultation, when Forman was called to a Mrs Roberts's house, he

[61] Forman only occasionally recorded a sum owed or paid in the casebooks. Between Mar. and May 1596 he records four sums received (Snewinge, 24 Mar.; Merriat, 10 May; Midnole, 13 May; Lydyard, 20 May 1596).

[62] Rowse, *Forman*, 145–50; *DNB*. Broughton consulted Forman on the following dates: 27 July, 25 Sept., 22 Oct. 1596; 18 Feb., 6, 18 (twice), 22 Mar., 8, 10, 12, 13, 19, 21, 24 Apr. 1597.

concluded that Allen was suffering from a false conception, or pregnancy. He noted, 'But yf thou means to cure her cut her off for 6 days for she is unfortunate to herself and is the cause and augmenter of her own sickness by taking of many unprofitable and mighti medisons which have done more harm than good & she harkneth too much to the councel of som unlucky person'. The entry concluded with details about her husband's infidelities. For the next three entries Forman's notes were sparse. On her fifth visit, she asked whether she would get better or not, 'mend or peir', and Forman recorded a lengthy judgement. The stars 'showeth she will run into ill her self for she will not be ruled to doe as she is bid but will forsake thee [i.e. Forman] shortly and goe and seke to som other body or fellowe som others councell, & she will urge thee moch & stand in her owne light, & wilbe ruled but for a season'. This was confirmed by the presence of Saturn in the fifth, sixth, and seventh houses, then Forman continued,

> her diz is by constellation of the heavans & naturall & hath bin long on her, and she will have a sore fit of sicknes very shortly and the moste pain is in the back head & matrix & syd [side] stom[ach].
>
> The rententive vertue is to strong by too moch naturall melancholy in the head belly matrix and she is to cold and dry . . .
>
> The remedi must be heate & moisture . . .

Her disease could be treated because it was natural, but she would become a difficult patient, and Forman would later add a note about 'unnatural melancholy' as a partial cause of her disease. The next month she consulted Forman again, having consumed too much sturgeon and Rhenish wine, and asked whether she was pregnant. Forman and Allen became friends and Forman recorded information that she conveyed outside of consultations. For instance, he noted that he had dined with her and promised her that she would soon be with child, then her husband returned home and 'colted' her.[63]

Margaret Altam, aged 28, contrasted with Brigit Allen in the severity of her condition, and the distance she maintained between herself and Forman. Forman kept particularly detailed records of her consultations with him, perhaps because she seems not to have been consulting him in person, perhaps because she was the daughter of Oliver Skinner, an alderman.[64] During this period she was in Forman's top twelve querents, between September 1596 and April 1597 consulting him seven times. In the first entry the secondary information is a

[63] Ashm. 234 (5, 6, 11, 18, 25 May; 12 June; 7, 15, 16, 19 July; 4 Aug. 1596); 226 (14, 28, Apr. 1598).

[64] Altam, or Altham, was the first wife of Sir James Altham (d. 1617), and they produced one child, Sir James Altham of Oxhey, *DNB*.

combination of Forman's inferences and the woman's complaints, beginning with the judgement that 'she is full of melancoly and the vains of her body be stoped', then listing her symptoms (her stomach hurts when she eats, and she is dry and drinks much; pained head, stomach, reins (kidneys) and matrix (womb)). Ultimately, Forman concluded from the stars that the cause was a change in the state of her body during the birth of her last child. Almost a month later, in October, she consulted Forman again. This time he received more information from her: 'She hath not bin well since her laste child which was 3 yers agoe'. The entry concluded with four phrases which might at first seem to be records of the woman's complaints, but were probably Forman's readings of the stars: 'she hath not her course corantly'; 'she is weke and hath byn long sick'; 'yt will cost her moch money before she be well'; 'she is somtims bettar and somtims worse'.

Almost two months later, in December, Altam again consulted Forman and he noted, 'at this tyme I was first with her', probably indicating that the first two consultations had been conducted by messenger: in them he did not note whether she had sent or come in person, though he did record her address in the second. Altam's third consultation commenced a set of three, weekly appointments. On the first of these, Forman explicitly recorded what she told him: 'This woman hath bin long sick & weke and she hath taken phisick that hath done her moch harm & mad her worse then she was as she saith herself'. Along with judgements of the causes of the disease ('she is moch stuffed with a tough kind of flem & hard of melancoly & red collor redy to stop her wind'), the entry included precise symptoms ('the flem cleaveth to her tongue and rofe of her mouth and is very sower & clammy and she can not speake mani tymes for it'; her meat came up and she passed water when she strained to bring up the phlegm). Forman then recorded a course of therapy in order to 'digest red coller & melancoly & purg yt, then bring downe her course & stop the consumption'. He also analysed the figure for additional information. On the previous occasion he judged that it would cost her much money before she would be well, but this time he concluded that her disease was 'hard or not at all to be cured, but will bring deth in thend'. Finally, he noted, 'she will leave me and take som worse phisisione'.

The next consultation, the second of the set of three, was again conducted by messenger: 'her self sent yt', meaning urine or a letter. This entry is brief. Her condition was the same, and Forman judged: 'yt seames ther wilbe som alteration in her shortly within 7 daies & she will die'. Ten days later she consulted him again. This time her questions conformed to one of Forman's standard formulas: what was the state of her disease, and would she get better or worse. Again, Forman's notes are brief. He recorded her present state, according to the stars, predicted that this would alter in four days, and concluded that she would die. Nine days later she seems to have consulted Forman via another woman, Susan Conyears. This time there were three components to the question: first, whether she should have any more physic; secondly, the state of her disease; and thirdly, whether she would live or die, a question which she had not posed herself before. Forman simply noted that the disease was strong of melancholy, and that there would be some alteration shortly. At the bottom of the entry Forman noted her death, nine months later. Altam's mother had consulted Forman on her daughter's behalf at the end of February, and his brief notes were not optimistic. Altam herself consulted Forman a last time at the end of April, though he did not record in what form or what she asked. He predicted that she would worsen, and would 'stand 5 wieks or 5 months at moste'. This time he was correct.[65]

Forman assessed the gravity of Altam's case, and when he judged an imminent decline, he did little or nothing to amend her condition. As with Brigit Allen, he seems to have prescribed her some physic, though the casebooks are unclear about this. He criticized Altam for having taken too much medicine before consulting him. He also seems only to have met her once, though he was probably familiar with her friend, Susan Conyears, and her parents were regular querents.[66] They both asked questions about their servants and Oliver Skinner occasionally consulted Forman about his own health.[67] In addition, five of the male servants in the Skinners' household consulted Forman in 1597.[68]

The casebooks were not meant to record the voices of Forman's querents. Most of his notes and treatises had an implied audience; the casebooks did not. They were for the use of Forman, and perhaps the young men such as Steven Mitchel, John Braddege, John Goodage, and Josuah Walworth who assisted his astrological and other pursuits, though Forman usually effaced them from his activities.[69] The casebooks were a product of the scribal component of the astrologer's art and Forman's thorough collection of information; as Lilly

[65] Ashm. 234 (10 Sept., 5 Oct., 1, 8, 18, 27 Dec. 1596); 226 (25 Feb., 30 Apr. 1597). Forman included Altam in a list of persons for whom he had correctly predicted death: Ashm. 219, fo. 134^{v}.

[66] Susan Conyears might have been related to Mrs Katherine Conyears, an older woman who consulted Forman six times within this period, and who, incidentally, also died in Nov. 1598: Ashm. 226 (28 Nov. 1597).

[67] Joan Waters, Ashm. 234 (18 Jan. 1597); Oliver Skinner, 234 (14 May 1596); 226 (23, 26 Feb. 1597).

[68] Ashm 226: Thomas Sharpe, (24 Dec. 1597), William Streate (24 Dec. 1597), Robert Steavens (29 Jan. 1597). Thomas Colman and an unnamed boy were also noted by Forman as having been part of the Skinner household.

[69] There are traces of Forman's assistants in the casebooks, such as the occasional entry in a different hand. See for instance Ashm. 219, fos. 213, 214, 216^{v}, 217, 224–6^{v}.

noted, Forman took 'indefatigable pains' in his judgements.[70] Forman studied his records to verify his astrological rules, and extracted cases to exemplify these in his guides to astrology. He also used them to ensure that he prescribed an appropriate course of therapy, if he prescribed one at all. This depended on the stars.[71] In the casebooks he documented the details of a case, headed with the name of the querent or patient, and he returned to these notes if he was consulted again. These records enabled Forman to provide continuity and consistency in his therapies, and he explained their significance in 'Astrologicalle judgmentes':

> some of them will take physic and some will take none. Sometymes again, the tyme doth not serve to give physick, for having their names on my booke, I can allways tell thereby what theyr diseases be, and what counsel I have given them. For suppose theire comes to me this day 3, 4, 5 or 6, 10 or 20, and to morrow as many more, & the next day as manie more, some of them will take physic and some will take none. Some tymes again, the tyme doth not serve to give physick, and sometymes men, or ye parties have no tyme to tacke it because of necessarie businesse and they com again 2, 3, or 4 dayes a weeke after. If I had not their names, and disease on my booke, how could I tell what thier diseases were, or what to doe unto them, or what to give them, but so soone as they tell me again their names I find it one my boack. There do I see the cause of their diseaze, and how they are troubled & what I must doe unto them. Els should I forget as many doe, and so give them chalek for cheese, and so perhaps give them that which will doe them more harme then good . . .[72]

Forman used astrology to determine what was wrong with the patient and whether or not to prescribe a course of therapy. He then had to persuade the patient of the validity of his decisions. Those who had come to him did not necessarily accept astrology, nor respect Forman's authority. His skill, he asserted, was in making correct judgements, and thereby winning the confidence of the patient. In order for him to heal, he had to be trusted.[73] He and his patients negotiated their different expectations and ideas about a diagnosis and the appropriate course of therapy, where necessary arranging an appropriate and convenient moment for administering medicines. These exchanges were not recorded in the casebooks, yet they are fundamental to understanding them.

The dynamic between the patient and the practitioner was integral to the treatment and accordingly the themes of the relationship between the physician and the patient, and whether the physician could do the patient any good, ran throughout Forman's astrological manuals. In theory Forman was especially concerned that the physician should not meddle with supernatural

70 Lilly, *Life*, 17. 71 Ashm. 1495, fo. 32; 363, fos. 159–63^{v}, 170^{v}–1. 72 Ashm. 363, fo. 3^{r-v}.

73 For the subject of trust in 16th-cent. Latin medical literature see Winfried Schleiner, *Medical Ethics in the Renaissance* (Washington, DC, 1995), 6–7, 25.

diseases and he illustrated this principle in the seventh chapter of 'Astrologicalle judgmentes', in a section on how to know whether the physician would profit the sick or not. In some cases it was not a propitious moment to cure the disease, and Forman told the patient to go away for a season or a year. In one case he refused to conduct a consultation with a woman for three years. She was housebound and sent for him frequently. He always refused to see her, telling her messenger that the stars were inauspicious; he judged that the finger of God was on her and 'that her punishment was supernaturall. I meane that god did punish her with that grievious disease for some affence she had done, for she was 9 yeares in this disease. And she had spent much mony on the phisitions and surgeons in that time, and could find neither ease nor remedie.' Despite her persistence, Forman refused to consider her case. Then one day he was having breakfast at the house of one of her neighbours when the persistent woman was carried in in a chair and placed so as to block the door. Forman could not escape and had to speak to her. She wept bitterly and said,

> Oh Lord! What have I done against thee that thou hast punished me so, and [am] I accused above other women that thou wilt not suffer this man to deale with me. And in all this not to come unto me, and now Lord that I am brought here unto him that he will not speake unto me.

Forman and the other breakfast guests were so moved that he promised to cure her, God willing, and within nineteen weeks she had recovered fully.[74]

In practice, Forman was not always so strict, and he, though reconciled to an inability to alter a divine affliction, might have given the patient some ease. For instance, in December 1597 he recorded the following: 'The sickness coms from god. And yt is entailed the seed of the partie & the ofspring shall have the same diz & ther is noe way but prayer unto god & repentance first. That the finger of god may be taken from her, or ells no medison will prevaille.' This was what he was reading in the stars. His notes continued, 'The diz hath been coming and going on the partie from year to year and will soe continue and ther is no perfect remedy for yt but ease may be found & remedy for a tyme but not for ever'.[75] Similarly, although Forman differentiated between the work of God and the devil, in practice discovering the cause of a disease could be difficult. If a disease deemed natural or unnatural did not respond to the appropriate therapies, then the causes had probably been misidentified, such as the case of Nicholas Chapman whom Forman initially diagnosed as suffering from a natural disease, but later determined to be afflicted by witchcraft.[76]

74 Ashm. 363, fos. 187–8. This was in 1579, probably in Salisbury.

75 Ashm. 226, fo. 271. This case is recorded on a separate piece of paper inserted into the casebooks.

76 Ashm. 195, fos. 210, 218.

The devil worked through nature to cause unnatural diseases, such as madness, and if the astrologer discerned the workings of the devil, he could attempt a cure. For instance, Forman recorded elaborate details of a case of melancholy.

> I knewe a woman named Susan ~~Crosbe~~ dwelling at westmester that was in this desperate melancoly dizease. And the dyvell wold speake often tymes within her, and byd her kill her selfe—drowne or hang herselfe—or kill her husband. And she could abid no knives nor pins nor sheres nor needles nor nailles, but she moste cut herself or thruste the pins into her fleshe. This woman was twise hanged, and yet cut downe still and saved. Once she was drowned & taken up before she was thorowe ded and hanged up by the heells, and broughte to lyfe again. And the dyvell did usually speak to her and her husband. And many tymes she wold praye very devoutly, as yt seemed.

Forman then noted the astrological configurations under which this woman had been born, explained how their motions had caused her disease, and described the course that it ran: 'And she remained in this disease 3 years & better and all the phisick in the wordle could not helpe her for she was thorowly purged often tyms & dieted & let blod but all wold not healpe.'[77] He similarly failed to help Elizabeth Brandan, whose fervent Bible reading prompted greater and greater doubts in God, but he helped a young woman who had visions of a man imploring her to kill herself and, with a strong purge, enabled Susan Cuckston to handle pins and knives without inflicting self-harm.[78]

The authority with which the astrologer determined whether a disease was supernatural, unnatural, or natural was the same authority that governed his other decisions. If a patient did not respect this authority, as in the case of Brigit Allen, Forman described her or him as unwilling to be ruled, a disposition that needed to be overcome before a treatment could be effected. Likewise in 'Grounds of arte' he explained that at certain times 'the verie presence of the physician aswel as the medison shall be verie comfortable to the sick and the sick shall rejoice in and have in great regard the phisisione and he shall doe the sicke more good'.[79] In the case of an apothecary's wife, Forman noted that 'he lyked well of my reasons and counsell & she was very desirous of my counsel & to follow yt', then he added in the margin, 'but yet I never gave her anything'.[80] In another case he recorded, 'She seamed to be self willed and not moch to regard me, but I gested it out with her. She folowed my councelle and in thend recovered her health'.[81] In some cases, Forman's mere presence provided ease. When he arrived to see Mrs Snelling, who had been constipated for nearly a

77 Ashm. 355, p. 129; cf. Forman's discussion of melancholy in 'Grounds of arte', Ashm. 1495, fos. 45–98^{v}.

78 Ashm. 355, pp. 127–30.

79 Ashm. 1495, fo. 477^{v}.

80 Ashm. 1495, fo. 486 (Tyke or Kyte, 12 Jan. 1596).

81 Ashm. 1495, fo. 486 (Mary Boies, 6 Jan. 1596).

week, 'as I toke her by the hand she rejoysed soe much of my comming to her that she presently went to stolle'.[82] About another woman Forman noted, 'she was ruled and I had all things to my owne mind'.[83] Another woman 'quickly was cured and thought well the physition and would not let him depart from her'.[84] Obviously, if the practitioner had a good rapport with a patient or her family, it did his reputation no harm. In one case Forman noted that he cured a man, and he 'caused me many patients and reported well of me'.[85]

In most cases, however, the physician's presence was not enough, nor was his authority necessarily respected. Forman noted three reasons why people did not want to take physic. The first was that they were too busy. The second was that it was against their complexion and did not agree with their nature. The third was that, although physic was neither good nor bad in itself, it was abused by physicians, and this caused people to fear it:

> they see that many physicians for want of art & knowledge have dealt so evill with them or their friends in former tymes making their bodies Apothecaries shops, & consume their substance and wealth, and use so much Physick unto them, that they bring them from better to worse. And where before they were a little out of quyet, they macke them sik. And where they be a little sicke, they retinewe [retain] them so, till in the end they dye, so that more in a yeare often perish through the follie of ignorant phisicions (for want of art and knowledge, to know the cause of the disease) then other wise.[86]

Later Forman noted,

> Alas how simple are physicians them that will take on them to minister any medicin to owne [one] that is sick. For to cure him of his disease, when he knowes not the cause therof, but giveth his medicins at all adventures, and perhaps gives him that which is cleane contrarie to his diseaze, and so mackes him worse than he was . . .[87]

The abuse of physic damaged the credibility of all medical practitioners, making many people fear it. Such abuse also made Forman's job difficult. If a patient did not accept the physician's judgement, a cure could not be effected. It was not enough for a patient to tell a practitioner what was wrong, and then to accept or to refuse the prescribed medicines. Based on when he was asked a question, the astrologer discerned the cause of the disease. As the stars revealed the disease, so they governed its cure and if a course of physic was required, it had to be administered at an appropriate time. If the time was not propitious

82 Ashm. 1495, fo. 486^{v} (29 Mar. 1596). See also Ashm. 234, fo. 8 for the casebook entry.

83 Ashm. 1495, fo. 500^{v} (Madeline Joice, 25 Mar. 1593).

84 Ashm. 1495, fo. 503 (Adrian Pain, 11 May 1593).

85 Ashm. 1495, fo. 486^{v} (Mr Watkins, 9 Feb. 1596).

86 Ashm. 363, fo. 5.

87 Ashm. 363, fo. 6^{v}.

for curing a disease, as when the cause was supernatural, the physician should decline to treat the patient until a season or a year has passed. In his experience, Forman noted, many did return, though having consulted other medical practitioners in vain during the interval.

Remedies were central to how medical practitioners defined themselves. Officially, surgeons ministered to the surface of the body, set broken bones, and might specialize in procedures to mend hernias or remove stones; physicians advised on a regimen to preserve health and prescribed therapies to maintain and restore the balance of humours, whether through diet, blood-letting, or prescribed purgatives, emetics, or cordials; apothecaries filled the prescriptions written by physicians, while barbers-surgeons performed the requisite phlebotomy.[88] These boundaries were more virtual than real. In addition to Forman, a range of medical practitioners in Elizabethan London challenged the ideas and practices defined in this hierarchy. They wrote books about a new medicine, often including alchemical remedies and occasionally Paracelsian ideas about the unity of physic and surgery and other matters. The College of Physicians objected to those without the necessary credentials practising physic, and many irregular practitioners defied their authority and prescribed and provided herbal and chemical remedies.[89] Particularly during outbreaks of plague, London was portrayed as teeming with empirics who posted bills throughout the city advertising a water, pill, or potion to prevent and cure the disease.[90] Forman, it seems, did not post bills and despite his portrayal of himself as prudent in his use of physic in his astrological manuals, the Censors of the College of Physicians collected information about his flagrant use of remedies. When they first interviewed him in March 1594 he 'claimed to have cured Mr Anize, Mr Nicholas and Mr Allen in Thames Street all suffering from a fever to whom he had given an electuary of syrup of roses with wormwood

[88] For a general discussion of remedies, see Wear, *Knowledge and Practice*, ch. 2.

[89] Forman mimicked this division in 'A discourse of the plague', and criticized physicians and surgeons alike in 'Astrologicalle judgmentes': Ashm. 208, fo. 132^{v}; 363, fo. 9. On the notion of the medical hierarchy, and challenges to it, see Pelling and Webster, 'Medical Practitioners', 165; Roberts, 'Personnel and Practice of Medicine', 219. For the distinction between medicine and physic see Harold Cook, 'The New Philosophy and Medicine in Seventeenth-Century England', in David Lindberg and Robert Westman (eds.), *Reappraisals of the Scientific Revolution* (Cambridge, 1990), 397–436.

[90] Dekker mocked such empirics who 'clapt up their bils upon every post (like a Fencers Challenge)'. Lodge said that he was inspired to write about the plague because amongst the '*Thessali* that have bestowed a new Printed livery upon every old post' was one of his neighbours who had forgotten to underwrite it with his name, and thus people mistakenly flocked to Lodge requesting the 'promised preservatives' and 'cordial waters'. Several decades later, Stephen Bredwell complained about 'a Fellow in Distaffe Lane, that disperseth Bills abroad' advertising a preservative drink for the plague attributed to John Banister, the Elizabethan surgeon and Bredwell's grandfather: Dekker, *Wonderfulle yeare*, sig. D3^{r-v}; Lodge, *Plague*, sig. A3^{r-v}; Stephen Bredwell, *Physick for the sicknesse, commonly called the plague* (1636), p. [54]; see also Pelling, *Medical Conflicts*, *passim*.

water, and twenty others he had cured in the same way'.[91] A decade and a half later, as noted above, the Censors heard evidence that Forman prescribed and sold medicaments and purgatives.[92]

Forman asserted his prerogative as an astrologer-physician to minister remedies to the sick and his prudence in so doing; remedies were central to the exchanges between himself and his clients. He told the physicians that he had cured twenty-three people of a fever with an electuary and the judgement of the stars, and in the psalm about his trouble with the College he recorded how he cured himself and others by lancing the plague sores then administering a precious water. Lancing the sores was a conventional, surgical method for treating the plague; Fioravanti, for instance, recorded recipes for poultices to 'break' the buboes and ointments to dress them. Ambroise Paré, the great French surgeon, recommended opening the buboes either with ointments or a knife, and administering a strong water. Forman described this same method, though he accidentally discovered the virtue of his strong water.[93] He did not describe this treatment in his plague treatises, instead focusing on purges to prevent or cure the plague.[94] His astrological manuals similarly omit details of his legendary method, though in 'Grounds of arte', for instance, he described dressing a plague sore on the groin of Ann Sands on 4 December 1593 after first administering a repulsative, then two days later he dressed a sore under the arm of one John Hart.[95] Late in his life he implied that he visited people with plague and brought them many 'medisons and potions', and was reprimanded for so doing.[96]

Mostly Forman noted his use of electuaries and strong waters. He made these himself, infusing herbs in wine and beer and releasing the powers of herbs and minerals through alchemical distillation. In May 1587 he had begun to distil many waters, in May 1590 he distilled a strong water for the stone, and in June

91 Annals, 8 Mar. 1593/4, pp. 84–5.

92 Annals, 9 Jan., p. 191; 30 Mar. 1607, p. 192.

93 Fioravanti, *Joyfull jewell*, 50–5, 37–8; Paré, *Plague*, 61–91, esp. 68–9. See also, Drouet, *New counsel*, sigs. E4^{v}–F1. Like Paré, though in more detail, Forman discussed plague sores as tokens of the type of plague: Ashm. 1436, fos. 131, 170–202.

94 Ashm. 208, fos. 111^{v}, 113^{r-v}.

95 Ashm. 1495, fo. 503^{v}. In the casebooks Forman occasionally recorded that a patient might be suffering from, or was soon to suffer from, plague: Ashm. 234, fo. 112 (Jeames Curties, 10 Oct.; Richard Snelling, 11 Oct. 1596), fo. 116 (Clemente Grene, 11 Oct. 1596), fo. 150^{v} (Thomas Tonpe, 11 Jan. 1597), fo. 151^{v} (Eliz. Lawe, 13 Jan. 1597), fo. 152^{v} (Willm Garten, 15 Jan. 1597), fo. 153 (Jone Bristowe; John Tomsen, 17 Jan. 1597), fo. 154 (An Serjeante, 18 Jan. 1597), fo. 155 (An Sothery, 19 Jan. 1597), fo. 155^{v} (Jerveis Lillies, 19 Jan. 1597); Ashm. 226, fo. 271^{v} (Agnis Sax, 13 Dec. 1597), fo. 272 (Katherin Cooper, 14 Dec. 1597).

96 Ashm. 1436, fos. 72–4, 'A caveat to phisisions, apoticaries and surgeons', e.g. 'Take heed I sai youe physisions, chirurgeons, apoticaries that goe to visit many with medisons and potions leste thes sickned jewes say unto youe as they said unto christ on the crosse and unto me in the day of battelle being shut up into my house save thyselves as thou haste saved others etc.'

Table 6.3. *Numbers of treatments and prescriptions, March–May 1596 inclusive*

	Recorded prescriptions and treatments	No. of medical consultations	% of female, male, total	% of total prescriptions etc.
Females	58	175	33	60
Males	38	102	37	40
Total	96	277	35	100

1589 he recommended infusing stibium in his strong water, a preparation that worked as a vomit for one Margaret Rich where hellebore had failed.[97] In summer 1592 he cured himself from the plague, in 1593 he 'stilled my strong water by the which I got motch money'.[98] In 1594 he cured himself of gout 'with the dregs of my strong water thorowe gods helpe', and was involved in an elaborate procedure for distilling *argentum vivum* (mercury), though it is unclear whether this was for alchemical or medicinal purposes.[99] In the late 1590s and 1600s Forman compiled a series of alchemical commonplace books in which he collected recipes for herbal, chemical, and magical remedies, documented his control of the production of these substances, and expounded Paracelsian ideas about purges to restore and substances to maintain the virtues of the spirits in the body.[100] In a section on 'Distillation', he defined the process and listed a dozen methods for distilling waters, liquors, and oils from herbs and minerals, including a note that a variety of strong waters, such as those made by himself and Dr Steavens, were 'distilled by a pot and alimbick on softe fier and after in a glasse in balnea maria or in ashes or sand'. These volumes are replete with instructions for making various pills and potions, and Forman occasionally noted that he had made and administered these remedies to good effect.[101]

The casebooks also contain records of Forman's use of remedies. In a minority of cases (35 per cent for men and women alike) Forman recorded a course of therapy, perhaps supporting his self-portrayal as prudent in his use of physic (see Table 6.3). He occasionally recorded that someone was reluctant to take physic or previously had taken much on ill advice, such as the man who 'hath taken evill drinks' and the woman who 'followes ill councle and takes all medisons'.[102] He also noted a sensitivity to it, such as the case of a woman who

[97] Ashm. 208, fo. 50; Sloane 2550, fo. 115^{r-v}. Forman recorded that he administered this remedy on Wed., 25 June, from which I have deduced the year. He also described many other preparations for stibium, on which see also Ch. 8.

[98] Ashm. 208, fo. 50.

[99] Ashm. 208, fo. 50^v; 1472, p. 56.

[100] Ashm. 1430, 1472, 1494, 1491, see Chs. 9–11 below and Bibliography.

[101] Ashm. 1494, pp. 448–54, quotation p. [451].

[102] Ashm. 234, fo. 33^v (Shorte, Pyme, 10 May 1595). The proximity of these cases suggests that Forman discerned this information from the stars.

Table 6.4. *Types of treatments and prescriptions, March–May 1596 inclusive*

	Prepare and purge and/or vomit	Let blood	Potion or pill
Female	46 (79% of treatments received by females)	12 (21%)	8 (14%)
Male	31 (82% of treatments received by males)	11 (29%)	3 (8%)
Total	77 (80% of treatments received by females and males)	23 (24%)	11 (12%)

Note: Some consultations recorded more than one treatment or prescription.

'can take noe phisick' but 'must be prepared strongly or ells a purge will not work'. In another case he noted, 'give her a gentill preparative and a gentill purge and noe more'. For a woman who was vomiting blood, Forman noted 'she is very weke take heed what youe giv her'.[103] Sometimes he wrote a follow-up report on the effects of a remedy and the course of the disease, and an occasional entry reveals the complexities of administering physic. In a rare message inserted into the casebooks in February 1600, the client wrote 'now desiring you to make the plaster for my back against ♀ or ♄ if posible you can, for I indure great payne. You may tel this bearer how I must use the oyle for hearing which you gave me whether I must take it whote or cold'.[104] But, as demonstrated by the case of Margaret Altam, little of Forman's correspondence with his querents survives.

Most of the prescriptions in the casebooks were to 'prepare and purge' or 'prepare and vomit' (80 per cent of total prescriptions; 79 per cent of prescriptions for women; 82 per cent for men). Only a quarter of Forman's treatments required bleeding, usually following a preparation and purge (21 per cent of female treatments; 29 per cent of male treatments) (see Table 6.4).[105] Occasionally Forman specified a potion or pill, such as his imperial water, strong water, an electuary, or diet drink, and sometimes he listed the ingredients (12 per cent of consultations).[106] In a few instances he recorded a magical remedy such as a sigil to harness the powers of the stars. He made his remedies himself, and in

[103] Ashm. 234, fo. 31 (Glover, 6 May 1596); fo. 23 (Burrels/Fild, 25 Apr. 1596).

[104] Ashm. 236, fo. 23.

[105] For a detailed discussion of blood-letting by Forman, including examples, see Ashm. 1494, pp. 305–20.

[106] For recipes for Forman's imperial and plague waters see his 'Treatise of purginge' (*c*.1589?), Sloane 2550, fos. 124–27^{v}. See also Sloane 2550, fos. 101^{v}–17^{v} for many herbal and chemical remedies. For recipes dated 1595 see Ashm. 1495, fos. 1–2. For recipes on the endpapers of casebooks see Ashm. 411, fo. 101, where he noted the diet drinks which he had prescribed to Mrs Jeffries, Mr Fardinando Clutterbag, Mrs Blague, and Mrs Cuer; also Ashm. 219, fos. 51^{v}–2 (Apr. 1599). For recipes within the casebooks see Ashm. 195, fo. 53 (2 June 1598); Ashm. 236, fo. 12 (25 Jan. 1600, for Mrs Bacon); Ashm. 236, fo. 87^{v} (20 Feb. 1600, for Anne Young, via various intermediaries); Ashm. 411, fo. 49^{v}, a recipe for sore eyes. For a list of herbs and minerals see Ashm. 219, fo. 182. See also a recipe for *aqua vitae* dated 9 June 1604 (Ashm. 1490, fo. 335^{v}) and numerous recipes and preparations in 'Of appoticarie druges'.

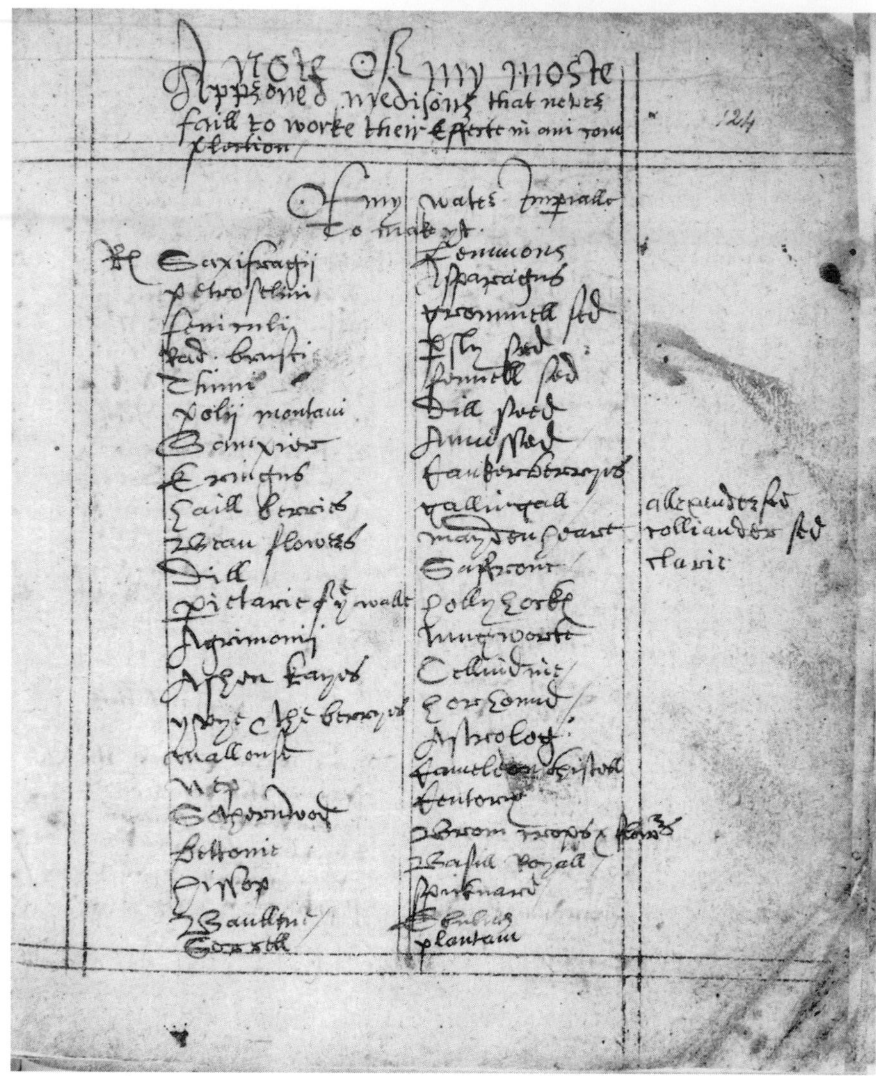

A note of my moste approved medisons that never faill to worke their effect in ani complexion

124

Of my water imperialle to make it

6.5. The first page of Simon Forman's recipe for his 'Water imperialle', Sloane 2550, fo. 124. By permission of the British Library.

general they were typical concoctions made from much beer and many herbs. More unusually, Forman controlled the timing at which the remedies were administered; without the knowledge of the stars, 'a man takinge the tyme will doe as moch with a preparative and 2 purges as with a wholl appoticaries shope'.[107] He selected from a congeries of remedies depending on the

[107] Ashm. 1436, fo. 143v.

complaint, and seems only to have prescribed therapies in a minority of cases.[108]

The impression of Forman's frugal use of remedies can be tested against his casebooks for 11 May to 5 September 1603. The original records for this period do not survive, but a fair copy of them includes numerous references to remedies.[109] Perhaps during this period Forman's recordkeeping changed, or perhaps he kept separate prescription books and this fair copy is a composite of the casebook and prescription book for the period. A comparison between August 1596 and August 1603 is instructive, as these records preserve comparable numbers of consultations (seventy-four and seventy-one medical consultations, respectively).[110] In August 1596 Forman prescribed therapies for 43 per cent of cases; in 1603 he prescribed therapies for 85 per cent of cases. In August 1596 three clients (4 per cent) were given strong water; in 1603 forty-nine people (64 per cent) were given strong water. If Forman's records of remedies in 1596 are incomplete, then perhaps he was not as frugal in his use of remedies as he portrayed himself. If these records are complete, then in August 1603 he prescribed twice as many remedies than in August 1596. Perhaps the outbreak of plague in 1603 explains this. In August 1603, Forman noted that forty-nine of the seventy-seven cases (57 per cent) had or would have plague; in August 1593 he identified only ten potential cases. These records raise more questions than they answer. Perhaps Forman prescribed more remedies than his casebooks record, or perhaps he prescribed more readily during an outbreak of plague. Whatever the answer, he did not send everyone away with a barrage of potions or a universal panacea.

Nor was there a trade in Forman's remedies or recipes, a testament, perhaps, to his prudence in administering physic. A couple of scraps of evidence document a limited circulation of Forman's recipes. Joshua Walworth, Forman's illegitimate son who had come to work as his assistant in 1602, kept a notebook which contained numerous remedies and may indicate that he was in charge of administering therapies to Forman's patients. In March 1603 Walworth recorded basic principles under the heading 'What physic is and what it doth comprehend and teach' along with recipes to encourage and discourage the growth of hair, also found elsewhere in Forman's notes. Walworth recorded the 'strong water my Mr made 1602 26 Sept', a drink that Walworth made for one Mrs Crooke on 21 March 1603, 'My Mr Forman's drinke of figs to comfort

108 Cf. Harold Cook, 'Good Advice and Little Medicine: The Professional Authority of Early Modern English Physicians', *Journal of British Studies*, 33 (1994), 1–31.

109 Ashm. 411, fos. 164–79. Only the beginning pages of these copies replicate the figures.

110 The records for the other seven months of 1603 combined contain only forty-five cases.

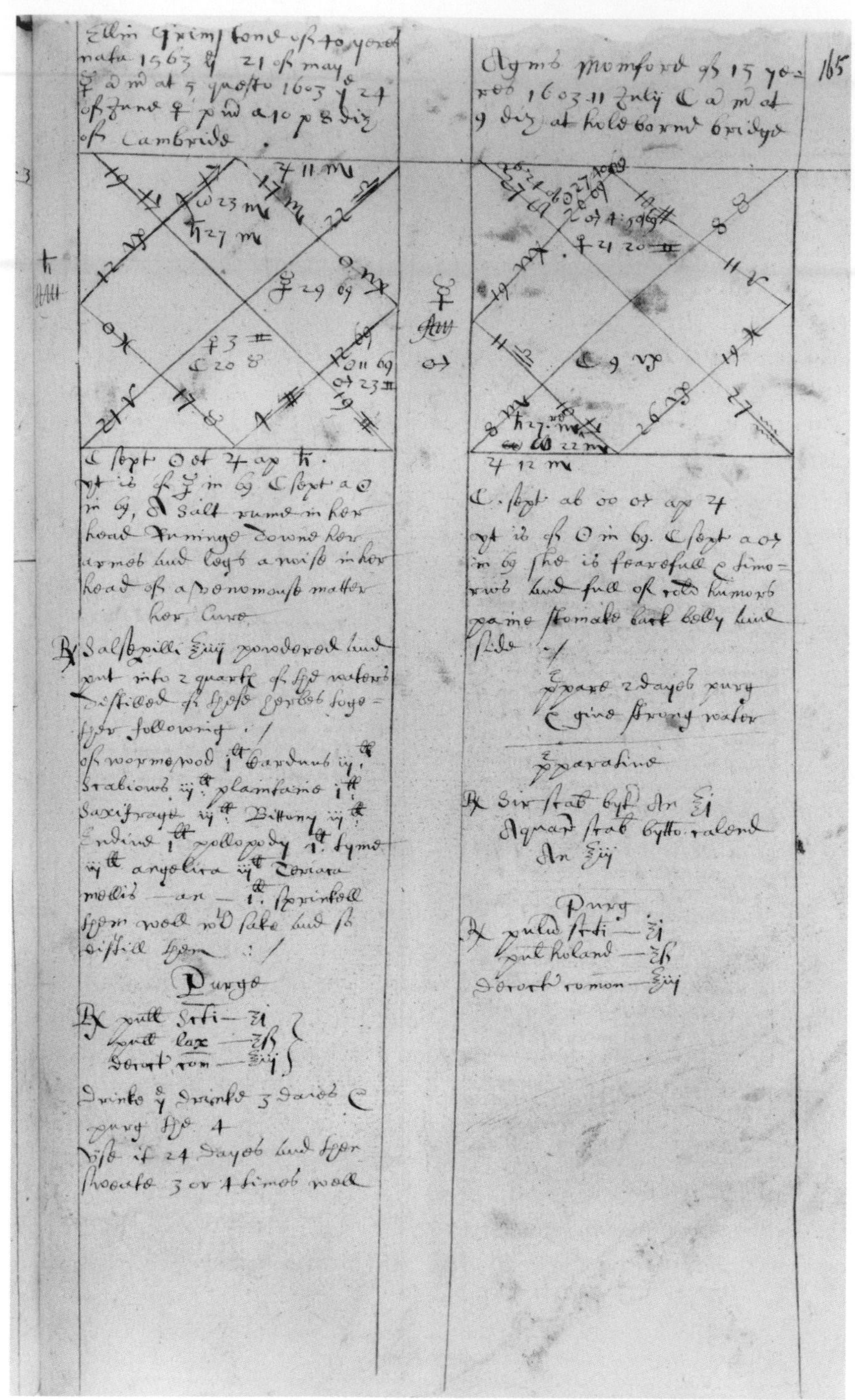

6.6. A page from the fair copy of Simon Forman's 1603 casebook, Ashm. 411, fo. 165. By permission of the Bodleian Library, University of Oxford.

and restore nature 1603 8 June', Forman's dietary drink and 'electuary rerum' dated 22 June 1603, and the recipe for a water which Forman invented in 1594.[111] Walworth had little opportunity to learn Forman's art or share his recipes, as, despite Forman's efforts, he died of plague in October that year.[112] Another notebook containing Forman's recipes and dating from 1615 is now lost. This was one of several hundred manuscripts which James Halliwell sold at Sotheby's on 21 May 1857, and it reputedly contained some notes on the diseases caused by the planets, on choler and melancholy, and on blood-letting, a diet drink dated 1615, Lodge's cure for the pestilence, recipes by Thomas Chayre, a remedy from 'a worthy man of Venice', Forman's strong water against the plague, and his medicine to renew age.[113] Forman's name did not adorn a product and his methods could not be bottled.

Forman had devised idiosyncratic and elaborate methods. A patient provided her name, age, perhaps address, and a question. Forman calculated the positions of the stars and planets and made a judgement, displaying his arcane expertise. Sometimes he provided an answer, sometimes a remedy, sometimes neither or both. This moment initiated a new dynamic between the astrologer-physician and his patient. Through his judgements he won the patient's trust, and only with that trust could he exercise his authority as an astrologer-physician. This tautologous dynamic of trust in the casebooks leads back to the question of gender: Forman had to win the trust of women because women did not tell him the truth. In each consultation he and his patients negotiated an exchange of trust for true judgements.

[111] Trinity MS O.2.59, fos. 121, 124, 141ᵛ, 142ᵛ, 145ᵛ, 146, 147ᵛ, 149. On grey hair see Ashm. 240, fo. 38. Richard Napier also noted this recipe, Ashm. 1457, fo. 59; Oxford, Corpus Christi College MS 169, fo. 95ᵛ.

[112] For Forman's account of Walworth's life and death see Ashm. 206, fos. 102–3; 240, fo. 31.

[113] *The collection of J. O. Halliwell*, Sotheby's sale catalogue, 21 May 1857, lot 154. This volume is reputed to have contained biographical information about Forman, *DNB*.

7
Gender, Authority, and Astrology

'<Never> trust a woman by her wordes | thoughe she doth wepe and cry'.[1] This was Forman's advice to the reader of 'Astrologicalle judgmentes', a manual that explained an art predicated on a series of exchanges, whether written or spoken, between a physician and his patient. Speech was suspect, women's speech doubly so; truth was recorded in the stars. Forman's ideas about femininity and female physiology were typical of Elizabethan London, a world in which sex and marriage were at the centre of gender dynamics played out in the language of chastity and honour and in the settings of the household and the city.[2] Throughout his writings, Forman framed the diseases of women according to notions of their sexual activity and moral accountability.[3] For instance, when discussing the causes of plague, he singled out the sins of women, beginning with Eve who acted as an agent of the devil when she deceived Adam. Like Eve, he extrapolated, 'women ar alwaies proud in theire conceighte, desirouse of content, and impaciente in adversities. And alwaies in extremities their love is without measure, and their hatred is dedlie & for ever inconstante.'[4] He portrayed the women of Elizabethan London who, like lawyers, clerics, and physicians, had brought the wrath of God to bear on England in the plague of 1592–3:

> Howe many lacivious Jessabells that live in pleasure enjoyinge the luste of the fleshe most filthely makinge a pastime therof . . . O it is a wonder to see howe demurely manie fine & proper women will goe in the streets, howe solemly they syt at tables, howe devoutly they com to the church, as thoughe they were religious, and yet verie strumpets, and those that a man would thinke of great honestie & credite. And yet moste common in silence of their bodies, they paint theire faces and set out their broidred heare with periwigs, and get them a gowne with a great hope on their taille, lyke one makinge a hobby hors in a morrishe daunce. Moste filthie to loke upon and hatefull before god and man.[5]

1 Ashm. 389, fo. 2. This is the only extant copy of the verse preface to 'Astrologicalle judgmentes' and it is badly damaged, hence my inference of the word 'never'. This echoes contemporary proverbs, e.g. George L. Apperson, *English Proverbs and Proverbial Phrases: A Historical Dictionary* (Toronto, 1929), 442, 703–7.

2 Laura Gowing, *Domestic Dangers: Women, Words, and Sex in Early Modern London* (Oxford, 1996).

3 Cf. Boorde, *Breviary of healthe*, sig. 82^{v}, on why woman is called woman, cited by Forman, King's MS 16, fo. 84^{v}.

4 Ashm. 208, fo. 116^{v}.

5 Ashm. 208, fo. 121^{v}.

These were women on display, parading a false virtue, masking deceit with urbanity.

There is an irony in an astrologer complaining that women could not be trusted. Astrologers, as Melton and others explained, masked deceit with the trappings of learning and art. The College of Physicians denigrated Forman's practices in these terms, and he defended himself with all of the personal credentials and institutional authorities that he could muster. But the facts were against him: the hundreds of people who consulted him in his study, and his particular renown with women, confirmed that he was a quack. Perhaps in a self-conscious effort to dispel the association of popularity with false practices, throughout his writings Forman stressed the truth and rigour of his methods. He dwelt particularly on the complexities of dealing with the female physiology and psyche, and he documented his expertise in these matters. Astrology, as he practised it, was not a tool to cozen the gullible masses and frivolous gentlewomen; it was the only true method for judging disease. Only an astrologer was fully equipped to understand women and to minister to their ills; only an astrologer could be trusted.

An understanding of women's diseases, according to Forman, began with an ability to diagnose pregnancy. Even if a woman reported on her sexual activities, she was not to be trusted. A lack of menstruation was not necessarily a sign of pregnancy, and vice versa. And urine was useless. Only the stars revealed the truth, as Forman noted, 'we have throughe longe experience observed by our astrologie thes rulles to be moste true and certaine which we have here set downe to judge by'. That is, if a woman had milk or water in her breasts, she might or might not be pregnant. But one thing was certain: she had been with a man, and his seed had caused a conception in her womb, which might be 'perfect' (meaning genuine) or false, as could be judged astrologically.[6]

In 'Grounds of arte' Forman specified that the third question to ask a patient, if a woman, was whether or not she was married:

> for then yf she be within yeares, shee maie be with childe oftentymes, or she may have impedments in her matrix by child bearinge the which maids have not. Againe yf she be yonge shee may have the grene sicknes by reason of the stoppinge of her menstrues. And many tymes alsoe a womane a child a maid is stopte and hath not her termes at all or hath them not in due order and course. And then they have paine in the reins in the side and stomacke and ar often lyke to vomite and have moch paine with all in the heed. And this never faileth.

Forman later added the phrase 'or verie seldome' to the end of this passage.[7] In the subsequent versions of this treatise he was more cynical, and marriage ceased

[6] Ashm. 390, fo. 190^{r-v}. [7] Ashm. 1495, fo. 29.

to be the defining factor in a woman's sexual activity. Forman, as a medical practitioner, required the truth about a woman's sexual activity, but it was difficult to obtain:

And yet as a man examine them [women] and tell them they are with child they will denie it utterly & say they are exceding honeste, when God knoweth no such matter. But some of them have had a bastard or 2 before & manytimes doe lie 3 or 4 times in a weeke with a man & yet they would be thought honest maides, wifes, or widdoes.

Forman continued,

And for because I have seene so much falls hoode in them, I have written this chapter for thy farder ayde & assistance in this behalfe. That when thou lookest in the chapter of the 5 house to see whether they be with child, thou maiest first looke to this whether she ever lay with any man or no or deserved for it.[8]

Forman recommended that, as pregnancy was not possible without sexual intercourse, the astrologer should consult the stars to see if a woman was a virgin, then whether she was pregnant. Women's diseases were bound both to their reproductive capacity and their sexual activity. In order to assess the one, the physician needed information about the other. Women, however, were seldom forthright or frank in the matter. At the end of his account of 'Macbeth' Forman noted, 'observe howe Mackbets quen did rise in the night in her slepe, & walked and talked and confessed all & the doctor noted her words'.[9] Doctors discovered the secrets of women.

Forman's distrust of women was coupled with an interest in female physiology and morbidity. He repeated the humanist account of the model of the womb and ovaries as an inversion of the penis and testes and he was particularly concerned with the womb as a seat of disease.[10] For instance, in a transcription of a medieval manuscript describing the life of Adam and Eve, Forman inserted a list of diseases from which humankind would suffer after the Fall. Because Eve 'harkened the serpent', women suffered more than seventy diseases specific to their sex, though Forman only recorded fourteen of these. These all related to the womb or the breasts, and were conditions that Forman encountered amongst his patients.[11]

[8] Ashm. 363, fo. 198v. [9] Ashm. 208, fo. 207v.

[10] Ashm. 363, fo. 100; Ian Maclean, *The Renaissance Notion of Woman: A Study in the Fortunes of Scholasticism and Medical Science in European Intellectual Life* (Cambridge, 1980), 31–3. On notions of anatomical differences between the sexes, see also Thomas Laqueur, *Making Sex: Body and Gender from the Greeks to Freud* (Cambridge, Mass., 1990); Londa Schiebinger, *The Mind has no Sex? Women in the Origins of Modern Science* (Cambridge, Mass., 1989); and a challenge to their dating of such distinctions to the 18th cent. in Michael Stolberg, 'A Woman Down to her Bones: The Anatomy of Sexual Difference in the Sixteenth and Seventeenth Centuries', *Isis*, 94 (2003), 274–99, printed with replies from Laqueur and Schiebinger.

[11] Ashm. 802, fo. 23. This text is discussed in Ch. 9.

The casebooks document Forman's focus on female reproduction. Although only 5 per cent of the women who came to him asked if they were pregnant, in 44 per cent of women's medical cases he mentioned factors concerning reproduction. He used the word 'matrix' to mean womb, and usually simply noted 'in matrix', or 'pain in matrix', whether or not she has her course (period), or 'taken in childbed'. Like most of Forman's writings, his notes on the diseases of women were astrological. His sources are elusive, though he drew extensively from Guido Bonatti's *De astronomia tractatus X* (Basel, 1550) for general questions such as whether or not a woman would conceive.[12] He also noted rules of his own devising. Although diseases of women were not yet the subject of a specialized literature written in English, Forman extracted passages on women from vernacular medical texts, adding his observations, for instance, that menstruating women appeared 'lancke betwen the eyes and the nose & blueshe as though she had wept moche'.[13] He also wrote a distinct treatise on the diseases of women, 'Matrix and paine therof', which was empirical as well as astrological.[14] He composed this in 1596 and revised it in 1599, the period when physicians in London were debating whether mental vexations specific to women had natural or supernatural causes, though he seems not to have engaged with these controversies.[15]

'Matrix' describes Forman's treatment of the stopping of the matrix due to congealed humours. He wrote it because

> we have seene and knowene manie women of all ages old and yonge in this predicament, we have moch considered herof, and by experience thorowe the grace of god, our industrie, and paines takinge in serchinge the cause by astrologie, and by the examination of diverse women that have bine trobled herwithe we have found that the distemprature of the matrix thorowe the causes above saide hath bine the cause of all their grife. Wheupon I have writen this lyttle treatise to showe the remedies therof.[16]

Women had problems with their wombs if evil humours congealed in them and were not properly evacuated. Three things made this happen: first, sexual intercourse too soon after the birth of a child; secondly, a false conception or some after-birth left behind; and thirdly, the midwife leaving the woman's womb open for too long after delivering the child. The physician's job was to

12 Ashm. 390, fos. 202–3ᵛ; Bonatti, *De astronomia tractatus X*, fo. 430.

13 MacDonald (ed.), *Witchcraft and Hysteria*; Schleiner, *Medical Ethics*, 112. King's MS 16, fos. 78ᵛ–80ᵛ; Edmond, 'Forman's Vade-Mecum', 56 (source of discussion and citation).

14 'Matrix and the pain thereof', ed. Traister (hereafter 'Matrix'). The MS is Ashm. 390, fos. 161–8, and although it is a fair copy, it is bound amidst Forman's astrological notes relating to the diseases of women, fos. 161–205. Forman included sections on diseases of women in his guides to astrology, though he either excised them or left them incomplete, Ashm. 363, fos. 102–10ᵛ; 1495, p. 506.

15 MacDonald (ed.), *Witchcraft and Hysteria*, p. xii.

16 'Matrix', 441.

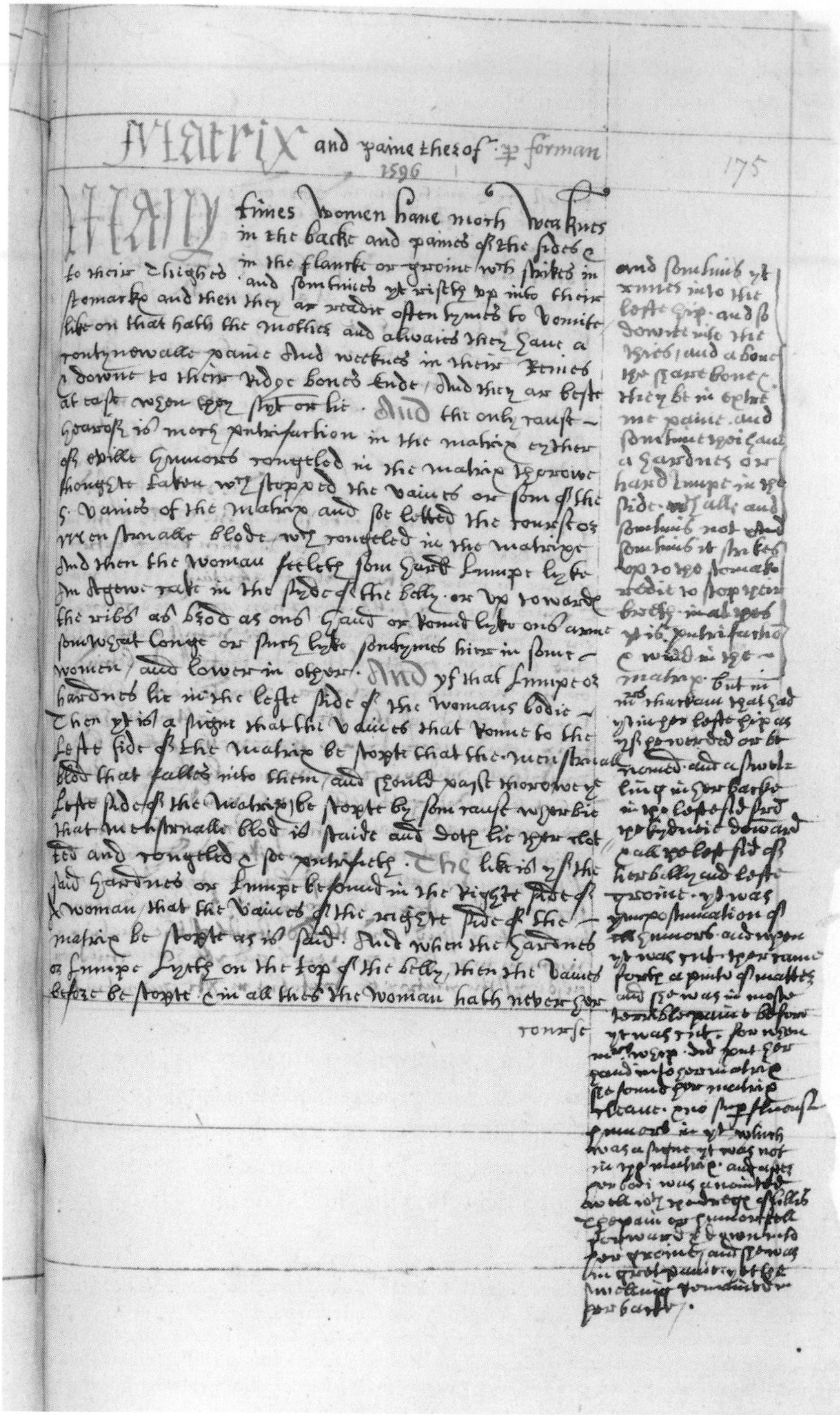

Matrix and paine therof ♃ forman
1596
175

Many times women haue moch weaknes in the backe and paines of the sides in the flanke or groine wth strikes in to their thighes

7.1. Simon Forman, 'Matrix and paine therof', 1596, Ashm. 390, fo. 175. By permission of the Bodleian Library, University of Oxford.

evacuate the womb of evil humours, as he evacuated the body with purges and emetics.[17] Medicines taken orally or rectally were no good for this. The matrix required special attention. In order to discover whether in practice this was possible, Forman noted,

> I have made diligente inquisition amonge grave matrons and midwifes and others to knowe wher the matrix doth exempte himself of any thinge that yt receyveth of man more then once in a month or noe. And they have told me yea, that yt doth exempte yt selfe of any thing that yt receyveth of man and dothe vomite out the nature and sperme of man received by divers coitions, and will alsoe belche out wind (like as the stomacke doth) at the vulva.[18]

As the menstrual cycle followed the moon, so these lesser evacuations of the womb followed the tide.[19] These were natural evacuations, in contrast to medicines that purged the womb violently and artificially. For best effect, the physician was to 'joine arte and nature together', and to prescribe physic to purge the womb at times which corresponded with its natural evacuations. In order to find the appropriate moment to administer a remedy, 'First youe muste learne the tyme when their [a woman's] menstrualle course doth use to com, and som thre or 4 dais alwaies before they have their course youe shall make them a lotion to washe their bellies as hote as thei can suffer yt all over.'[20]

'Matrix' stood apart from Forman's other texts in its blend of empiricism and astrology. He appealed to his experience of correct and false astrological judgements throughout his writings, but in this case he explained how he had gathered information to confirm his ideas and he provided vivid accounts of his observations and therapeutic procedures. More explicit than the casebooks, the cases in 'Matrix' reveal the boundary between Forman and his female patients. This boundary was generally traversed by other women, the grave matrons and midwives from whom Forman had obtained his information. In particular, Forman described how a midwife, Mrs Whip, inserted her hand into Mrs Chackam's womb, and he also recommended Mrs Whip's ointment.[21] These women, like Forman's male servants, do not appear in the casebooks, with the possible exception of one Mrs Cuer, who might have been a go-between for Forman and some of his patients.[22] On one occasion Forman noted, 'I with my owne hands did minister a cataplasme to her lower parts of

17 'Matrix', 443. 18 Ibid.

19 For the influences of the moon on the uterus, see Maclean, *Renaissance Notion of Woman*, 41.

20 'Matrix', 444, 442.

21 Ibid. 441, 445. See p. 442 for another description of a skilful midwife inserting her hand into the matrix.

22 See Ashm. 234, fo. 33^v (10 May 1596); 226, fos. 35, 193^v, 208^v, 232^v, 300^v (14 Mar., 26 Aug., 12 Sept., 12 Oct. 1597; 4 Feb. 1598). She and her husband attended Forman's wedding in July 1599 (Ashm. 219, fo. 111). For Mrs Cuer as a patient, see Ashm. 236, fo. 183 (6 Aug. 1600); 411, fo. 101 (May 1601).

her belly', but this was probably not the norm.[23] His expertise encompassed the skill of midwives under the rubric of astrology. Some women trusted Forman, a man and an astrologer, to recommend therapies conventionally controlled by women.[24]

Although Forman diagnosed some of his male patients as suffering from venereal diseases, he did not display an interest in conditions specific to men. He did observe male problems, as illustrated by the following note:

> I have knowen divers men that have had great pain in their yard [penis], especiali when their yard did stand, as thoughe thei had had a ston in their yarde, & somtims as thoughe the top of the yard wold burste, & thei could scante make water. And their water wold burne their yard and smarte wonderfulle, and matter [splatter] with all and all to matter their shirtes. And in the bottom of the urinall after the urin was setled ther wold ly a gret deall of thick residence.[25]

The cause and the treatment were simple: too much heat in the kidneys could be addressed with a syrup made from cooling herbs. Men's diseases were more straightforward than women's.

Forman's study of the diseases of women was predicated on an assumption that women were untrustworthy. However candid a woman might have been about her sexual activities or lack thereof, he insisted on verifying her words according to the stars. Occasionally he recorded a narrative in which a patient described the state of her body, such as the woman who thought she might have been pregnant and who had intermittent contractions and bleeding.[26] Forman also revealed the balance of physical observation, astrological calculation, and personal assessment in making judgements when he advised Napier, who had asked how to know if a woman was a virgin, 'I answere youe, when the velme or stringe of her virginity is broken. Yf youe will knowe otherwise then muste yt be upon a question & by sight of the partie.'[27] Since any woman of reproductive age might have been suffering from an ailment whose cause was seated in the womb, her sexual activity was paramount in observing and treating her disease. Forman and his women patients talked about sex, and whether Forman verified what a woman told him or discovered her activities in the stars, these discussions fostered trust. The casebooks are the product of these conversations, but almost nothing remains of the dialogues that generated them.

[23] Ashm. 1495, fo. 503^{v} (Sisseli Burton, 6 Dec. 1593).

[24] Pelling, 'Compromised by Gender', 107; cf. Monica Green, 'Women's Medical Practice and Medical Care in Medieval Europe', *Signs*, 14 (1989), 434–73.

[25] King's MS 16, fo. 82.

[26] Ashm. 234, fo. 23^{v} (Braddeden, 27 Apr. 1596).

[27] Ashm. 1488, fo. 89.

Dialogues, histrionic and bathetic, populate 'Astrologicalle judgmentes'. These are case histories, typical of the narratives found in learned medical texts, often concerning young and genteel women and containing moral and sexual overtones.[28] They demonstrate how Forman exercised his authority as an astrologer-physician, an authority that he attributed to the veracity of his judgements and the virtue in his therapies. One case concerned Isabel Williams, aged 25, who told Forman that she was unwell and asked him about the state of her body. He drew a figure, and prompted by it he

> asked her whether she was a maid or a wife, or neither. Sir said she I am a maide, yea said I, and a good one to[o]. What meane you Sir by that quoth she. Marry said I, thou art as good a maide as he left thee that lay last with thee. Sir, said she, I never laid with any man in my life.

The banter continued until Forman told Williams that she was pregnant. She denied it, was offended, and went home and complained to her mistress. This is the only case history in 'Astrologicalle judgmentes' that was set in Forman's consulting room; most of them were about gentlewomen who called him to their houses. Williams's mistress came to Forman, bringing Williams with her, and asked what he had said. He repeated that the maid was with child. The woman feigned offence, vouched that the maid was honest, and asked Forman to give her some physic. He agreed, on condition that she, the mistress, would take responsibility for the danger. She consented, insisting that her maid never knew what belonged to a man. Forman suspected the 'humour' of the mistress and the knavery of the maid, perhaps because he thought the maid was trying to procure an abortion, and he prescribed a physic that revealed all.[29] Within six weeks Williams was delivered of twins, proving Forman's judgement and Williams's deceit. According to Forman, he was consulted in such cases many times.[30]

The case of an unnamed gentlewoman contains elaborate details about the process of negotiating a therapeutic relationship. She had undertaken a lengthy journey to London to consult Forman and had high expectations of his abilities. He called at the house where she was staying, 'When I came to her, our

[28] Laurinda Dixon, *Perilous Chastity: Women and Illness in Pre-Enlightenment Art and Medicine* (Ithaca, NY, 1995); King, *Hippocrates' Woman*, ch. 10; Nancy Siraisi, 'Girolamo Cardano and the Art of Medical Narrative', *Journal of the History of Ideas*, 52 (1991), 581–602. On medical cases in a legal context see esp. Pomata, *Contracting a Cure*.

[29] For attempts to procure abortions from physicians see Schleiner, *Medical Ethics*, 34.

[30] e.g. Ashm. 363, fo. [199]: 'The like I did by another at the pickeldhearinge whoe denied it strongly yet at last was delivered of a mayde child contrarly to the expectation [of] her mistress. The like I did by one at the stockes the father of whose child was her mister. The like of an other gentlewoman belonging to a Lady in this land, & diverse others of the which I could tell there deeds have manifested their folly'.

selves beinge lefte alone, she showed me her urine, accordinge to the ordinary custome, and desireth my judgemente.' He had cast a figure before leaving his house and it showed that 'the course of heaven yielded no disease, but some paine of her head and eyes'. He reported this judgement to the woman, and she more insistently asked whether he had found any disease at all. He said no, he could not find any disease at all in her body. Then,

She saide she was troubled with a greater matter thee which, if I could not finde, she thought my skill was not sufficient to give her remedie for it: And therefore she saide further I am sorry that I have taken so greate a journy to come so farre unto you, thee which I perceive is not such in respecte of your skill, as is reported to be. And I am also sorry that I have troubled you so much, and againe that it is not my good fortuine to find that good and knowledge at your hands as others have done.

Forman asked for two hours to see if he could discover anything else. She agreed.

Forman went home, looked at the figure he had cast, consulted many books, 'sifted her mind', and came to the same conclusion: the disease was in her head. He returned to her house for dinner, after which she retired to her room and sent for him: 'and I told her as before, I found no other disease in her body, but only in her head. And [I] keept the rest of the secret matter to my selfe, because she seemeth to deel so coningly with me, and thought to overretched me, and to try my skill so deeply.' The woman thanked Forman and said, 'Sir, you are note the man that I looketh for, or did hope to finde that can no better discerne my greeve. I am very sorry, I have troubled you'. He replied,

Yea gentlewoman, quoth I, and I am very sorrie also that you should be so troublesome both to me and to yourselfe, to the which need not have been, if the greeve of your mind, were noe greater then the greeve of your body. But because the disease of the mind are not seene in a pisspotte, it pertaines not to me, but rather to a dynnie [divine] that can give goode counsell, of the which at this time you have more neede thereof than of medicine to cure any disease of your body. You had little need of either of them at thise present. And so I leave you . . .

He turned around and stepped quietly out of the door. He had reached the street by the time she had recovered from the shock of what he had said, but she caught up with him, grabbed his cloak, and begged him to return to her chamber. He declined, resisted, then gave in and returned with her. Once in her chamber, she shut the door and sat down in front of it.

The denouement followed. She asked what he meant when he said she was more sick in her mind than her body. He replied,

Well gentlewoman, quoth I, because hereafter you shall not saye that you have found lesse in me then was reported unto you, I will now unfould my mind more largly unto you because yourselfe shall not saye your journy hath bene in vaine, and againe, because I will not have arte blemished. This it is you come unto me with a pisspott to knowe your disease of your body or rather the disease of your mind, but how should the greefe of the mind be discerned therein, when the disease of the body cannot be seene therein. I never saw a gentlewoman of your vocation having so deepe occation to use good counsell, to mocke a man of arte with a pispott. Thou shouldest have delt plainly with mee and not fraudulently if you ment to have any succour at my hands, and have told me the greefes of thy mind for the which cause you are come to me . . .

As it transpired, Forman had discerned a romantic scenario, which he recounted to the woman as follows. The woman had been 'familiar' with a man who was not her husband. She and her lover had fallen out, and he had threatened to reveal the affair to her husband. This was the source of her disease: 'for feare hereof thou art much proplexed in thy mind, which made the[e] come unto me for good councell to prevent the mischeefe and harme that may and is like to inssue hereof. For thy creadit and whole estate dependeth thereon, if it once come to thy husbands eares.' When Forman recounted this tale, the woman was amazed and ashamed. She did not know what to say, and burst into tears, 'sayinge Sir it is true, it is true, and I am so much ashamed of my follie herein that I am hartely sorry for provoking you so much'. Then she told him the whole story and asked for his advice. He concluded, 'So I adviseth her so wisly that wee stopt the gentlemans mouth, and made them frinds againe, but in such sorte that thay should never come together againe as thay had done before, and so saved her creadit and cureth her disease.'[31]

Forman used this case to illustrate the importance of distinguishing between diseases of the mind and body, a distinction that he thought it best to demonstrate through examples. Because the mind had more power over the body than the body over the mind, Forman explained, if the mind was disrupted the body would 'languish long in a small disease' and these diseases might distract from an assessment of the root of the problem.[32] The case of the adulterous gentlewoman accordingly demonstrated Forman's version of psychology and illness at the same time as crystallizing the problems of gender, astrology, and medicine. Forman's skill as an astrologer-physician enabled him to see the secrets hidden in the cosmos and in his patients' minds, a skill especially important in discerning the causes of a woman's disease. After the secret had been discovered, then Forman and his patient talked, about truth, about honour, and about sex. In each consultation, Forman enacted and affirmed his authority.

[31] Ashm. 363, fos. [138ᵛ]–[40ᵛ]. [32] Ashm. 363, fo. [138ᵛ].

These conclusions are based on Forman's casebooks and treatises. I have not found a single patient's account of a consultation with him. The casebooks are themselves a tenuous clue to how his services as an astrologer-physician were perceived. In the thousands of records they record, and as physical objects, they were central to representations of him in the pamphlet literature that surrounded the murder of Sir Thomas Overbury. One account described Forman as 'the fiend in human shape, | That by his art did act the devil's ape', portraying him as 'poring over his blasphemous books, | making strange characters in blood-red lines'.[33] One of his books was reputed to have been brought into the trial as evidence for his meddling in the illicit romances of those at court. Forman allegedly had made his querents write their own names in this book before he would practise his art.[34] This was the procedure for engaging in a contract, and it contained diabolic overtones. This book, if indeed it ever existed, has not been positively identified. It was probably a casebook. Whether demonic or, as he thought, divine, Forman's astrological physic was controversial. It required a complete faith in the physician. Some people objected; some complied; and many were convinced.

[33] R[ichard] N[iccols], 'Sir Thomas Overburies vision' [1616], *The Harleian Miscellany*, 7 (1810), 178–88, quotation, 184.

[34] W[eldon], *Court and character of King James*, 110.

IV

ALCHEMY, MAGIC, AND MEDICINE

Around 1606 Forman began to write a treatise on the philosophers' stone. At the outset he explained that 'the science of philosophi de lapide philosoco et de transmuatione metallorum' was the lower, terrestrial astronomy and the influences of the planets was the higher, celestial astronomy. He was writing in order to preserve this knowledge for posterity, but after a brief description of the transmutation of metals he moved on to the higher astronomy, then left off.[1] He had begun drafting this tract on pages which contained an unfinished copy of a treatise attributed to Hermes Trismegistus, and this likewise remained incomplete.[2] Whatever Forman's intentions, he did not produce a coherent account of the philosophers' stone, nor of the relationship between alchemy, magic, and medicine. But he devoted several reams of paper and dozens of quills and bottles of ink to the study of alchemy and magic, and, sometimes because of the astrological significance of the moment, sometimes as a record of his expertise, and sometimes out of habit, he chronicled his alchemical and magical activities throughout his notes. These papers constitute about a quarter of Forman's extant manuscripts. Through them I have recovered Forman's pursuit of the secrets of nature in ancient texts, the alembic, and the streets of London. He amalgamated numerous alchemical, magical, and medical traditions in a quest that his contemporaries would have called chymical, hermetical, Paracelsical, philosophical, iatrochemical, or spagyrical physic, and that we might call Paracelsianism. Forman did not define his activities. Each of the following chapters dwells on a set of texts that he copied, augmented, appropriated, extracted, and recopied. By following the paths of these processes of reading and writing, I assess Forman's alchemical and magical activities, their relationship to each other, and their bearing on his practices as an astrologer-physician.

[1] Ashm. 1433, ii, fo. 21. See p. 56 above for Forman's account of why he wrote this tract, and see Ashm. 1490, fo. 352^{v} for a fragment of a preface to an alchemical work by Forman.

[2] Ashm. 1433, ii, fos. 1–34. This contains the Emerald Tablet with Hortulanus' commentary (4^{v}–10^{v}) and other texts, interspersed with the figures that Adam McLean has identified as 'The crowning of nature' <www.levity.com/alchemy/crowning.html>.

8

'Of Cako', or the Medical Uses of Antimony

An alchemist needed time, money, and space, and Forman was not born with any of these. In the mid-1580s he filled two notebooks with copies of alchemical texts and began two others. During this period he lived in Salisbury, spent a few years without a fixed address, then settled in London in the early 1590s. He had distilled strong waters since at least 1587 but it was not until 1594 that he began to 'practise the philosophers stone'.[1] Thereafter he associated the production of alchemical remedies and the pursuit of the philosophers' stone. At Lent 1595 he 'began ye philosophers ston & befor mad my furnes and all for yt, as in my other bock yt aperes. I mad many sirups & drugs & distilled many waters & bought stills.'[2] The following September he 'drempt of 3 black cats, and of my philosophical powder which I was distiling'.[3] In October 1595 he dreamt that a man wrote some words about the philosophers' stone on Forman's coat and gave him two kinds of white powder.[4] The following December he complained about being unlucky, having broken 'two glasses and lost the water'.[5] Three months later, in March 1596, in another dream a friend gave him some of the philosophers' stone in liquid form. Forman cupped it in his hand, but before he could find a glass to hold it, it ran through his fingers.[6] His pursuit of the philosophers' stone continued, and in March of 1596, 'In subliming of ☉ & ☿ my pot & glasse brokee & all my labour was lost per lapidem'.[7] In November 1598 Forman was more successful. He and an unnamed associate made an amalgam of gold and silver, then philosophical mercury, iron, and 'cako'. This went through several operations, and a few days later was put into 'our ege', a sealed glass vessel.[8] The mysterious cako provides a key into the ways in which Forman studied alchemy and how these studies informed his medical ideas and practices.

Alchemy was both a textual and a practical tradition, and an alchemist might have intended to use the philosophers' stone to transmute base metals into

[1] Ashm. 208, fo. 50.

[2] Ashm. 208, fos. 53ᵛ, 54. I suspect that the other book to which he referred was an early alchemical commonplace book, now missing or subsumed into Ashm. 1472.

[3] Ashm. 208, fo. 54ᵛ.

[4] Ashm. 1472, p. [809]. Cf. Siraisi, *Cardano*, 175–6.

[5] Ashm. 208, fo. 55.

[6] Ashm. 1472, p. [809].

[7] Ashm. 208, fo. 57.

[8] Ashm. 195, fo. 203ᵛ.

gold, heal disease, preserve health, prolong life, achieve spiritual enlightenment, or some combination thereof. Alchemical texts recorded procedures, recipes, and principles of operation encoded in tropes and other devices. While the astrologer needed to draw a figure in order to make his calculations, an alchemist could conduct experiments without keeping records, though a few intractable experimental notebooks survive.[9] Forman's industrious pursuit of the secrets of the philosophers' stone fell into two phases, the periods from the mid-1580s to 1594 when he made alchemical remedies, and after 1594 when he began a practical pursuit of the philosophers' stone. During the first phase Forman filled ten notebooks and began two others with copies of more than a hundred alchemical texts.[10] Later he purchased numerous printed alchemical books, either because he began to be able to afford them or they became increasingly available from the London booksellers, or both.[11] The second phase was marked by the compilation of a series of alchemical commonplace books.[12] There are three of these, though one is briefer than the other two.[13] Forman's first volume dates from around 1597, when he began synthesizing his alchemical notes under subject headings arranged loosely alphabetically in 'Principles of philosofi gathered by S. Forman', a volume containing more than 200 entries flanked by a list of authors cited and a verse preface at the beginning and a table (or index) at the end.[14] Forman typically used the word 'philosophy' to designate alchemical activities.[15]

[9] Donald R. Dickson (ed.), *Thomas and Rebecca Vaughan's* Aqua Vitae: Non Vitis (*BL MS Sloane 1741*) (Tempe, Ariz., 2001); Betty Jo Teeter Dobbs, *The Foundations of Newton's Alchemy, or 'The Hunting of the Greene Lyon'* (Cambridge, 1975); William R. Newman and Lawrence M. Principe, *Alchemy Tried in the Fire: Starkey, Boyle, and the Fate of Helmontian Alchemy* (Chicago, 2002).

[10] These are contained in twelve notebooks, now bound in Ashm. 208, 1423, 1433, and 1490, for which full details are listed in the Bibliography. On the circulation of alchemical MSS see Webster, 'Alchemical and Paracelsian Medicine'; contrast Debus, *English Paracelsians* and Kocher, 'Paracelsian Medicine'. For recent works on MS culture see David Carlson, *English Humanist Books: Writers and Patrons, Manuscript and Print, 1475–1525* (Toronto, 1993); Harold Love, *Scribal Publication in Seventeenth-Century England* (Oxford, 1993); Arthur Marotti, *Manuscripts, Print, and the English Renaissance Lyric* (Ithaca, NY, 1995); Henry Woudhuysen, *Sir Philip Sidney and the Circulation of Manuscripts, 1558–1640* (Oxford, 1996).

[11] e.g. Joseph Duchesne, *The practise of chymicall, and hermeticall physicke, for the preservation of health*, tr. Thomas Tymme (1605); Paracelsus, *Operum medico-chimicorum sive paradoxorum, tomus genuinus undecimus*, tr. Zacharias Palthen, xi (Frankfurt, 1605).

[12] Forman was not formally trained in keeping commonplacc books. Cf. the commonplace books of John Dee and his Cambridge contemporaries: Sherman, *Dee*, 59–65. See also Ann Moss, *Printed Common-Place Books and the Structuring of Renaissance Thought* (Oxford, 1996); Sharpe, *Reading Revolutions*. Forman's commonplace books were paginated or foliated through at some point, and according to this pagination each has had roughly a third of its pages extracted, either by Forman as part of the process of compiling and recopying or by a later reader.

[13] Ashm. 1430. This volume seems to have been written at the same time or later than 'Of appoticarie druges', *c.*1607–10. [14] Ashm. 1472.

[15] Cf. *OED*. Forman used the terms alchemy (alchymy) and philosophy, e.g. Ashm. 1433, ii, fo. 21; iii, fos. 5–15. He did not use the terms chymia, spagyry, or iatrochemistry. On terminology, see William R. Newman and Lawrence M. Principe, 'Alchemy vs. Chemistry: The Etymological Origins of a Historiographic

Between around 1607 and at least 1610 Forman compiled an even larger alchemical volume, 'Of appoticarie druges', in which he incorporated most of the information from the earlier volume and added more references to printed books and more details about magic.[16] This work fills two huge volumes, runs to at least 700 folio pages, and contains around 300 entries. Some pages were removed, perhaps by Ashmole, and are now in the Sloane collection, others seem to be missing, and there are blank pages throughout.[17] Forman organized it alphabetically, partially indexed it, and noted many cross-references. The entries range in length from nothing more than a heading to fifty-odd pages and they combine extracts from other texts with Forman's ideas as developed through his studies and practices of alchemy, astrology, magic, medicine, and natural history. There are substantial, uniform entries for the major alchemical processes of calcination, digestion, fermentation, distillation, circulation, sublimation, and fixation, and the alchemical substances, salt, sulphur, mercury, antimony, gold, and lead. Each of these begins with a description and definition of the substance and concludes with experiments and recipes. There are also lengthy entries on more general natural philosophical topics such as 'anima mundi' and 'microcosmos'.

'Of appoticarie druges' was the repository of Forman's alchemical pursuits and their medical applications.[18] He gathered information from sources ancient, medieval, and modern; artisanal and natural philosophical; and from printed and manuscript texts and by word of mouth. The volume is eclectic, and it is not clear which words are Forman's, which copied, and what he collected and advocated. For instance, in an account of the great elixir attributed to Raymon Lully, a passage concluded, 'and herin is seen the great force of arte, but yet I thinke yt be not so gret as this Author saith'.[19] Although the headings are typically alchemical, the volumes are especially rich with medical preparations. This is reflected in the title, perhaps echoing a passage from a book that Forman drew on extensively, Thomas Tymme's 1605 selection and translation of writings by Joseph Duchesne (or Quercetanus), *The practise of*

Mistake', *Early Science and Medicine*, 3 (1998), 32–65; Hereward Tilton, *The Quest for the Phoenix: Spiritual Alchemy and Rosicrucianism in the Work of Count Michael Maier (1569–1622)* (Berlin, 2003), chs. 1, 6; Trevor-Roper, 'Court Physician and Paracelsianism', 87–8.

16 Forman kept these notes in two volumes, now bound as Ashm. 1494 and 1491 respectively, with some pages now in Sloane, 3822, fos. 6–19, 68–102ᵛ. I am indebted to David Pingree for assembling a copy of these volumes in which most of the pages from Sloane 3822 are reinstated, and to Carol Kaske for providing me with a copy of this document and initiating a project to edit it.

17 Most of the item is paginated, not foliated. The pagination runs to 1422, but there are currently 639 pages excluding the excised pages now in Sloane 3822.

18 Perhaps its purpose was spelt out in a prefatory section that is now missing. The first volume has sixteen blank, numbered pages at the beginning, some of which bear the numbers 10, 30, 32, 34, 42, 44, 50. The title and Forman's name appear at the top of the page of the first entry.

19 Ashm. 1494, p. 469.

chymicall, and hermeticall physicke for the preservation of health.[20] Duchesne (*c.*1544–1609) was one of the foremost French proponents of alchemical and Paracelsian medicine and this book concluded with a discussion of the need to teach apothecaries to follow the prescriptions of true physicians; because most apothecaries only sold trash, many practitioners had their remedies made in-house.[21] Forman did this and 'Of appoticarie druges' might thus be read as a record of his study and practice of 'chymical and hermetical physic', a compendium of his expertise in using alchemy, astrology, and magic in his medical and related practices, complete with advice about which shops in London supplied the best materials.

In November 1598, shortly before he made the amalgam of gold and silver that involved 'cako', Forman had transcribed a short treatise 'Of cako' and interpolated his alchemical experiences and observations throughout the text.[22] Although Forman did not know the identity of its author, this text was to become well known in the next century as Alexander von Suchten's 'Second treatise on antimony'. Suchten (1520?–1590?) was a Polish follower of Paracelsus and his two treatises on antimony were printed in German in 1570, Latin in 1575, and promptly translated into English and circulated in manuscript.[23] The ore of antimony (stibnite) was generally referred to as antimony, the metal extracted from the ore was called regulus (metalline antimony), and when further refined with other metals it became star regulus or quicksilver.[24] For some alchemists antimony was a crucial ingredient in the production of the philosophers' stone, specifically in transmutational alchemy.[25] Suchten and others

[20] Debus, *English Paracelsians*, 87.

[21] Duchesne, *Chymicall physicke*, sigs. BB3^{v}–4. For other practitioners who had their remedies made in-house, see for instance Pelling, *Medical Conflicts*, 240 n.

[22] Ashm. 208, fos. 78–93^{v}. Parts of a rough copy, and parts of another fair copy of this text in Forman's hand are bound in Ashm. 1486, fos. 7–11, 12–20. Some of these pages are damaged.

[23] For the early edns. see J. R. Partington, *A History of Chemistry*, ii (1961), 156. Thomas Robson dated his English copy of the text 1575, the year of the Latin publication: Ashm. 1418, iii, fos. 17–30. Ashmole in turn copied Robson's text: Ashm. 1459, fos. 136–61^{v}. Robson also copied Forman's 'Of cako', without noting the similarities between it and the Suchten text: Ashm. 1421, fos. 29–34^{v}. I have not compared Forman's text with other extant English versions in the Sloane Collection, the Hartlib Papers, or the Library of the Royal College of Physicians. For a later, printed translation see Alexander von Suchten, *Of the secrets of antimony: In two treatises* (1670).

[24] Newman and Principe, *Alchemy Tried in the Fire*, 50–6.

[25] Most notably in *The triumphal chariot of antimony*, a work attributed to a 15th-cent Benedictine monk, Basil Valentine, but written much later and first printed in 1599. For the suggestion that this work was indebted to Suchten, see John Read, *Prelude to Chemistry: An Outline of Alchemy, its Literature and Relationships* (Cambridge, Mass., 1966 [1936]), 187. For further discussion of works attributed to Basil Valentine, see Principe, *Aspiring Adept.* Antimony has featured throughout most studies of early modern alchemy, e.g. Dobbs, *Foundations of Newton's Alchemy*, and it, and Suchten's influence, are receiving increasing attention in studies of the chymical experiments of Starkey, Boyle, and Newton: William Newman, *Gehennical Fire*, 135–41; Newman and Principe, *Alchemy Tried in the Fire.*

8.1. Simon Forman's copy of 'Of cako', an anonymized and altered version of Alexander von Suchten's 'Second treatise on antimony', Ashm. 208, fo. 78. By permission of the Bodleian Library, University of Oxford.

advocated its medical use while many traditional physicians denounced it. The debates reached a crisis in 1566 when the Faculty of Medicine in Paris forbade the internal uses of antimony.[26] According to some Paracelsians, antimony contained salt, sulphur, and mercury, the three constituents of all things.[27] It could be applied topically or taken as a purge; and it could be used to make a form of *aurum potabile*, a panacea central to English alchemical debates early in the seventeenth century.

Francis Anthony (1550–1623) was internationally renowned for his potable gold and in 1598 he and the College of Physicians debated the legitimacy of his methods in the College's chambers and in print.[28] Antimony was also a problem for the College and they encountered several practitioners who administered it, particularly in the 1610s, but it became most controversial in the 1630s and 1640s with the case of John Evans, best known as William Lilly's astrological tutor.[29] Evans's *The universall medicine* (1635) promoted a 'new' method for taking antimony, an antimonial cup that conferred its properties to wine and prompted gentle purgations of 'preternatural' humours. The first edition of the work was burnt by the College at the instruction of the archbishop of Canterbury, and the 1642 edition included endorsements of Evans's methods from numerous physicians, gentlemen, and others, including Richard Napier, who noted that it was at times useful, 'Although I needed not by reason of my long practice and moch experience, seek out the experiments of new Medicines'.[30] James Primrose, a member of the College, challenged Evans's claims while upholding the purgative virtues of antimony and other chemical remedies. Evans's cup, Primrose argued, was made from the regulus of antimony sold by apothecaries though it should have been made from stibium, its shape was a mere token of its efficacy, and it was overpriced; Evans was a quack who had misread his sources and exaggerated the authenticity and novelty of his methods.[31]

Forman thought he was copying an old treatise on cako, not a modish text

[26] Allen Debus, *The French Paracelsians: The Chemical Challenge to Medical and Scientific Tradition in Early Modern France* (Cambridge, 1991), 21–6, 46–101.

[27] Duchesne, *Chymicall physic*, sig. I1^{v}.

[28] Debus, *English Paracelsians*, 142–5. Anthony consulted Forman on 18 Sept. 1599, though it is unclear how well they knew each other: Ashm. 219, fo. 155.

[29] Lilly, *Life*, 31. Debus, *English Paracelsians*, 170; Pelling, *Medical Conflicts*, 69 n. The College first accused an 'empiric' of using metallic remedies in 1569: Webster, 'Alchemical and Paracelsian Medicine', 324–5. See also the case of Peter Piers, accused in 1587 of using an antimony pill: Pelling, *Medical Conflicts*, 312 n.

[30] Evans, *Universall medicine*, sig. C3. On the medicinal uses of minerals prior to Paracelsus, see Robert Multhauf, 'Medical Chemistry and the Paracelsians', *Bulletin of the History of Medicine*, 28 (1954), 101–25.

[31] James Primrose, *The communal antimonial cup wide cast, or a treatise concerning the antimonial cup* (1640), esp. pp. 2, 4, 11, 31.

on antimony. Its author was simply identified as 'authoris incogniti' and where Suchten's treatise referred to antimony, Forman's 'Of cako' referred to cako. I have not located this word in other versions of Suchten's text, nor in other alchemical works, though a contemporary work, 'A treatise on cachelah', circulated amongst people associated with Dee's circle in the 1580s and 1590s and probably related to the manuscript that Forman copied.[32] The word 'cako' derived from the Hebrew 'kochav', meaning star, perhaps indicating the star regulus of antimony.[33]

In addition to anonymizing the treatise and substituting cako for antimony, the text that Forman copied had been subjected to two major alterations. Variant introductions and conclusions framed it, launching the discussion of cako with the florid language typical of medieval alchemical texts, perhaps drawing on an older source in describing the life and death of cako. Suchten's original text, in contrast, began with an epistle that stressed that he would write about common antimony in a plain style, describe the manual operations for preparing antimony, and leave it to the reader to decide if this was the medicinal arcanum of which the old magi and Paracelsus had written.[34] Forman's text concluded with a lengthy section headed 'Opus magnum', again in florid language, containing more preparations for cako. Finally, the references to Paracelsus had been omitted from Forman's copy, though the attacks on 'Galenists' were preserved. Suchten's 'Second treatise on antimony' had become an anonymous treatise on a mysterious substance, subsumed within an older alchemical tradition.

Forman's tastes in alchemical texts were unrefined and his transcriptions informed more by happenstance than deliberation. He copied texts reputedly ancient and modern, English and Arabic, transmutational, medical, and spiritual. 'Of cako' explicitly praised the medicinal virtues of alchemical preparations. When cako (crude antimony in Suchten's text) was taken from the mine, the author (Suchten) explained, it needed to be purged and cleansed in a series of four operations in order to reduce or mature it into progressively purer

[32] Kendal, Cumbrian Record Office, MS WD Hothman 5, fos. 77–95, cited in Penny Bayer, 'Women's Alchemical Literature 1560–1616 in Italy, France, the Swiss Cantons and England, and its Diffusion to 1660', Ph.D. thesis, University of Warwick, 2003, 225.

[33] Forman noted that 'Cakob in hebrue is asmoch to say, mercury and Cakos in greke is asmoch to say crud or rawe indigested Antimony as yt coms newly out of the earth or myne', though this passage follows various accounts of the relationships between antimony, stibnite, and mercury (Suchten often called the regulus of antimony its mercury): Ashm. 1494, pp. 52^{v}–53. This word probably does not relate to the Greek 'caco', meaning bad, and commonly used as a prefix in early modern English to designate an ill use or effect, such as in cacochymist, cacodemon, cacophony: *OED*. I am indebted to David Katz, William Newman, and Peter Forshaw for advice about this word.

[34] Ashm. 1418, iii, fo. 17^{r-v}.

substances, and ultimately into gold. In a section on 'what medicine ther is in vulgar Cako' he noted that, although many men had prepared antimony and used it in medicines, none had perceived its medicinal secret. This was because the antimony of physicians was not the same thing as the antimony of philosophers (i.e. alchemists):

For in the cako of philosophers ar all the medicins potentiall and for that cause it is called quintessence. But in the Cako vulgar is not the quintessence medicinalle but the elemente and the matter only of the Quintessence. The which essence is a medison againste all diseases which proceed of the fier of the lyttle wordle.

An analogy elucidated this:

Ther is a fier within the wood, which we must have in our kytchens for to dress our meate. Soe ther is a fier in Cako, by which we dresse our medison, the which by it receyveth the essence, and by the same essence extinguishethe the elementalle heate in our diseases.

The cako of physicians was an ordinary and crude substance, philosophical cako rendered substances medicinal, purifying them, making them essential, and an essential substance restored health.

This was contrary to the practices of Galenic physicians. They did not believe in the virtue of purity and were forever combining substances in juleps and masking their natures with honey. Furthermore, the alchemist differed from the Galenist in his theory of medicine: 'The Gallienestes doe boaste them selves to doe awai the heate [of diseases] with endive and poppie and nightshade and with other cold simples, which they cannot doe, unlesse the heat doe naturally cease of it self.'[35] The virtue of preparing medicines with cako was that it caused the body to purify itself by the natural means of sweating, not by altering the balance of the humours with purges or emetics.[36] In these passages Suchten described the composition of the body from the constituents of salt, sulphur, and mercury; correlated these substances with the liver, heart, and brain; and stressed the importance of opening and enforcing the virtues of these organs with restoratives and expulsives. These were tenets of Paracelsian medicine.[37]

Forman signalled the importance of cako in the verse preface to 'Principles of philosofi', his *c.*1597 alchemical commonplace book. In allegorical language

[35] Ashm. 208, fo. 83^{v}. [36] Ashm. 208, fo. 83.

[37] Pagel, *Paracelsus*; Massimo Bianchi, 'The Visible and the Invisible: From Alchemy to Paracelsus', in Piyo Rattansi and Antonio Clericuzio (eds.), *Alchemy and Chemistry in the Sixteenth and Seventeenth Centuries* (Dordrecht, 1994), 17–50.

typical of alchemical poems, Cako played a leading role.[38] Forman also included an entry for cako in this volume, incorporating 'Of cako' within it. I will refer to 'Of cako' as Text A and the entry for cako in 'Principles of philosofi' as Text B.[39] Forman also altered 'Of cako' as he transcribed it, replacing the opening section of Text A with a more lucid definition:

Of this Cako coms the great secreate of philosophers. For from Cako commeth Regulus, and well yt may be called soe for yt ruleth and governeth all the reste. For by this regulus is drawen forth the Sulfur of all mettalls apt to the philosophers stone, and with out the which yt cannot be done.

Forman then, perhaps referring to the opaque description at the beginning of Text A, explained that the secret of cako was transmitted by tradition from generation to generation, not in texts. When it had been written about, endless tropes had been used to obscure it from posterity. He knew this through his own experience:

I cam to the knowledge therof and with my owne handes and eyes. I sawe and proved the experience ther of at my owne coste and charges secretly. For yt was the will of god yt should be soe. For in all my practizes and workings I never came to any knowledge, but only by the will of god and by my owne industry & coste. Neither had I any frinds that ever gave me 40s. in all my life. Not that they could not—but because they wold not, but put me to live and shifte for my selfe when I was but 12 years old. Yet when they all forsoke me for that I was soe moch bent to my bocke—god toke me to his grace, and delivered me from hunger penury and mysery, and from imprisoments sclanders death & sicknes, and from infinit of other trobles and from many enimies which wer very mightie and strong as from Lawiars Councellors Justics Judges bishops and many others.[40]

Forman signed his name at the bottom of this passage. He also altered Text A by removing the final section headed 'Opus magnum' and omitting passages that he had interjected in his initial copy, thereby effacing the traces of his reading of the text. In other words, Text B is almost the same as Text A except Forman presented himself as its author.

A second major alteration was the introduction of a section of 'notes' which sympathized with the anti-Galenic sentiments in Suchten's text and

[38] Ashm. 1472, fo. 6, e.g.: 'And Mars in Cako his Musick doth sounde | And diana [silver] also and none but shee | doth seperate Cako with mercurie | for when saturne mars hath plaied his parte | and in strivinge with Cako hath lefte his harte | dyana to seperate and set them aparte | Conjoyneth with Cako to enter this arte | Agreing to gether like man and wife | Till ☿ passeth and endeth the strife | And 3 in on doth then agre | And with ☿ from ☾ awaie doth flee | Caryinge with him bothe Cako and mars . . .'

[39] Ashm. 1472, pp. 200–[11].

[40] Ashm. 1472, p. 200. Cf. the 'on simple fellow' discussed above, p. 57.

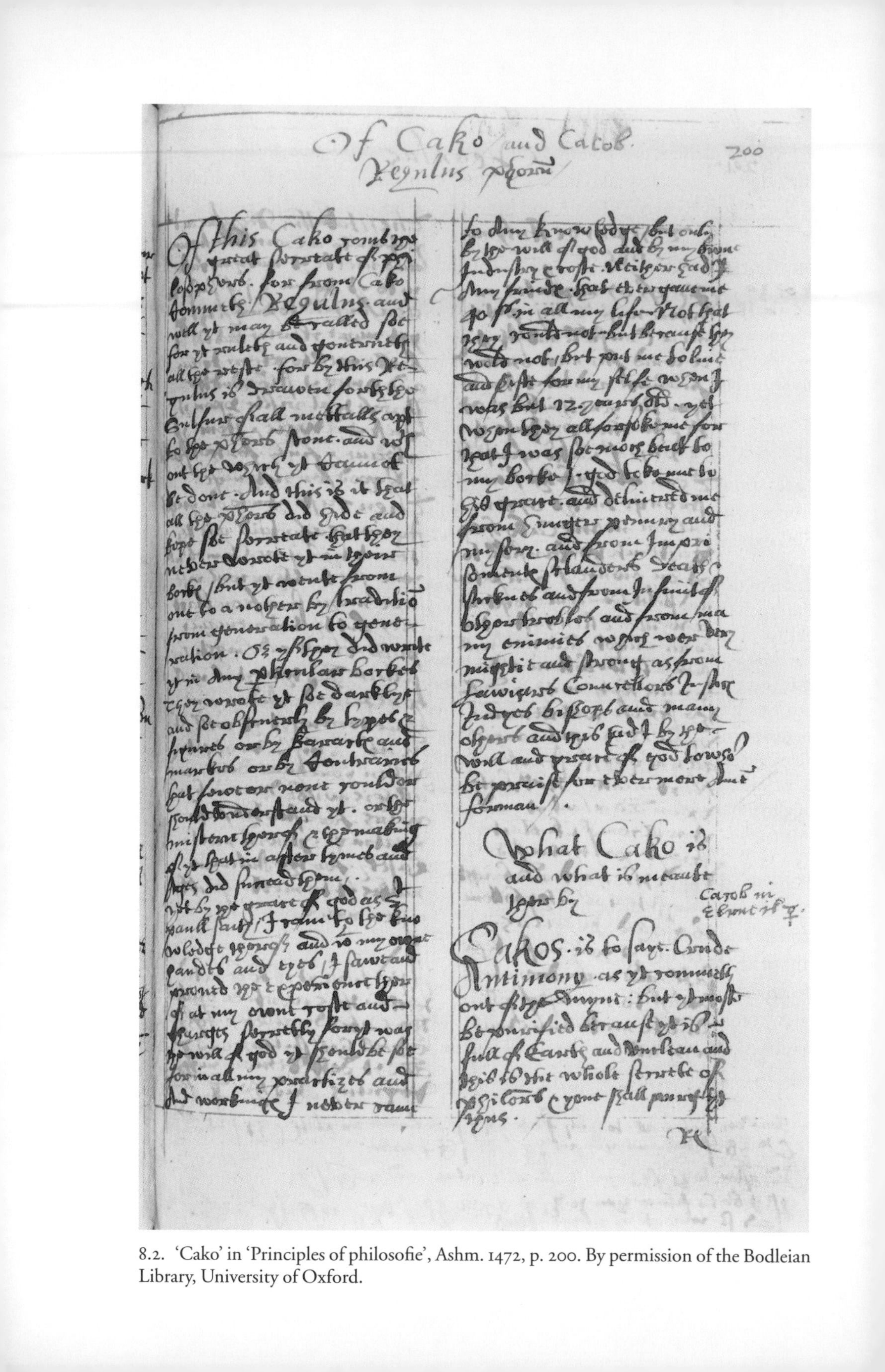

8.2. 'Cako' in 'Principles of philosofie', Ashm. 1472, p. 200. By permission of the Bodleian Library, University of Oxford.

embellished a discussion of philosophical medicine with an account of the vital principles of all things in nature. Forman described how the life of a substance could be revived, 'of and in the multiplication of the forme and not of the matter of mettalls': 'for all the mistery of nature doth issue out of on fountaine & ar on essence, but miraculosly severed, according to the will of god, the which is a specifica of all his creatures which is not comprehensible more then god is'.[41] No dead thing could be raised without the addition of this soul, and anyone who taught to the contrary was not a complete philosopher.[42]

And yt followeth that in a lyving thinge ther be a nature & fashion of the thinge which should be raised again. For yt is the will of god that all things shall dye and that is the specifick of nature, the which after the death is multiplied infinitly. For his mortalytie doth put one ymmortallity and his corruption doth put one incorruption and his mortall body after his resurrection, is becom a glorified body able to give life to ded things . . .[43]

He elucidated this with an organic metaphor:

As youe see that a grain caste into the earth is made quicke by the water, vz that in the grain is a ded water by which the water becommeth again a lyvinge water and it is a ferment of waters. Vz. yt giveth to the water his nature specifick, thus of on[e] grain then groweth other infinite. So moste youe understand in this worke the ☿ of cako in ♄ was his death . . .[44]

Perhaps unwittingly, it seems, Forman restored the vitalist, Paracelsian dimensions of this text while deliberately strengthening its anti-Galenic sentiments and presenting himself as its author.

Forman copied this text again, this time into 'Of appoticarie druges', his *c.*1607 commonplace book, and again he transformed it. Although in Text A the word cako directly replaced antimony, there is no evidence in Texts A or B that Forman equated these substances; indeed at times Forman seems confused. For instance, Suchten's version of this text explained the process of purifying crude antimony into the regulus of antimony, while Text A described the same sequence in terms of changing cako into regulus.[45] Then in Text B Forman replaced this passage with an account of changing cako into antimony, then regulus, evidently in an attempt to relate cako and antimony.[46] Moreover, 'Principles of philosofi' included separate entries for cako and antimony,

41 Ashm. 1472, pp. 206, [205].

42 Ashm. 1472, p. [205]. In a later version Forman extended this stipulation to include divines, physicians, and astrologers as well as philosophers: Ashm. 1494, p. 56ᵛ.

43 Ashm. 1472, p. [205]. This is elaborated on in Ashm. 1494, p. 59.

44 Ashm. 1472, p. 206.

45 Ashm. 1418, iii, fo. 17ᵛ; 208, fo. 78. Forman did not specify that this was the regulus of antimony.

46 Ashm. 1472, p. 200.

neither mentioning the other, while 'Of appoticarie druges' combined this material under the entry for antimony (Text C).[47] Here Forman subsumed and revised Text B, noting that from antimony was made cako, and from cako, regulus, thus reversing the relationship between antimony and cako as described in Text B.[48]

The progression from 'Of cako' to the entry on antimony in 'Of appoticarie druges' was as follows: in the first stage Forman copied an anonymous text, while adding notes of his experiments (Text A); in the second stage he recopied the text, altered it so that he appeared to be its author, and added a section on philosophical medicine (Text B); in the third stage he reclassified cako under the entry for antimony, though he continued to define them as distinct substances (Text C). Somehow Suchten's treatise had been stripped of its author and dressed up as a medieval text. Forman appropriated its expertise, and unaware of its provenance from the pen of a prominent Paracelsian physician, he modernized it, infusing it with a vitalism typical of Paracelsian texts and strengthening its anti-Galenic sentiments. Later, perhaps drawing on his own experience, he rectified his apparent confusion about the substances of antimony and cako.

Forman copied, appropriated, and revised 'Of cako' throughout the pages of his commonplace books because his alchemical pursuits were informed by Paracelsian doctrines and practices. Paracelsian alchemy provided a cosmology to explain the processes of disease and healing and the practices to effect a cure, combining philosophical (meaning alchemical) and medicinal information. Mercury prepared with strong water, Forman explained, produced 'perfect ☉ good for all workes of the gould smithes and other imperfecte bodies, but not for mans body'.[49] Instructions for how to dissolve gold in strong water specified that the product 'is holsom for the bodie and for phisick or to putrifie and make ferment for the stone or to make aurum potabile therof'.[50] Similarly, some sorts of vinegar were used for cooking, some for philosophy, and some for

47 Ashm. 1472, pp. 136–[41]; 1494, pp. 52–70. The incorporated text begins on fo. 53. Ashm. 1430 does not contain entries for antimony or cako. These entries for antimony do not incorporate Forman's earlier notes on stibium, 'a certain kind of poisone in his kinde, and some saie yt is made of antimonie': Sloane 3822, fo. 115.

48 Ashm. 1494, p. 53. It is clear that the notes on cako in 'Of appoticarie druges' (Text C) were copied from Text B and not Text A because the marginal notes in Text B were subsumed directly into Text C. In Text C there was a recipe for the oil of antimony which did not appear in Text B, but which was in the section on antimony in 'Principles of philosofi': Ashm. 1494, p. 67; 1472, p. [137]. Forman made two significant changes between Texts B and C, changing the sequence of recipes and inserting a drawing of the 'altitude of antimony', a figure of a man with various properties described in the margins around him: Ashm. 1494, pp. 63, 57^v (sic). Forman recorded his name and the year 1607 at the end of this entry: Ashm. 1494, p. 64.

49 Ashm. 1494, p. 239^v, following Raymond Lully.

50 Ashm. 1494, p. 136.

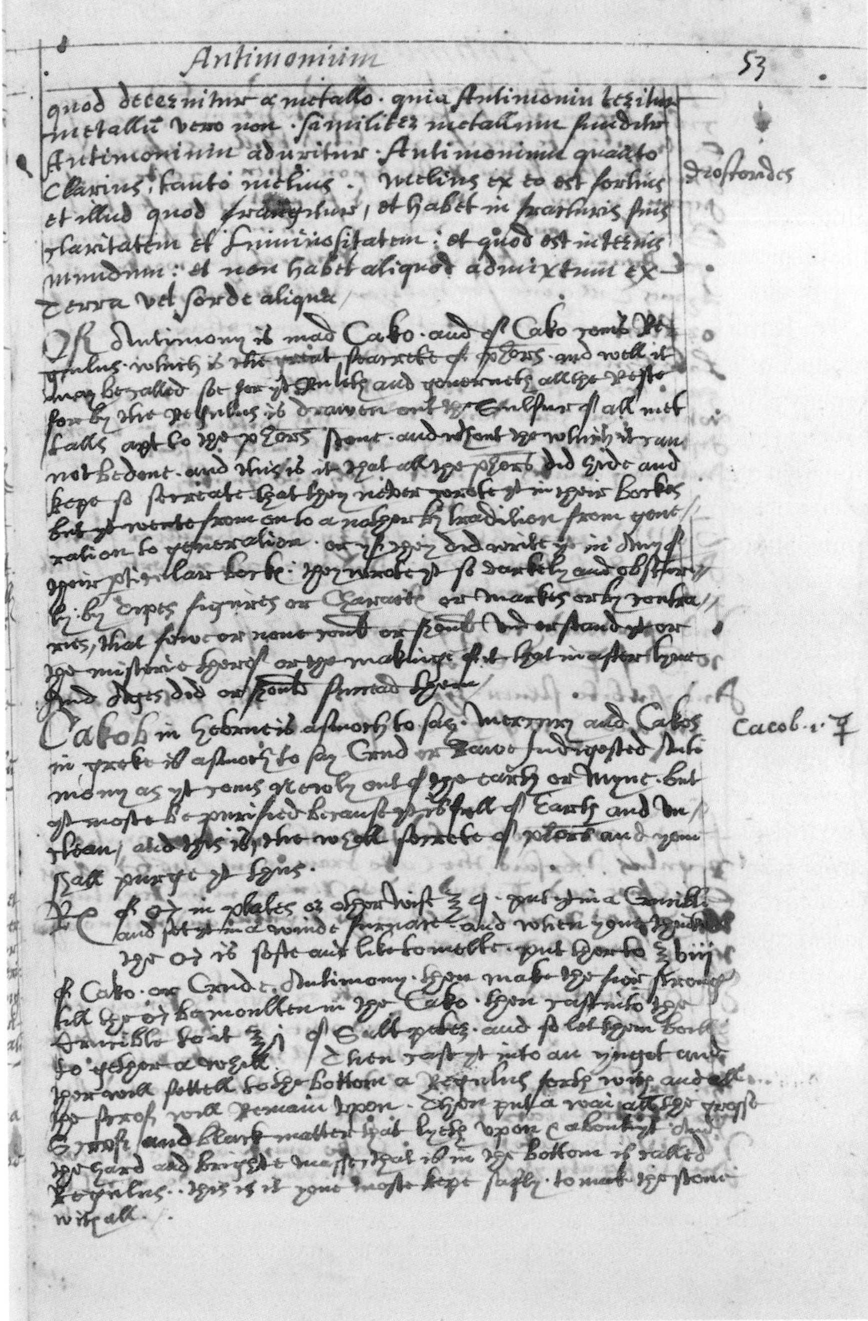

Antimonium 53

quod decernitur a metallo. quia Antimonium texitur metallum vero non. similiter metallum funditur Antimonium aduritur. Antimonium quanto clarius, tanto melius. melius ex eo est fortius et illud quod frangitur, et habet in fracturis suis claritatem et luminositatem: et quod est internis mundum: et non habet aliquod admixtum ex terra vel sorde aliqua/ Dioscorides

Of Antimony is mad Cako. and of Cako com the regulus which is the most secret of stones [illegible]

Cakob in Hebrew is as much to say [illegible] Cacob. 1. 7

[illegible]

8.3. 'Antimony' in 'Of appoticarie druges', Ashm. 1494, p. 53. By permission of the Bodleian Library, University of Oxford.

medicine.[51] Honey could be used to dress wounds, sweeten food, or make syrups, as apothecaries did, and its quintessence would dissolve gold, iron, and other hard metals.[52] But the 'saffron of iron', or crocus of Mars (iron), crokefer, was not 'allowed' in the art of philosophy though Forman included it as an ingredient in a remedy against the green sickness.[53] The entry for antimony in 'Of appoticarie druges' contained various procedures to refine it for both philosophical and medicinal purposes, including an elaborate recipe to make the oil of antimony into a sweet, red, potable powder which taken in a dose of two or three grains 'will serve againste all extreme sicknes'.[54]

For Forman antimony was not a singular remedy, nor remedies the singular product of alchemy. His study of cako and antimony illustrates the heterogeneity of his alchemical pursuits, combining doctrines and practices old and new, chymical, magical, and medicinal. 'Of appoticarie druges' was the culmination of this process of collection and compilation and preserves Forman's doctrinal and practical eclecticism. His sources were diverse, ranging from the tomes of Andreas Libavius and Oswald Croll to less weighty items such as *The secretes of the reverende Maister Alexis of Piemont* and 'an old writen bocke'.[55] He gathered information by word of mouth, such as the various preparations that one Henry King had given to an unnamed friend.[56] Someone called Grant and Mr and Mrs Young informed him about chemical preparations, Mr Coxen and Mr Corkesdean advised him about gardening, and he watched Bromall make a verdigris that looked like gold.[57] A man called Simon helped him to preserve roses and he instructed Willian Cassan in how to make artificial pearls. From Cassan in turn Forman learnt about a mercurial preparation that purged upwards and downwards and was good against the pox and 'depe diseases'.[58] Elsewhere Forman noted that he had heard about a man who had found three buried chests of lead, and that he 'made such frindes that I gote the quantity of one drame thereof and it loked like browne clay dried hard'. He tested it by

51 Ashm. 1494, pp. 168–72.

52 Ashm. 1494, p. 544.

53 Ashm. 1494, p. 395. A yellow or red powder obtained from calcinations, *OED*.

54 Ashm. 1494, p. 67. See also p. 62 for other medicinal recipes.

55 Ashm. 1491, p. 871; 1494, p. 174 (Libavius); 1491, p. 918 (Croll); 1494, p. 116; 1491, pp. 1131–3 (Alexis); 1491, p. 834 (old book). Forman was probably citing Libavius' *Alchemia* (Frankfurt, 1597) and Croll's *Basilica chymica* (Frankfurt, 1609). Except on the occasions where Forman specified a page or folio reference, it is difficult to be certain which edn. he was using. For references to knowledge of dyers, curriers, metalworkers, cooks, masons, soldiers, painters, scriveners, surgeons, etc. see Ashm. 1494, pp. 116, 123, 130, 138–9, 156, 220–31, 402, 413, 422, 455–9, 504, 514, 570–2, 636–40; 1491, pp. 910, 1140, 1146, 1131–3, 1208, 1210, 1294–7, 1366–7, 1386–7.

56 Ashm. 1494, pp. 284, 337–40.

57 Ashm. 1494 and 1491, pp. [147] (Grant); 446, 424, 493 (Youngs); 1073 (Coxen); 1084 (Corkesdean); 1285 (Bromall).

58 Ashm. 1494 and 1491, pp. [94^{v}], 870 (Casson); 861 (Simon).

taste, reporting that it was gritty, neither sweet nor salty, and made the roof of his mouth itch.[59] For some ingredients he recommended the apothecaries, for others, such as the hard iron supplied by 'the needlemaker at bartholomewe lane end ner the exchange and I have yt for 3d a pound', he directed the reader elsewhere.[60]

Most of the entries for the major minerals included medicinal applications, and many of the references to purges were drawn from Tymme's 1605 translation of Duchesne's works. Duchesne outlined 'the knowledge of the internal anatomy of things' and 'the assured science of their beginnings', combining traditional and innovative methods to restore the true composition of medicine.[61] All things, he explained, whether animal, vegetable, or mineral, had three beginnings, salt, sulphur, and mercury.[62] According to this principle some substances worked to open the flow of vital spirits and restore the health of the body. Forman followed Duchesne's expositions and remedies. The best purgations were made from mercurial substances, including antimony and the loadstone, because they were so corpulent and gross.[63] Philosophical salts had their beginnings in salt, sulphur, and mercury; 'Salte is necessary for the Cueringe of dyverse diseases for yt hath vertue to clense to open to cut and to make thin, and to move sweets & to farder urin & to provoke vomit.'[64] Less philosophically, Forman noted Duchesne's description of a purgative pill that could be reused for twenty years, each time passing through the body intact.[65]

Forman also included a diverse range of non-mineral preparations in 'Of appoticarie druges', perhaps because the three mineral constituents were present in all things, but probably because he was collecting information without recourse to a philosophical rationale. For instance, Forman specified an extensive list of herbal remedies against the scurvy; the extraordinary powers of mistletoe that grew on oak trees to heal diseases, protect its bearer, and compel spirits; and ypocras, a mulled wine which was a variation on 'Dr Steavens water'.[66] Vinegar was a corrective to opium, and if a medicine had caused too much purging, vomiting, or sleeping, the effects could be reversed by rubbing vinegar on the palms of the hands and the soles of the feet.[67] In other cases

59 Ashm. 392, p. 576. This was 14 Apr. 1608.

60 Ashm. 1494, pp. 491^{v}, 624, 1235.

61 Duchesne, *Chymicall physicke*, sigs. M3^{v}, Z2^{r-v}.

62 Ibid., sigs. B3, J1^{v}, T3^{v}, P4^{v}.

63 Ashm. 1491, pp. 1124–8; Duchesne, *Chymicall physicke*, sigs. L4–M1.

64 Ashm. 1491, p. 1036; cf. Duchesne, *Chymicall physicke*, sig. E4.

65 Ashm. 1491, p. 864. See also p. 1176 on the use of the cream of tartar in 'purgative physic' and Ashm. 1494, p. 158 for a note about the bitter salt found in the galls of animals that purges wonderfully, following Duchesne, *Chymicall physicke*, sigs. M2^{v}, U3.

66 Ashm. 1491, pp. 1088–96, 1278–80, 1346.

67 Ashm. 1494, p. 168.

Forman drew more on magical than alchemical traditions, such as 'If you anoint a leper such as on as was begotten on a woman when she had her course with the menstrues of a viergin or young woman clear from infirmities he shalbe healed'.[68] Similarly, to cure someone who was frantic, put some of his or her blood into an egg shell, bury it for a month, mix it with porridge, feed it to a pig or dog, thereby transferring the disease to the animal, then kill it.[69] Various substances conferred powers when used externally. For instance, electrum

was good againste poison, vessells or rings being made therof, and against Enchantments and witchcraft and against sprites. A ringe made herof and worne of the harte finger, helpeth the cramps, launces and falling evill, also yf a man were such a ringe, yt changeth his collour yf any sicknes or evill be towards the man.[70]

A sort of white iron could be 'buried for a certain space in a vessell either of wine or milk, yt remedieth diseases in the splene'.[71] St John's wort (hypericon) worked against haunting and frenzy if worn around the neck.[72] Some varieties of the ashes, or calces, of plants and animals, following Pliny, Aetius, and Aegineta, as cited in Duchesne, could be used for a host of medicinal purposes.[73]

Forman gathered this information and he put some of it into practice. He compiled extensive notes on ♄ (lead), recording its power to nourish and 'encreaseth the blod in man & vitall & vegitable poer in man, destroieth the leprosie, palsie, gout, and all naturalle diseases caused of ♄ naturally', and noting 'To drawe the salte of ♄ as I my selfe did it 1607'.[74] He recorded various methods to make an oil of gold, or *aurum potabile*, which 'healeth all manner of diseases in man whatsoever and Encreaseth youth and reneweth a mans age'.[75] One method was to dissolve it in salt and salt petre, a recipe that Napier admired in the margin; Forman specified what then needed to be done to this if it were to be used for the 'health of mans body'.[76] He also recorded another method:

I have used to quentch the beste gould red hote in the beste Clarret wine and to give yt to drink to weke sick persons in many notable diseases. Quentch it 50 tymes, and drink a good draughgt therof every dais 7 or eight days togther, and the gold will be soft and pliable like wax . . .[77]

[68] Ashm. 1491, p. 738. Forman attributed this to himself.
[69] Ashm. 1494, p. 184.
[70] Ashm. 1494, pp. 483–4.
[71] Ashm. 1491, p. 491ᵛ. Forman cited John Maplet's *A greene forest, or a naturall historie* (1567) as his source.
[72] Ashm. 1494, p. 568.
[73] Ashm. 1494, pp. 349–50; Duchesne, *Chymicall physicke*, sig. A4ᵛ.
[74] Ashm. 1491, pp. 955, 970.
[75] Ashm. 1494, p. 153. The definition of the oil of gold as *aurum potabile* appears on p. 145. See also p. [139].
[76] Ashm. 1494, pp. [145]–6.
[77] Ashm. 1494, p. 123, repeated on pp. 124, 135.

In 1610 Forman made a medicine for himself that included coral, amber, and pearl.[78] In 1606 Sir Michael Sands had told him about a fool who had eaten a snake, lost his hair, recovered it, and become wise and wealthy. A couple of years later Forman did 'boill 2 snakes in my strong water when I distilled it. And after I drank that water and yt made me loke fresh and toke away all my gray hairs when I was 56 years old and many toke me not to be above 40 or 42.'[79] Forman also included an elaborate recipe for metheglyn, a spiced, medicinal mead made with honey, and for *rosa solis*, a cordial made with aniseed, liquorice, raisins, figs, cinnamon, cloves, etc.[80] He stressed that he had made this often, and 'yt digesteth and consumeth all reumatick humors & encreaseth and strengthneth nature yt helps digestion healeth the lyver and is good against a cold stomach and breketh winde & comfortethe the wholl bodye.'[81]

Through Forman's appropriation of Suchten's treatise on antimony, and through the traces of his medicinal practices in 'Of appoticarie druges', I have begun to recover the alchemical components of Forman's medicine. His pursuit of chymical remedies was textual and practical, local and international, old and new. 'Of appoticarie druges' embodied his engagement with numerous alchemical, natural historical, medical, and magical traditions, tacitly guided by a Paracelsian programme for the reform of medicinal preparations.

[78] Ashm. 1491, p. 942. [79] Ashm. 1491, p. 938. [80] Ashm. 1491, pp. 684, 944.
[81] For Napier's copy of this recipe see Ashm. 1488, fo. 275.

9
The Food of Angels

Nine hundred years after Adam and Eve were expelled from Paradise, Adam lay on his deathbed, called his numerous children before him, and told them the story of the Fall. Because he and Eve had eaten the forbidden fruit, God had expelled them from the Garden and proclaimed that they and their offspring would suffer seventy diseases from the crowns of their heads to the soles of their feet forevermore. Genesis did not record this part of the story, but the 'Vita Adae et Evae', or 'Life of Adam and Eve' (hereafter the 'Life'), did. This was part of a tradition of pseudoepigraphical texts collectively known as the Book of Adam and Eve, dating from between the first and third centuries AD.[1] Versions of the 'Life' circulated throughout medieval and early modern Europe, in Latin and the vernacular, and in 1599 Forman transcribed and augmented an English version of it.[2]

Forman's copy of the 'Life' is unique. Versions of this text, in English and Latin, survive from the late fourteenth and fifteenth centuries, and it probably circulated widely in sixteenth-century England, but Forman's copy is the only known sixteenth-century example of English origin, in English or Latin.[3] The first part (A) recounts the creation of Adam, then Eve, and their expulsion from Paradise. This section is not present in the standard Latin version of the 'Life'.

[1] H. F. D. Sparks (ed.), *The Apocryphal Old Testament* (Oxford, 1984), 141–67 and R. H. Charles (ed.), *The Apocrypha and Pseudoepigrapha of the Old Testament in English* (Oxford, 1913), 123–54. Recent scholarship on this text has been summarized by Michael E. Stone, *A History of the Literature of Adam and Eve* (Baltimore, Md., 1994).

[2] Ashm. 802, ii. I follow the title used by modern scholars. Forman's earlier interest in Adam and Eve is documented in his 'Argument between Forman and death' (1585), which concluded with details about Adam and Eve being in Paradise for seven hours, and with the Fall creating death: Ashm. 208, fo. 248.

[3] On medieval copies see M. E. B. Halford, 'The Apocryphal Vita Adae et Evae: Some Comments on the Manuscript Tradition', *Neuphilologische Mitteilungen*, 82 (1981), 417–27; J. H. Mozley, 'The "Vita Adae"', *Journal of Theological Studies*, 30 (1929), 121–49. The English versions are as follows: Bodleian, Bodley MS 596 is a prose version of the late 14th or early 15th cent.; Trinity R.3.21, fos. 249–57, is virtually identical to Bodley MS 596 (and was owned by John Stowe); BL Additional MS 35298, fos. 162–5, is also in prose; Oxford, Trinity College MS 57, fo. 157^{v} is in verse. Early modern MSS on biblical themes are difficult to locate except in well-catalogued collections. There are numerous 16th-cent. copies of the 'Life' on the Continent: Stone, *Literature of Adam and Eve*, 9. The 'Life' was printed in Latin in the late 15th cent. and in 1518. For suggestions that the 'Life' circulated widely in 16th-century England see Sparks, *Apocryphal Old Testament*, 143; Charles, *Apocrypha and Pseudoepigrapha*, 124; Halford, 'Apocryphal Vita Adae et Evae', 417. For current research on the 'Life' see Gary A. Anderson and Michael E. Stone, <http://www.iath.virginia.edu/anderson/>.

The fifteenth-century versions of English provenance began with the creation of Adam and Eve, but did not contain as much detail as Forman's text.[4] The remaining sections of Forman's text are consistent with the other English and Latin versions. The second part (B) 'showeth what became of Adam after he was caste out of paradice'. The third and final part (C) narrates 'Howe Adam calleth together all his children and enformeth them of many things, and also telleth them that he is nere his death'.[5] Here Forman's version contained elaborate details about the afflictions that man and woman had suffered since the Fall and listed the diseases by name. In all cases except one, Forman's text had more detail than either the English or Latin versions.[6]

Forman not only copied the 'Life', he read it closely.[7] This is evident from his marginal notes, in this case interjections extracted from one text and aligned with another. The majority of these annotations concerned either the genealogy of knowledge or the nature of Adam and Eve before the Fall, and I will consider each in turn. Forman wrote these marginalia by leafing through and juxtaposing pages in the 'Life' and numerous other texts, many of which were alchemical. The result was a conglomeration of ideas about the creation of the world and the macrocosm–microcosm analogy with a Paracelsian emphasis on the causes of disease.

Forman read the 'Life' as a history of disease and healing and filled its margins with mythical details about the genealogy of knowledge. The 'Life' described how after the Fall Adam and Eve had lost the knowledge of how to nourish themselves and became hungry and ill; then 'god did replenishe him [Adam] with all kinds of wisdom Arte and Conninge and in the Science of Astrologie and knoweledg of the stars'. Next to this passage, Forman noted that

[4] Forman's text closely resembles two 15th-cent. MSS of the 'Life', Bodley MS 596 and Trinity R.3.21, and he was probably copying a related MS. Moreover, the way in which Forman ruled his text with wide margins, rubricated it, and wrote in a upright hand, might indicate that he was mimicking a 15th-century MS. For details on the creation of Adam and Eve in other versions of the 'Life' see Halford, 'Apocryphal Vita Adae et Evae', 420 n.; S. Harrison Thomson, 'A Fifth Recension of the Latin "Vita Ade et Eve"', *Studi medievali*, NS 6 (1933), 271–8; Sparks, *Apocryphal Old Testament*, 161 n. A tradition, known as the Arundel class, of English MSS has these details at the end, including descriptions of the eight substances out of which Adam was made, and his naming after the four cardinal points: Halford, 'Apocryphal Vita Adae et Evae', 419; Stone, *Literature of Adam and Eve*, 17.

[5] I have divided Ashm. 802, ii into the following sections: A, fos. 1–8^{v}; B, fos. 9–20; C, fos. 20–30.

[6] Forman's text does not contain Satan's description of his rebellion, 'Life', chs. 14, 15. This is present in the English versions and the Latin 'Life'.

[7] My discussion is restricted to a textual analysis of the 'Life'. This text demonstrates a recording and transforming of legendary elements, particularly aspects of the Holy Rood. There is some evidence that versions of the 'Life' persisted in Cornish Creation plays through the 16th cent. (Stone, *Literature of Adam and Eve*, 16), and John Aubrey seems to have suggested that Forman was involved in creation plays in Salisbury: 'My grandfather Lyte told me that at his Lord Maier's shew there was the representation of the creation of the world, and writ underneath, "and all for man."' Aubrey, *Natural history of Wiltshire*, 79.

the angel Raziel gave Adam a book of astronomy and magic, and he described more angelic books alongside details of the trials of Adam and Eve after the Fall.[8] Solomon discovered these books:

> When Cabrymael the Angell byd him [Solomon] loke secretly in the Arke of the testament of god in the which he found all the boockes of Moyeses and Aron, and the bocks of Noah and of Jerimy and of the other profets the which Sallomon had long tyme sought for, and therin alsoe he found the boock which was called Raziel, the which god gave unto Adam, by the Angell Raziell, when Adam was dryven out of paradice. And he found also therin on another bocke named the Semiphoras which god alsoe gave unto Adam in paradice. And also he found therin another bocke that god gave unto Moyses in the Mounte Synay after Moises had fasted 40 dais & 40 nights. Therin did he find alsoe the rod of Moyses which was changed into a serpente and from a serpent again to a rod . . .[9]

This time capsule also contained the tablets on which the commandments were written, a square, golden table inlaid with fourteen precious stones, and a box inscribed with the seven names of God. Forman cited a variety of sources, including Josephus, Augustine, and the popular fifteenth-century world chronicle, Werner Rolevinck's *Fasciculus temporum*; perhaps he consulted these texts himself, or extracted references to them from the standard histories that prefaced magical and alchemical texts.[10]

The genealogy of knowledge was a common theme amongst alchemists. For instance, in a text that Forman transcribed and claimed to have corrected, Bernard of Trier explained that 'The firste inventers of this arte . . . was Hermes Trismegistus: for he made and composed the boocks of the 3 kinds of naturall philosophie, that is to say, vegitable, minerall & animall.'[11] Forman also copied a text by another medieval alchemist, Aegidius de Vadis, who conceded that God made 'the first mane Adam perfecte in all naturall things, and didest endue him with sufficient knowledge'. This knowledge was imparted to the rest of mankind throughout the ages, beginning with Bezaleel and Aholiab, the first metalworkers, endowed with the wisdom to build and furnish the tabernacle of the congregation of the Israelites.[12] Forman also collected information about the history of different types of the philosophers' stone. Conventionally it came in three sorts, animal, vegetable, and mineral. In 'Of appoticarie druges' Forman recorded a fourth type and defined each according to its history. Hermes had the animal, or angelic stone; Solomon had the

[8] Ashm. 802, ii, fo. 3^{v}. [9] Ashm. 802, ii, fo. 14^{r-v}.

[10] See also Ashm. 802, ii, fos. 15^{v}–16, 28^{v}, 29.

[11] Bernard of Trier, 'The most excellent and true booke', Ashm. 1490, fo. 222^{v}.

[12] 'A dialogue of Egidius de Vadius', Ashm. 1490, fos. 28–36^{v}; Exod. 31: 1–11.

vegetable, or growing stone; Lully, Ripley, and others had the mineral stone; and Moses had a magical, or prospective stone. Forman concluded, 'The angellical stone is true medison to mans bodie against all infirmities and makes a man live longe and by that stone he obteined wisdom and knowledge of thinges in dreams & otherwise.'[13] I will return to the magical and angelical stones below.

While Forman garnered details about the genealogy of alchemical knowledge, sixteenth-century authors debated the history of the subject. All accounts agreed that this knowledge was divinely imparted, but when and to whom was uncertain. Some people argued that Adam was the first alchemist.[14] Conrad Gesner (1516–65), the Swiss physician and natural historian, mocked this idea in a book of recipes and distillations that was translated into English in 1559 as *The treasure of Euonymus*. He jeered at the suggestion that Adam might even have invented alchemy, and questioned whether Solomon, Aristotle, Plato, Thomas Aquinas, Albertus Magnus, Rhazes, and Avicenna knew anything about the art.[15] Two and a half decades later, in the earliest theoretical alchemical text printed in English, *The difference betwene the auncient phisicke . . . and the latter phisicke* (1585), Richard Bostocke, a lawyer and friend of John Dee's, wrote a history of alchemy, 'the true knowledge of God and the Science of Chymia (from which *medicina* may not be separated)', beginning with Adam, Abraham, and Hermes Trismegistus.[16] He challenged the notion that Paracelsus promoted a new physic; medicine had become corrupt since the Fall, Galenic medicine perpetuated this corruption, and Paracelsus had restored the original, true, and ancient physic.[17] The year after Bostocke's text was published, a similar work appeared, *A coppie of a letter sent by a learned physician to his friend*, under the initials I.W. He, like Bostocke, argued that the Paracelsians were not 'a new sect'. Rather,

[13] Ashm. 1494, p. 623. For Forman's assessment of a substance in terms of the three conventional types of the stone, see Ashm. 392, p. 578.

[14] Arnold Williams, *The Common Expositor: An Account of the Commentaries on Genesis, 1527–1633* (Chapel Hill, NC, 1948), 82; cf. Nick Jardine, *The Birth of History and Philosophy of Science: Kepler's* A defence of Tycho against Ursus *with Essays on its Provenance and Significance* (Cambridge, 1984), ch. 8.

[15] 'Some also ascende higher, and make the first men by and after the beginning of the world, authors therof.' Conrad Gesner, *The treasure of Euonymus*, tr. Peter Morwyng (1559), sig. A1^{v}. In Ben Jonson's *The Alchemist* there is a joke about Adam writing a treatise of the philosophers' stone in High Dutch, *Ben Jonson*, ed. Herford *et al.*, v, II. i. 84–6. See also David Katz, 'The Language of Adam in the Seventeenth Century', in Hugh Lloyd-Jones, Valerie Pearl, and Blair Worden (eds.), *History and Imagination: Essays in Honour of H. R. Trevor-Roper* (1981), 132–45.

[16] Bostocke, *Difference betwene the auncient phisick . . . and the latter phisicke*, ch. 10. For edited selections, see Allen Debus, 'An Elizabethan History of Medical Chemistry', *Annals of Science*, 18 (1962), 1–29. For biographical information about Bostocke, see Harley, 'Rychard Bostok'.

[17] Bostocke, *Difference betwene the auncient phisicke . . . and the latter phisicke*, sigs. F4, F8. For arguments that Bostocke's text was an anomaly see Debus, *English Paracelsians*, ch. 2; Kocher, 'Paracelsian Medicine in England', 465.

it had his beginning with our first father Adam, and so from that time to time hath continued untill this day: but indeed so amplified and enlarged of late, and brought unto every mans sight (that hath both his eies) by the long labour and infinite paines of *Paracelsus*, that it seemeth to be borne a new with him.[18]

These treatises were printed during the period when Forman was copying as many alchemical texts as he could find and he might have read, and perhaps even owned, copies of them.

The question of whether or not Adam had scientific knowledge (conventionally defined as astronomy and natural history, not alchemy) had theological importance. When knowledge was imparted to Adam and what this knowledge constituted (the fall of angels, the fall and redemption of man) had ramifications for the existence and nature of free will. The significance of Adam's knowledge for alchemists was that it potentially contained the secrets of the relationship between the microcosm and the macrocosm. The Fall resulted in the corruption of life, the perpetuation of disease, and the loss of the prime substance. For Paracelsus and his followers, the universe was made from philosophical salt, sulphur, and mercury, and the search for the philosophers' stone was the pursuit of these prime substances. Accordingly, the theme of creation prominent in hermetic and related texts became a constant point of reference for alchemists, especially Paracelsians.[19] As God created the world, so the alchemist created the philosophers' stone.

Although some alchemists discussed creation, few English authors seem to have turned from the analogy between creation and the production of the philosophers' stone to a general exposition on Genesis.[20] Forman did this in notes 'Upon the firste of Genesis'.[21] He structured his discussion like a biblical

[18] I.W., *A coppie of a letter sent by a learned physician to his friend* ([1586?]), sig. A1^v. It is possible that these initials denote the person who sent the letter to press, not its author. For a possible attack on this treatise, as noted Ch. 5, n. 25, see *The whole worke of the famous chirurgion Master John Vigo*, George Baker's preface to the reader, sig. ¶3.

[19] Webster, *Paracelsus to Newton*, 49. See also Norma Emerton, 'Creation in the Thought of J. B. van Helmont and Robert Fludd', in Rattansi and Clericuzio (eds.), *Alchemy and Chemistry*, 85–101.

[20] For conflicts between theologians and alchemists on the subject of Creation see Williams, *Common Expositor*, 46.

[21] Ashm. 802, i. This is now bound alongside the 'Life', which began with an account of creation similar to that in this text. 'Upon the firste of Genesis' is in two parts, which are inversely bound. The original foliation makes it clear that in its initial form this text began with 'Upon the firste of genesis' (now fos. 3–12), and was followed by 'the heaven and the earth and what the heavens are that were first created' (now fos. 1–2). In the original foliation the first item is fos. 1–6, and the second fos. 9 and 10; pp. 7 and 8 are missing. The hand and inks are consistent throughout, and the catchwords support this reading. It is unclear whether this is the introduction to what was intended as a long tract, or if it is complete except for the two pages. Some of Forman's related notes, in rough format, are now bound in his copy of *The hystory of Kyng Boccus and Sydrack*, St John's College, Oxford. These are on the birth of Lucifer, which figures in Forman's creation tract as the beginning of supercelestial time, fos. 5–6. For a printed version of these notes see Philip Bliss, 'Extracts'. For

commentary, quoting a verse and expanding on it with citations from diverse authorities, including Augustine, Nicholas de Lyra, the fourteenth-century Parisian exegete, and, less conventionally, the Picatrix, an Arabic magical compendium. Forman narrated how God had created something out of nothing, which was God's prerogative.[22] He spoke the word 'fiat' and

> of this word fiat came the chaos. For as the breath in cold weather goinge out of a mans mouth becommeth thicke and is seen: and is condensate to a cloud or water which riseth like a miste from the mouth of a man and after dropeth downe and ys seen which before was nothinge: soe lykewise of that worde fiat beinge once pronounsed cam firste an Invisible Substance by power Imperiall of the Creator . . .[23]

This was more than a simile. With a word God created an invisible substance, chaos. From this chaos He made 'The heavens firste as chife and principalle Agente and father of all thinges superioure, and the Earth as principall passive mother of all thinges inferioure.'[24] The art of alchemy was analogous to God's creation.

> Then was the sprite of the Lord borne upon the face of the waters which was the liquide forme of thinges and the moste apteste to make moste formes shapes and creatures of. As for example a man taketh a great pote & filles yt with water honni oylle wine verjuce milke and such lyke lyquid thinges, and he setes yt on fier to distill howe many sortes of water may he drawe out of this smalle Chaos, & every on better then other. And yet in thend ther is dregs lefte, which may be Congealed into a thicker or harder masse, out of which again also, a man may drawe or make divers other thinges, and formes.[25]

Forman noted the word 'chaos' next to passages about creation in the alchemical texts that he copied.[26] And under the headings for 'Chaos' in his alchemical commonplace books he described creation, much as he had in 'Upon the firste of Genesis', though in verse.[27] Genesis, as Forman explained, was 'The trewe knowledge, wherof to many is rare which moch may healpe thee in tyme of need'.[28]

Forman's interest in other demonic progeny, see also his copy of 'The parlamont and consultation of the devils and their decre about the beginning of Merlin', Ashm. 802, fos. 66–82. For another 16th-cent. MS commentary on Genesis, bound alongside alchemical notes, including some by Forman, see Ashm. 766, vi.

22 See Williams, *Common Expositor*, 44–5.

23 Ashm. 802, fo. 4^{v}; see also fo. 8.

24 Ashm. 802, fo. 1.

25 Ashm. 802, fo. 2.

26 See his transcripts, in chronological order from 1585: Ripley (Ashm. 1490, fos. 114–36^{v}), Bernard of Trier (Ashm. 1490, fos. 221–36^{v}), J. J. (Ashm. 1490, fos. 277–89), Henry Lock (Ashm. 1490, fos. 294–325), Aegidius de Vadis (Ashm. 1490, fos. 28–36^{v}), Blomfild (1490, fos. 167–70^{v}).

27 Ashm. 1430, fos. 26–33; 1472, pp. 178–88; 1494, pp. 473–8. For a version of this in verse see Ashm. 240, fos. 33–5, printed in Schuler (ed.), *Alchemical Poetry*, 49–70. See also Sloane 2550, fo. 4, for an earlier, briefer verse on chaos by Forman *c.*1589?.

28 Ashm. 1430, fo. 26. This phrase also appeared in Forman's creation tract, Ashm. 802, fo. 8.

Even more profound secrets lay in the creation of Adam.[29] The 'Life' recounted how God made Adam out of nothing, like him in holiness, image, and eternity, 'for he breathed into his nostrels the breath of life, and made him a lyvinge soule, to live for evermore'.[30] The similarities between God and Adam corresponded to the three parts of the soul, animate, sensitive, and rational, and to the ingredients of Adam, the red earth, the slime of the earth, and the quintessential substance.[31] In the margin next to this account Forman spelt out the analogy to include the composition of the body, soul, and spirit, paraphrasing a passage in his essays on the 'Heavens', the writings akin to those that he promised to publish if *Longitude* had been well received.[32] In the bottom margin he glossed this with details of the three parts of the body of man, natural, animal, and vital, and the same parts of the soul of man; thus Adam shared being with inanimate things, life with plants, sense with animals, and mind and intelligence with angels.

These annotations echoed passages in 'Of appoticarie druges' under the heading 'Anima & spiritus'.[33] The entry began with a discussion of whether man had only a soul, or a soul and a spirit. In a passage that was almost identical to the one which flanks the composition of Adam in the 'Life', Forman explained that every man was composed of three things, body, soul, and spirit, concluding with a quotation of most of a chapter from Agrippa's *De occulta philosophia* on the joining of man's soul with his body (bk. 3, ch. 37).[34] Agrippa described how, according to the Platonists, God infused (or breathed) the soul into man's body with an astral vehicle, thereby joining

[29] Under the heading 'Sulfur' in 'Of appoticarie druges' next to an analogy between an alchemical operation and human procreation, Forman added a 12-page marginal note that continued the analogy, explaining that women are most fertile when young, men when older and so forth. Forman explicated the analogy, 'And as of on man came all men so of on bodie or simple mineralle most all springe. The woman Eva was hid in Adams side and ther wer 2 in one, and in them 2 was a third person, a sonn moch like to his father. So in our bodie on which we most worke is hid both ☿ and sulfur malle and femall. By ☿ here is understod the woman which was taken sulfur out of her husbands side with sulfur her sonne, for sulfur firste signified the sonn, although he was agent in the father.' He concluded that as Adam had been 30 years old when he was created, and Eve was a little younger, it was important that metals were used at the correct ages: Ashm. 1491, pp. 1022–[5]; see also p. 1034^{r-v} (sic).

[30] Ashm. 802, ii, fo. 1^{r-v}; cf. Philip Almond, *Adam and Eve in Seventeenth Century Thought* (Cambridge, 1999), 15–19; Williams, *Common Expositor*, 77.

[31] Ashm. 802, ii, fo. 1^{v}; see also fos. 2^{v}–3 where Adam is described as made of nine things, the slime of the earth, the sea, stones, clouds, winds, sun, light of the world, the holy ghost, and fire.

[32] Ashm. 244, fo. 37. On the 'Heavens' see Ch. 2.

[33] See also Ashm. 1472, pp. 64–7; 1494, pp. 190–200, 218.

[34] Ashm. 1494, pp. 190–200, 218. Agrippa's previous chapter was about the creation of man, after the image of God. There were some similarities between this and the beginning of Forman's entry on 'Anima & spiritus', though here Forman was not following Agrippa directly. Forman's notes on Cabala, which include extracts from Agrippa, were also written in 1610 and, perhaps coincidentally, are now bound with his essays on the 'Heavens' in Ashm. 244.

the ethereal body to the gross body. The heart was the receptacle of the soul, from which it was diffused throughout the body. If disease (or 'mischief') impeded this motion, the soul retracted to the heart and when the heart failed, the soul left the body.[35] It seems that Forman, like Thomas Vaughan (1622–66), a Welsh cleric and alchemist, read Agrippa's *De occulta philosophia* as a text sympathetic to and informative about alchemy.[36] With these passages Forman introduced a number of alchemical procedures, then he effected an abrupt transition from man to minerals, noting 'Now we com to speak of the soulle and sprite in mineralles and metalles and metal, animals & vegitable philosophically'. Following Paracelsus, the spirit was mercury, the soul was sulphur, the body salt.[37]

In the margins of the 'Life' Forman drew on an eclectic range of sources in order, it seems, to constitute a Paracelsian cosmology. In the entry on 'Microcosmos' in 'Of appoticarie druges', for instance, he began with an account of creation and concluded with an exposition of natural magic, drawing on Hermes, Paracelsus, the Picatrix, and other sources.[38] In this essay, as in Forman's other alchemical and related notes, Paracelsus was given no special authority; in the margins of the 'Life', however, his name was prominent and Forman cited him at length in annotations on the subject of the nature of Adam. Above the description of Adam's creation, Forman noted:

> Paracelsus: The materiall seed of microcosmus was taken out of all the elements from all the places of the whole wordle into on place, and created man out of it and yt was don upon the water (which was matrix majoris mundi) and out of all thes did god mak man even of the vertu of all things.[39]

Next to the description of God breathing into Adam's nostrils Forman added definitions of the divine and animal souls that he attributed to Paracelsus.[40] The divine soul was eternal, only man's imagination could kill it; the animal or elemental soul died with the body. At the bottom of the page Forman added a description of Adam as born with eternal life, power over all creatures, and 'altitude':

> that is the heighte and glory of all thinges. For when he was created ther was noe creatur in beuty shape and wisdom like to Adam. For the upper parte of Adam from the girdle upwards was in heaven in respecte of his purity and beinge. And the lowar parte from the girdle downwards was on earth, till he had broken the commandments.

[35] Cf. Hannaway, *Chemists and the Word*, 27–8.

[36] William Newman, 'Thomas Vaughan as an Interpreter of Agrippa von Nettesheim', *Ambix*, 29 (1982), 125–40.

[37] Ashm. 1494, p. 196.

[38] Sloane 3822, fos. 68–75; cf. Ashm. 244, fos. 35–60.

[39] Ashm. 802, ii, fo. 2.

[40] Ibid.

9.1. A page of the 'Life of Adam and Eve', transcribed and annotated by Simon Forman, Ashm. 802, ii, fo. 2. By permission of the Bodleian Library, University of Oxford.

And before his fall he had no genitors, but after he was put forth of paradice, his genitors began to growe forth of him.[41]

In these annotations Forman was drawing on the pseudo-Paracelsian 'Liber Azoth'. This text appeared in the eleventh volume of Zaccharias Palthen's edition of the works of Paracelsus, printed in 1605, which Forman seems to have owned.[42]

The annotations continued. Forman flanked the naming and composition of Adam with a note which glossed the story of creation, beginning with Adam and Eve as created 'Angelically with the necrocomish soulle, that is with a soulle puer righteouse & undefiled & ymortalle'. They had 'a peculiar and dyvine Lymbus which was separated and did differ from the Lymbus of the earthy Adam'. Limbus, a margin between the eternal and the concrete, was a gnostic concept which pervaded Paracelsian texts.[43] When Adam and Eve were in the Garden,

they did feed and eate angelically of divine food, wherin ther was noe corruption poison nore infection of mortallity nor eternall death. For they eat of all the trees of the garden that wer good, ∧ after their nature, ∧ and ther was noe tre evill nor infected with dedly poison, but the tree of good and evill. For Adam & Eve were made good and did knowe nothing but good . . .

God had put a commandment on this tree:

youe shall eat of all the fruits of the garden but only [not?] of this tre. For in this tree is good and evill life and deth, honny and galle, good meat & poison that will infecte thee with a contynuall sicknes and diseas therfore take heed of yt. So Adam & Eva did eat good fruite in which was noe poison nor evil to troble their bodies, as men use to eat good and holsom meats & never feell sicknes nor diseas, nor distemper of their bodies. But yf they eat the appell colloquintida or som rubarb ellebor agarick or som such thinge wherin ther is a poisoned substance (although yt show well) then theyr stomakes, bowells and whole bodi is sick & sore trobled, by which they presently knowe they have eaten som poysoened & evill thinge, wherby they presently knowe that ther ar bad meats as well as good . . .

But one could not know that there were poisonous as well as wholesome meats by being told. This knowledge had to be learnt through experience. Adam could not have understood poison until he had tasted it.

41 Ashm. 802, ii, fo. 2; cf. Forman's notes on giants, 802, iii, fos. 51–9ᵛ; 244, fos. 179–86.

42 Paracelsus, *Operum medico-chimicorum sive paradoxorum, tomus genuinus undecimus*, tr. Zacharias Palthen, xi (Frankfurt, 1605), 66–110.

43 Pagel, *Paracelsus*, 83, 228.

But then yt is to late. The poison & venom hath taken hould and root in them and they most die or be deformed or become monsters, for then their bodies swell and becom full of sore botches and blains and soe they ar altered and presently from their firste form & shape, as Adam was, which was first dyvine and had a heavenly form, but after he had eaten he was poisoned with sinn and felt the operation of the apple in his hart & body wherby he knewe he had don evill . . . For his bodie being poisoned wth sinne he becam monstrouse and lost his first form and shape divine & heavenly and becam earthy full of sores and sicknes for evermore. And soe as a leprose man is chased or expelld out of the company of good hole and sound men leste they should be infected by him, even soe was Adam cast out of paradice . . .[44]

A similar passage in the 'Heavens' extrapolated the consequences of the Fall for future generations, explaining that after Adam had eaten from the tree of knowledge and become mortal,

both his bodie and soulle were defiled and infected with an incurable disease and leprosye of eternalle death and mortality, the which hereditarius morbus doth remaine to this daie and shall do for ever as long as the wordle endureth upon seade and offspringe without remady were yt not for Christe Jesus that good and true phisision of our soulls . . .[45]

At the moment that Adam and Eve forsook the food of angels, they learnt disease and death, initiating the suffering and redemption thereafter enacted by humankind.

Forman's annotations to the 'Life', his essays of the 'Heavens', and some of the entries in 'Of appoticarie druges' contained the same blend of alchemy and the Fall. He was looking for the secrets of creation, knowledge of the microcosm, and the causes and cures of disease. Following alchemical and Paracelsian traditions, he sought these secrets in texts on Genesis. In pseudo-Paracelsus' 'Liber Azoth' Forman found the words to articulate the history of life and death, but his pursuit of the food of angels had led him through numerous other texts and traditions, alchemical, magical, theological, historical. Forman mapped these forays in the pages of the 'Life', a text itself rich with the significance of disease.

When Adam summoned his children to his deathbed, Seth asked if he could bring him anything (ch. 30). Adam replied, 'Sonne I desier nothinge but I wax full sicke and have greate sorowe and penance in my bodie.'[46] Seth said that he did not understand. So Adam recounted the story of the Fall and reported the words that God had spoken in anger: 'I shall caste into thy bodie seventy wondes ∧ & too ∧ of divers sorowes, from the crowne of the head unto the soule of

[44] Ashm. 802, ii, fos. 2^{v}–3. [45] Ashm. 244, fo. 38^{v}.

[46] Ashm. 802, ii, fo. 21. I am following the chapter designations in Sparks, *Apocryphal Old Testament.*

thy feete, and all in divers members of thy bodie, be they tormented with soe many sicknises thou and thyne offspringe forevermore'.[47] Food had a particular bearing on Adam's and Eve's well-being. When they were expelled from Paradise, they built a tabernacle where they stayed for seven days lamenting their Fall, 'for losinge and wantinge their naturalle foode'.[48] They had nothing to eat and were very hungry, so Adam began to look for food, but could find none; they looked together, argued, and still could find nothing except herbs and grass such as beasts ate. And Adam said to Eve, 'Our lorde god delyvered meate to beastes but to us he delivered meate of angells, the which he hath nowe deprived us of: and given us over to feed with the beastes of the filde.'[49] After Cain and Abel were born, God sent Michael to teach Adam to 'worke & to till ye lande, and to provide fruite to live by' ('Life', ch. 22). Forman's text continued with details absent from the Latin and English versions. Adam's descendants lived by tilling the ground until after the flood. They ate herbs and fruit and roots but not flesh. It never rained, and the ground was moistened with mist.[50] At the end of the 'Life', Adam told Seth that 'I had my knowinge and my understandinge of things that is to com, by eatinge, that I eate of the tree of understandinge.'[51]

The food of angels, as a phrase or a concept, appeared throughout medieval religious texts.[52] In the sixteenth century food was central to interpretations of the Fall. The eating of the fruit and the necessity to work for bread were integral to theological definitions of free will and knowledge. Questions about what man ate before the Fall and when meat (flesh) began to be eaten, and discussions of the meaning of the necessity to till the ground and the longevity of the patriarchs figured, for instance, in the printed English commentaries by two Elizabethan divines, Gervase Babington and Nicholas Gibbens. In *Certain plaine, briefe, and comfortable notes, upon every chapter of Genesis* (1596), Babington discussed 'How dooth God appoint man foode before his fall':

Man is appointed heere his foode of God that he should eate, and some moove the question how that shall be. For if man were created immortall if he sinned not, what

[47] Ashm. 802, ii, fo. 21^{v}. Some versions of the 'Life' gave the number as seventy, some as seventy-two.

[48] Ashm. 802, ii, fo. 9. [49] Ashm. 802, ii, fos. 9^{v}–10. [50] Ashm. 802, ii, fo. 15^{v}.

[51] Ashm. 802, ii, fo. 18^{v} ('Life', ch. 24). Another medicinal theme in the 'Life', this of Christian origin, was the oil of mercy: Ashm. 802, ii, fos. 23^{v}, 25^{r-v}; 'Life', ch. 36. Forman's text contained additions about the Tree of Mercy, probably drawn from the gospel of Nicodemus.

[52] The phrase appeared in verses, 'Christ's affliction', following one of the English versions of the 'Life' in a contiguous script: Bodley MS 596, fos. 12^{v}–13. On the eucharist as food, see Caroline Walker Bynum, *Holy Feast, Holy Fast: The Religious Significance of Food to Medieval Women* (Berkeley, Calif., 1987). On food, medicine, and the Fall in medieval scholastic texts see Joseph Ziegler, 'Medicine and Immortality in Terrestrial Paradise', in Peter Biller and Joseph Ziegler (eds.), *Religion and Medicine in the Middle Ages* (Woodbridge, 2001), 201–42.

needed he any meate to be appointed for him, since yet he had not sinned. Answer is made by some, that there be two kindes of Immortall, one that cannot die but ever live, an other that may live for ever, a condition being observed, and die also if that condition be broken. One imortall after the first sort needeth no meate, but he that is immortall after the second sort dooth neede, and such was Adam: if he had not sinned he had not dyed, but sinning he was so made, that he might die, and therefore his flesh and nature not such that could live without meate. Others answer that this appointment of meate was made by God in respect of their fall, which he knew would bee. Howsoever it was, curiositie becometh us not: but this comfort we may rightlie take by it, that what the Lord hath made, he will maintaine and nourish, and casteth for them his providence ever to that end.[53]

Likewise, Gibbens's *Questions and disputations concerning the holy scripture* (1602) discussed the significance of food and the longevity of the patriarchs. Gibbens asked whether God showed his liberality as much in providing food for Adam and Eve as in creating them.[54] He argued that they did not eat flesh before the Fall because when their bodies were immortal, meat 'was no convenient foode to nourish them'.[55] He answered the question 'wherein consisteth the punishment of Adam?' with an exposition of 'in sorrow thou shalt eate thereof [the ground]' (Gen. 3: 17), explaining that Adam became proud, and God, like a physician, administered 'a potion of humilitie, wherby man being dailie emptied of his old corruptions, might with hunger and thirst, gaspe for the death of Christ, which is the fruit of life'.[56] He then outlined Adam's tripartite punishment, 'the curse of the earth; the miserie of life; and the end therof by death'. Whereas before the Fall the earth had brought forth fruit of its own accord, it had been corrupted by sin. Where once wheat had grown now grew weeds. This curse was man's misery: working the soil bridled him from waxing proud. Other afflictions accompanied work, including diseases of the body and vexations of the mind.[57]

Gibbens elaborated these final points in response to the question of why the patriarchs lived so long. The answer was that it was 'of the wisedom of the Lord for the disposition of his counsailes, for our sinnes, and the weakenes of our bodies, that we cannot now live so long as they'. Over time, he explained, the human body has become increasingly corrupt and unable to resist disease. The patriarchs had lived so long, first, 'because they were of temperate and sober diet, not given so much to fleshlie appetite, nor mixing their meat with such

[53] Gervase Babington, *Certain plaine, briefe, and comfortable notes, upon every chapter of Genesis* (1596 [1591]), 14–15.

[54] Nicholas Gibbens, *Questions and disputations concerning the holy scripture* (1602), 39–42.

[55] Ibid. 39. [56] Ibid. 161. [57] Ibid. 162–3.

varieties, but content with simple food, which the aboundance of the earth brought forth unto them'. Secondly,

> because the fruits of the earth were much more nourishable and healthfull before the floud, then afterward they were, either thorough the waters of the sea, bringing barrennes and saltnes to the earth, and to the fruits therof; or for that the Lord had given unto man more libertie of food, the fruite of the field was not so necessarie.[58]

Although Forman did not necessarily read these commentaries, they demonstrate a long-standing theological association between food and disease that was still current in Elizabethan England.[59]

The prolongation of life and the Fall of man also featured in medieval alchemical traditions, especially in the writings of Roger Bacon. Paracelsus and his followers adopted these associations and expounded a cosmology that associated food, disease, and the Fall.[60] According to the doctrine of 'Tartar', food consisted of parts which were pure and impure, and the body could only use those which were pure. Impurities remained in the body, causing obstructions and resulting in disease.[61] The 'Life', like Paracelsian histories of disease, explained how disease originated with the Fall. In the Garden Adam and Eve had consumed the food (or meat) of angels, but once they had tasted the forbidden fruit their bodies and souls were corrupted and man had thereafter suffered disease. Bostocke and I.W. clearly formulated these ideas; Forman did not.

In a chapter on 'the originall causes of all diseases in the greate worlde, and the little worlde, which is man', Bostocke recounted the story of the Fall in order to demonstrate that the binary principle of Galenic medicine, predicated on opposites, was corrupt. The serpent, 'Binarius', had persuaded Adam and Eve to eat the apple, 'Whereupon by the curse of God impure Seedes were mingled with the perfect seedes, and did cleave fast to them, and doe cover them as a garment: and death was joyned to life.' This impurity was in all

[58] Nicholas Gibbens, 218–19; for antediluvian vegetarianism ibid. 361–5 and Almond, *Adam and Eve*, 118–23.

[59] On food and medicine in early modern England, see Pelling, *Common Lot*, ch. 2.

[60] Roger Bacon, *Opus Maius*, ed. John H. Bridges (Oxford, 1900), 204–13; William Newman, 'The Philosopher's Egg: Theory and Practice in the Alchemy of Roger Bacon', *Micrologus: Nature, Sciences and Medieval Societies*, 3 (1995), 75–101. See also Faye Getz, 'To Prolong Life and Promote Health: Baconian Alchemy and Pharmacy in the English Learned Tradition', in Sheila Campbell, Bert Hall, and David Klausner (eds.), *Health, Disease and Healing in Medieval Culture* (New York, 1992), 141–51; Michela Pereira, '*Mater Medicinarum*: English Physicians and the Alchemical Elixir in the Fifteenth Century', in Roger French *et al.* (eds.), *Medicine from the Black Death to the French Disease* (Aldershot, 1998), 26–52. Forman cited Bacon extensively throughout his writings, and he probably owned, for instance, a copy of *Libellus Rogerii Baconi Angli . . . de retardandis senectutis accidentibus* (Oxford, 1590).

[61] Pagel, *Paracelsus*, 153–8.

things, depending on the nature of the soil in which they grew or the food on which they fed, as experience showed.

> But the foode and nourishments for mans body, though they have in them mingled, venemous, sickly or medicinable properties, yet for all that, by reason of that mixture with their good seedes, as long as unitie and concord is kept betweene them, they be tempered, seperated, resolved and expelled out of mans body.

If this did not work, 'the seedes of diseases do then take roote in mans body'. Man knew by ancient art and by experience how to separate the good from the bad and the life from the death in all things. Thus, diseases proceeded from the breach of unity, and only in unity could they be cured.[62]

I.W. repeated many of these ideas alongside condemnations of the practices of Galenic physicians, noting that 'before the fall of *Adam* all thinges were good, all things came unto him and were bred unto his hand without his labour. But afterward part of it was joyned to poison, part of it so fast lockt up, that without great sweate of browes he should not eat of it.' Traditional physicians were too conservative and lazy to separate the poison from the bread: 'And in these our latter dayes sloth is growen so strong & idlenes hath gotten such masterie, that there are very few which will let one drop fal from their browes to seeke this bread, but indevour by all methodicall meanes to maintaine this idlenes'. They sat on cushions in their chambers and wrote prescriptions for apothecaries to fill.[63] The original food, or 'bread', was the philosophers' stone, the ultimate aspiration, he argued, of a true physician. He continued, 'If you had bestowed but half of your study in the first booke of Moses, which youe spent in the foolish Philosophie of *Aristotle*, you had espied your errors long agoe'.[64] Genesis taught good medicine.

Food, disease, and the Fall had been prominent in English theological and alchemical texts for several centuries, but references to the food of angels in sixteenth- and seventeenth-century texts were distinctive.[65] A manuscript compilation of astrological rules and recipes that Forman owned listed the afflictions of man and the discoveries of the knowledge to remedy them. In the year 3613 after creation God had given Moses the commandments, and had struck those who would not obey them with numerous infirmities, none of which could be helped with medicine. Obedient people in turn were fed with

[62] Bostocke, *Difference betwene the auncient phisicke . . . and the latter phisicke*, sigs. B4–6ᵛ. For the use of the term 'Binarius' by Agrippa, then Vaughan, see Newman, 'Thomas Vaughan', 132 n.

[63] I.W., *Coppie of a letter*, sig. B6ᵛ. [64] Ibid., sig. B7v.

[65] Bishop Joseph Hall (1574–1656) used the phrase in a sermon printed in 1624, cited in *OED*, 'frequence'.

'mana or angells food'.[66] Manna, the food from heaven that sustained the Israelites in the wilderness, was referred to in alchemical texts as a spiritual food, like the food of angels.[67] For instance, an alchemical text entitled 'Manna', probably dating from the late sixteenth or early seventeenth century, described the healing virtues and magical uses of the philosophers' stone.[68] Another sixteenth-century English manuscript, 'The epitome of the treasure of all welth', written in 1562 by one 'Edwardus Generosus Anglicus Innominatus', specified that a form of the philosophers' stone was the food of angels.[69] According to this text, St Dunstan, the tenth-century archbishop of Canterbury, had departed from the standard description of a tripartite philosophers' stone.[70] Conventionally the mineral stone could be used to transmute base metals into gold, usually through a process called projection. The vegetable stone had the power to improve plants and animals and to make them grow. The animal stone was often called the elixir of life and healed man's body. St Dunstan, according to Edwardus, renamed the animal stone as the angelic stone and added the magical stone, a substance providing exceptional temporal and geographical vision and an ability to understand the language of animals. The angelic stone was 'preservative to the state of mans body', and 'by this stone shall mans body bee kept from corrupcon alsoe he shalbe endued with divine guiftes & foreknowledgee of thinges by dreames and revealations'.[71] It was invisible, aromatic, and flavoursome, '& therefore in St Dunstans workee itt is said that Solomon King Davids sonne doth call itt the foode of Angell, because a man may live a long time without any food having some ∧ but the ∧ tast of this stone'.[72] A similar substance that prolonged life and had 'neyther culler nor forme' was described in 'The revelation of the secret spirit', a text that Agnello, the alchemist whom Drouet had encountered in London in the 1560s, saw

[66] Ashm. 1429, fo. 77. [67] Exod. 1: 15–35.

[68] King's, Keynes MS 33; Glasgow, Glasgow University Library, Ferguson MS 9, fos. 14–24; Ferguson MS 199, pp. 72–8 (partial copy); Sloane 2194, fos. 77–84^{v}; Sloane 2222, fos. 128^{v}–36; Sloane 2585, fos. 90–105; Ashm. 1419, fos. 45–56; printed in John Frederick Houpreght (ed.), *Aurifontina chymica: Or a collection of fourteen small treatises concerning the first matter of philosophers* (1680), 107–43. See Principe, *Aspiring Adept*, 199 for a discussion of this work.

[69] Ashm. 1419, fos. 57–82^{v}. I am indebted to William Newman for identifying this text for me. Other copies are King's, Keynes MS 22; Ferguson MS 199, pp. 19–70; Sloane 2502, fos. 54–69v, 70–81^{v} (two copies). For the history of this text see Lauren Kassell, 'Reading for the Philosophers' Stone', in Marina Frasca-Spada and Nick Jardine (eds.), *History of Science, History of the Book* (Cambridge, 2000), 132–50; Principe, *Aspiring Adept*, 197–200.

[70] Ashm. 1419, fos. 63–4^{v}. [71] Ashm. 1419, fo. 63^{v}.

[72] Ashm. 1419, fo. 64; Ashmole, *Theatrum chemicum Britannicum*, sigs. A4^{v}–B1^{v}. On Ashmole's reading of Edwardus' 'Epitome', 'Manna', and other texts, see Kassell, 'Reading for the Philosophers' Stone'; Principe, *Aspiring Adept*, 197–200.

through a London press in Latin with an Italian commentary in 1566.[73] Forman knew this text, having acquired a manuscript of it in Agnello's hand, and Forman described St Dunstan's four-part scheme, as described by Edwardus, though he did not identify its source.[74]

In whatever text or in whatever form Forman encountered the description of the angelic stone as the food of angels, he read the 'Life' as part of a project to explore an alchemical tradition concerned with health. Before he covered the margins with alchemical notes, he added a list of diseases in the section of the 'Life' that described Adam's deathbed scene (ch. 34), elaborating on the theme of corruption internal to the text. Adam had announced that God had inflicted seventy-two diseases on him and his offspring at the Fall. In the Latin and English versions the narrative continued with Adam's expression of sorrow and pain to his children (ch. 35). Forman interrupted the narrative and inserted a list of diseases, divided according to physiology and sex.[75] Twenty-one diseases afflicted men and women alike, and might occur in all parts of the body, twelve diseases occurred only in the head, three diseases affected the throat, four diseases each were of the breast and stomach, two diseases affected the left side, four diseases were of the heart, three of the bowels, twelve of the kidneys, and fourteen diseases afflicted only women. That Forman inserted this list into his transcript of the 'Life' is clear from his changes to the numbers of diseases, and the shifts in format and script.[76]

73 *Espositione . . . sopra un libro intitolato Apocalypsis spiritus secreti* (1566). This was tr. into English by one R.N.E. and printed in 1623. Latin MS copies are Ashm. 1467, fos. 202^v–8^v; 1490, fos. 15–17^v; London, Wellcome MS 1700, pp. 217–27. English copies are King's, Keynes MS 67, fo. 7^v; Sloane 3738, fo. 3b.

74 Ashm. 1490, fos. 15–17b is Forman's copy, and I am indebted to Deborah Harkness for confirming that it is in Agnello's hand: private correspondence 5 Nov. 2001. On Agnello see also p. 108 above. Although Forman did not record reading Edwardus' treatise or St Dunstan's work on the angelic stone, he evidently encountered St Dunstan's definition of it. He did have a copy of an alchemical text on the mineral, not the magical stone, attributed to St Dunstan which he recopied in 1608: Ashm. 1433, i. The date of Forman's initial transcription is uncertain. This text might be related to the text that Edwardus attributed to St Dunstan. Of the handful of extant copies of Dunstan's alchemical tract those of Forman, Thomas Robson, and Ashmole are in the Ashmole collection. Ashmole noted that Sir Thomas Browne had a Latin copy, which was confirmed by a letter from Brown to Ashmole in 1659: *Ashmole*, ed. Josten, ii, 755 n. Josten identified the Dunstan text as possibly Sloane 1255, ii. See also Sloane 1744, 1876, 3738, and 3757. Oxford, Corpus Christi College MS 128 is the only medieval copy identified. It may have been owned by John Dee, and is listed in Roberts and Watson, *Dee's Library*, DM [129].

75 Ashm. 802, ii, fos. 21^v–3.

76 The number of diseases listed, for instance, adds up to seventy-five, not seventy-two. The list began: 'Of thes diseases ther be 21 that be generalle both to man and woman'. The '1' of the '21' was crossed through and a '2' was inserted so that it read '22'. Twenty-three diseases were then listed, though the twenty-second and twenty-third extended into the margin. Forman's hand became less neat as the list proceeded, and he left blank spaces for the numbers of diseases to be inserted. The following subsets are uniform and tidy, though the hand began to slant and sprawl with the second. In the next section there was a space for the number of diseases to be filled in: 'In the brest there commeth _ diseases'. Four diseases were listed and numbered, and a symptom was listed next to them: 'a stinking breath'. The next subset, diseases of the stomach, also left the

Whether Forman devised this list or derived it from another text, it might not have been a coincidence that two similar lists appeared in tracts published in England around this time. The first was in *A coppie of a letter* by I.W. which explained that causes of disease were not 'humors intemperie & obstructions', as humours were 'the fantasticall inventions of an idle head, having no foundation or ground in nature'. A list of twenty-nine diseases followed, unlike Forman's, using Latin terminology and describing less specific diseases. I.W. concluded:

> This is the cause that man dieth such sundry deaths, because hee eateth in his bread the death of all other things, which when perfect separation is not made, bringeth foorth fruit according to his kinde. Over these deaths hath the Physician power, and not over that which was injoyned to the body of man particularly.[77]

He listed diseases that could be cured because they were produced by the natural world, grown in nature and 'transplanted' into the bodies of men and women.

The association between disease and the Fall in the late sixteenth century was evident in a work of another genre, Guillaume Saluste Du Bartas's creation epic, *La sepmaine; ou, creation du monde* (Paris, 1578). Josuah Sylvester's translation was printed in 1599, the same year in which Forman copied his treatise on Adam and Eve. In the third part of the first day of the second week, 'The Furies', Du Bartas recounted how after the Fall man was beset by three furies, sickness, war, and death. Sickness attacked Adam in a mock-heroic battle, beginning with diseases of the head and moving down his body.[78] Du Bartas, however, did not describe Adam's deathbed scene, though the 'Handicrafts' concluded with Adam near death, overwhelmed with a vision of the future.[79]

Whether or not Du Bartas or I.W. influenced Forman's taxonomy of disease, their texts demonstrate that there were precedents in Elizabethan England for cataloguing the diseases which afflicted man after the Fall, though I have not located another instance of Adam rehearsing a list of diseases on his deathbed.

number blank and included symptoms. After this the diseases were not numbered and the format became less formal. The final category was the diseases of women, on which see Ch. 7.

[77] I.W., *Coppie of a letter*, sig. B7^r–v^.

[78] *The Divine Weeks and Works of Guillaume de Saluste Sieur du Bartas*, ed. Susan Snyder, tr. Josuah Sylvester (Oxford, 1979), 378, ll. 736–68; *The Workes of Guillaume de Salluste*, ed. Urban T. Holmes, John C. Lyons, and Robert W. Linker (Chapel Hill, NC, 1935–40), 733, ll. 305 ff. The tradition of using medical and scientific material in Hexamera was present in St Ambrose, who probably drew on Cicero's *De natura deorum*: Siraisi, *Medieval and Renaissance Medicine*, 7–8. Ashmole described an old Latin text, owned by Dr Barlow, Bishop of Lincoln, which he thought Du Bartas translated and published as his own: Ashm. 826, fo. 119.

[79] 'Heere sorrow stopt the doore | Of his sad voice, and almost dead for woe, | The prophetizing spirit foresooke him so.' 'The Handicrafts', ll. 772–4, in Du Bartas, *Divine Weeks*, ed. Snyder, 379.

Du Bartas, Forman, and the elusive I.W. probably drew on similar sources and traditions and their lists suggest an association of the Fall, disease, and alchemy across a spectrum of literature, medical, alchemical, literary, and moral, in sixteenth-century Europe. Forman perused this material in pursuit of information about man, the cosmos, medicine, and disease. He documented what happened when Adam and Eve ate the fruit of the tree of knowledge and sowed the seeds of disease within their bodies. Banished from Paradise, they kept free will and the knowledge of good and evil, the two vehicles by which humankind had thereafter tried to return to the tree of life, once again to eat the food of angels and achieve eternity.

10
Magic and Medicine

Anno domini 1599 the 17 Aug ♀ an m [Friday morning] very early I drempt that I and Jhon Ward our clarke and another were in the chauncell of a church together and Jhon Ward was calling sprites for me thought he had powar in calling of sprites, and stod by loking on him to see the sprites but I could not see them but by glimpsinge and then me thought I sawe a white sprite. And I byd him aske the sprites what wold mak me to see and he determined to doe yt but we could not bring them to speake and talk to us. And I loked up and sawe the church dore open, and I went to shut yt leste any body should com in and as I came to the dore ther cam in a talle long old woman with exceading black hallowe eyes and too daughters with her. And I asked them sayinge what ar youe and wherfore com youe heather. And the woman said I com heather to learne som of thy conninge for thou art calling of sprites heare. And my daughter here is a witch and she by her skille dyd knowe yt & brought me heather to have som of this sprites. And she cam that she might have some alsoe. And her daughter was the uglieste creature that ever I sawe & black with a long face yll favored & she had mad contracts me thought with the dyvell. And me thought with that the body of the church was full of sprites flying up and downe. And I sayd unto the woman, doste thou and thy daughter think that my conninge and hers is like? I bind thes sprites by poware divine, and soe mak use of them to gods glory and youe mak contracts with the dyvell and give him your soulls to worke mischefe for youe. A waye youe evill disposed creatures god hath noe fellowship with the dyvell. And with that I waked.[1]

This dream is set in a church, enacted Forman's desire to be able to call spirits, and insisted that this art was divine not demonic. It also documented the connections between these themes and Forman's divinatory services. Forman recorded his dreams because they foretold the future, and this dream, he thought, presaged a visit later that day from one Mrs Riddelsden, 'for my Lady Hayward to learne her future lyfe, &c.' Frances Hayward (usually Howard) was the 21-year-old daughter of Thomas Howard, soon to became Mrs Henry Pranell, then countess of Hertford. She frequently consulted Forman, though it is not clear whether he associated the foul women in the dream with her and her messenger, or whether divination in general linked the dream and a concern for Lady Howard's future. Natural magic was a component of chymical and hermetical physic and the Paracelsian cosmology that linked the

[1] Ashm. 219, fo. 136. For other dreams about calling spirits see Ashm. 1472, p. [813] (19, 23 Aug. 1594).

microcosm and macrocosm, and enabled the adept physician to heal the body. But in drawing on a congeries of magical traditions Forman risked accusations of witchcraft and heresy.

Forman seldom noted his presence in a church. From 1584–9 he lived opposite St Thomas's Church in Salisbury, and St Thomas's was perhaps where he was caught at morning prayer with a book containing unorthodox prayers and images, probably a book of magic.[2] St Thomas's was also where, again in 1587, Forman reputedly had sex with Anne Young on the freshly laid tomb of his enemy, the sheriff Giles Estcourt.[3] In 1589 he had had another dream set in a church. This time God appeared to him and his friends in the form of an extremely bright light, and one of his friends, who had been dead for sixteen years, prophesied that there would be war between great nations.[4] In 1592 Forman predicted that the stinking graves in the yard of St Magnus's Church near London Bridge indicated an impending plague; which it did, afflicting him and his unnamed companion that summer.[5] Church windows recorded family history and in 1606 Forman noted that he had seen the arms of Sir William Forman, lord mayor of London during the reign of Henry VIII, 'in St Andrewes church in filpot Lane in London. In the glasse windowe in the south syd about the middle of the windowe in the bodie of the Church.'[6] In his casebooks he also recorded the incidental details of other people's lives that took place in church, such as the woman who lost her apron, the man whose purse was stolen, and the friends who met at morning service, though he did not record his habitual attendance at services. For him churches were places where one might pray, defile the memories of one's enemies, trace the past, and invoke spirits.

Forman's mentions of churches betray his silences about religion. He complained that priests had not objected to the pulling down of churches, he described magical abilities conferred by the church (as well as those conferred by nature or by God), and some of his friends, including Avis Allen with whom he had a turbulent relationship in 1593–7, were recusants.[7] Other friends, such as Thomas Blague and Richard Napier, were Protestant clerics, and in Forman's

[2] *Complete State Papers Domestic*, reel 81, 10 Mar. 1587; Ashm. 208, fo. 42ᵛ; 390, fo. 125. For Forman's residence in St Thomas's churchyard, see Ashm. 390, fo. 60.

[3] Salisbury record office, Bishop of Salisbury deposition books no. 10, fos. 46ʳ⁻ᵛ, 57; no. 11, fos. 17ʳ⁻ᵛ, 25ᵛ, 26. See also p. 35.

[4] Ashm. 1472, p. [811] (26 July 1589).

[5] Ashm. 1403, fos. 18ᵛ, 30.

[6] Ashm. 208, fo. 217ᵛ. Forman used to pass this church on his way to a needle maker's shop 'beyond St Andres church by Philpot Lane, going to Towar Street': Ashm. 1491, p. 872. William was elected lord mayor in 1538, *DNB*. For Forman's drawing of Sir William's coat of arms, as he found it in a book, see Ashm. 802, fo. 191.

[7] See for instance Ashm. 208, fo. 125ᵛ (against pulling down churches), 131ᵛ (against those who write that hell and devils do not exist). On magic and the church see Ashm. 1491, p. 1127, discussed below. On Avis Allen as a recusant see Rowse, *Forman*, 53; Traister, *Forman*, 151.

final years he served as a vestryman at St Mary's in Lambeth.[8] His readings of medieval texts, such as *The hystory of kyng Boccus and Sydrake* and the 'Life of Adam and Eve' (though its composition dated from earlier), informed his understanding of religious doctrine. But he did not address theological questions directly, instead embedding them in discussions about the causes of disease, such as in his plague treatises, and in his account of the relationship between man and the cosmos, such as in his essays on the 'Microcosmos' and the 'Heavens'. In his astrological tracts Forman distinguished between diseases caused by nature, by the devil, and by God. He blamed the plague of 1593 on the sins of his countrymen.[9] Against his many opponents he invoked the divine prerogative of his knowledge. God had overlooked the mathematical practitioners who denounced his method for calculating the longitude. Physicians, surgeons, and other medical practitioners were motivated by greed and practised according to conventions not wisdom. God had chosen him, Forman insisted, to do his work, blessing him especially with an aptitude for astrological physic and subjecting him to trials against adversaries who accused him of quackery and an allegiance to the devil. Suspicion of demonic magic probably fuelled Forman's dispute with Hood and perhaps informed his encounters with the College of Physicians. His reputation for demonic magic survived him, embodied in the papers and objects that were displayed at the Overbury trials.[10]

Forman distinguished between good and evil magic and worried that his divine pursuits might be mistaken for demonic, a concern realized when he was suspected of using necromancy to judge the cause of a disease without seeing a patient or her urine and probably prompting him in 1601 to cast a figure to decide 'Best to burn ye books'.[11] He aspired to the status of a magus. He was chosen by God to heal the plague. He read the fates of his clients in the stars and thereby won their trust. He cultivated a persona as a figure of opposition and power, a magician. His magic could be seen as a science with which to master the workings of nature, a perspective fostered by early modern natural philosophers who pursued magic, and perpetuated by scholars who have studied them.[12] His magic could also be seen as a subversion of

[8] *Lambeth Churchwardens' Accounts 1504–1645, and Vestry Book*, 1610, ed. Charles Drew, iii (1943), 210–14, 234, 237, 275. For ambiguous notes about his holding parish offices in 1599 see Ashm. 219, fo. 135.

[9] Ashm. 208, fos. 121–33^{v}.

[10] See the Introduction.

[11] Ashm. 403, fo. 81; 1495, fo. 486 (magic); 411, fo. 126^{v} (books). On demonic magic see Forman's translation of Artephius, 'Key of the greater wisdom', and his apparent denunciation of him: Sloane 3822, fos. 103–44; Ashm. 244, fo. 1^{v}. Artephius is reputed to have died in the 12th cent. after living for hundreds of years, and a number of fabulous alchemical and astrological texts are attributed to him.

[12] e.g. Dee, Boyle, and Newton: Yates, *Bruno*; Clulee, *Dee's Natural Philosophy*; Harkness, *Dee's Conversations with Angels*; Hunter, 'Alchemy, Magic and Moralism'; Principe, *Aspiring Adept*, ch. 6; J. E.

religion, the use of rituals to coerce demons and spirits, thus positioning Forman as an heir to medieval magical traditions.[13] Magic is often defined against science and religion, the precise relationship depending on whether one works with universal or historical definitions.[14] Forman was engaged in activities that for the most part had practical applications in terms of understanding and influencing the workings of nature, whether in calculating the longitude or treating disease. God's intentions and the threat of the devil were implicit in these concerns, and components of ritual were present in Forman's practices. Like a natural philosopher, he was systematic in observing the causes of disease; like a magus he harnessed the powers of the stars to improve his destiny; like a cleric, he prayed. Systematization and supplication cannot be so rigorously divided and components of magic, science, and religion were practical, operative activities in Forman's life. In the sixteenth and seventeenth centuries some scholars defined a magic which was not operative, but contemplative, allowing practitioners to achieve spiritual enlightenment through its practice. This is often referred to as spiritual magic.[15] Forman drew on similar traditions to these scholars, but he was not one of them. He summoned spirits, harnessed astral powers, and heard the voices of angels because as an astrologer-physician he was charged to divine things past, present, and to come, to heal disease, and to proclaim the sanctity of this work. For John Dee the magus could bring unity to a world riven by corruption, but Forman's ambitions were evidently more immediate, framed in the language of divine retribution, personal preferment, and wealth, not the progress of the commonwealth.[16]

In Forman's exposition of the 'Microcosmos' he drew on books espousing Renaissance Neoplatonism and Paracelsianism, traditions that since Ficino's efforts in the late fifteenth century had fostered discursive texts on magic. In medieval Europe magical books passed from hand to hand, sometimes excerpted into recipe books and other collections, sometimes copied in full.[17] Like books of secrets, magical books were cumulative endeavours, in part

McGuire and P. M. Rattansi, 'Newton and the "Pipes of Pan" ', *Notes and Records of the Royal Society*, 21 (1966), 108–43; Betty Jo Teeter Dobbs, *The Janus Faces of Genius: The Role of Alchemy in Newton's Thought* (Cambridge, 1991).

[13] Richard Kieckhefer, *Forbidden Rites: A Necromancer's Manual of the Fifteenth Century* (Thrupp, 1997).

[14] Richard Kieckhefer, 'The Specific Rationality of Medieval Magic', *American Historical Review*, 99 (1994), 813–36; Robert Scribner, 'The Reformation, Popular Magic, and the "Disenchantment of the World" ', *Journal of Interdisciplinary History*, 23 (1993), 475–94; Tambiah, *Magic, Science, Religion*.

[15] Walker, *Spiritual and Demonic Magic*; Webster, *Paracelsus to Newton*; cf. Clulee, *Dee's Natural Philosophy*, 128–42.

[16] Cf. Harkness, *Dee's Conversations with Angels*.

[17] Kieckhefer, *Forbidden Rites*.

practical and in part curious.[18] This was how Forman approached magic, as a practical, cumulative tradition. He most clearly articulated this in a treatise on geomancy written *c.*1590 and revised at the end of his life. Astronomy was the supreme form of knowledge and its operative components were 'astromagic' and 'alchemagic'. Astromagic was the use of amulets and other objects to harness the power of the stars, and alchemagic was the means of transmuting metals and making the philosophers' stone. The magus could employ his knowledge of the cosmos, through rituals and amulets, to make interventions in the workings of the world.[19] Forman considered the magical arts as akin to alchemy and astrology, and he copied magic texts and lodged magical information within his papers.

There were many traditions of magic and Forman's pursuit of it can be divided roughly into four sorts. He called spirits within a society of magic, then on his own with a scryer; he called angels; he practised astral magic, the use of amulets harnessing the powers of the stars; and he collected a diversity of magical material in 'Of appoticarie druges', therein depositing an invaluable record of the sorts of magic in circulation in early modern England. Beginning with 'Of appoticarie druges', then taking each of the other phases in turn, I will suggest that these magical activities were indivisible from Forman's work as an astrologer-physician.

'Of appoticarie druges' was a conglomeration of alchemical, astrological, medical, and magical information drawn from books learned and popular, experience, and hearsay. Thirty of its three-hundred entries mentioned magical operations or principles specifically and a handful ('magia naturalis', 'ars magnetica', 'homunculus') addressed it directly. A majority of these operations were to effect love magic or more malicious influences on a person's will and some were for healing. In the entry on 'Electrum', a mixture of two or more metals, Forman described the correlation between types of magic and metals: 'Quicksilver hath power of and over enchanting and enchanted. Led hath power over witchcraft. Copper hath power of binding. Tyne against thunder lightining and diseases. Silver dothe preserve and hath power in magik and enchantment. Yron doth bind and command and threaton.'[20] Under the entry for 'Spiritus' he described a hierarchy of spirits corresponding to the elements that could be used to bind, loose, curse, bless, and do harm.[21] Sometimes Forman appealed to occult forces in nature, sometimes to spirits; he never mentioned demons.

18 Eamon, *Science and the Secrets of Nature*; Long, *Openness, Secrecy, Authorship*, esp. ch. 5; Copenhaver, 'Tale of Two Fishes'.

19 Ashm. 392, fo. 46; see p. 52 above.

20 Ashm. 1494, pp. 483–4; on electrum see also Sloane 3822, fo. 7.

21 Ashm. 1491, pp. 1127–8. Forman also recorded this hierarchy of spirits in Ashm. 244, fos. 73^{v}–5.

Many entries described astral magic that worked through objects inscribed with images and words. Others described entities typically alchemical, such as the homunculus, mandrake, and speaking statue; classically occult natural objects (loadstone, poison from plants, spiders, snakes, and toads, and menstrual blood); images made from wax and metals; amulets made from metals, gems, stones, and herbs; potions in which such images were soaked or stones and minerals dissolved; human ingredients (urine, hair, blood, menstrual blood, turds, semen); animal ingredients (bones, snakes, and eggs); plants and herbs; and manufactured items such as nails, bells, and ink. Occasionally Forman recorded incantations and in quite a few entries he discussed the power of words and writing.[22] He designated some practices as traditional or old-fashioned, such as determining how well a garment would last according to the phase of the moon when it was first worn. Under 'Observances and old rulles' he discussed the meaning of thunder.[23] Very few operations were divinatory, except a brief account of hazel rods and a device made with a loadstone that could be used to communicate with someone hundreds of miles away. An entry on 'Prophetes and prophesyinge' described the need for a diviner to be physically pure.[24]

Forman also collected testimonials about the uses of magical objects and substances. Occasionally he had experienced these powers himself: he boiled snakes in a strong water and when he drank it his grey hair turned red again; he drew characters on his left arm and right breast in a semi-permanent ink in order to alter his destiny; and he had to give away the taffeta britches that he first wore during a waning moon.[25] Sometimes he noted gossip, such as when in 1603 a man in Westminster reported 'he sawe a mandrake of 7 inches longe with hair down to the feet and under the arm holes, like unto a man in form which was taken by on head a constable in turtell street from a witch which was carried to prison for bewitching of Sr Jhon Harizes sonn'.[26] But most of the information in these volumes does not contain verification or instruction. Forman did not privilege experience as a measure of whether or not a power or substance existed, and this compendium documents his collection of details about magic, informed through a lens of alchemical and Paracelsian medicine

22 See Ashm. 1494, pp. 398–404, 490, 586–96; 1491, pp. 1214, 1216, 1220–3, 1304–5, 1306–9.

23 Ashm. 1494, p. 272; 1491, p. 830.

24 Sloane 3822, fo. 90^v; Ashm. 1491, pp. 1358, 884. For evidence that Forman made such rods, see a record of his wife Jean (still a virgin) cutting eight hazel rods at the appointed hour which were then immediately whitened and inscribed on 8 Feb. 1598: Ashm. 226, fo. 303. The same communication device, constructed slightly differently, was described in a text appended to *Ars notoria: The notary art of Solomon*, tr. Robert Tanner (1657), 136–8.

25 Ashm. 1494, pp. 938 (hair), 586^v (tattooing), 272 (britches). For a recipe for the ink see Ashm. 1494, p. 402. Cf. Juliet Fleming, *Graffiti and the Writing Arts of Early Modern England* (2001), 111.

26 Ashm. 1494, p. 679.

refined in the final decade of his life. Forman's sources were ancient, medieval, Renaissance, Arabic, Jewish, Christian, and the traditions that he collected were natural, demonic, and angelic, designed to harm and to heal, and to divine the past, present, and future. This book contained information about calling spirits and angels and astral and sympathetic magic alongside details about chymical and hermetical substances and procedures. It was the culmination of three decades of work as an astrologer-physician, student of alchemy, and aspiring necromancer.

When he left Oxford in the mid-1570s, Forman studied magic along with astronomy, physic, and philosophy.[27] From the 1580s he pursued necromancy and other sorts of magic alongside his studies of astrology, alchemy, and medicine, drawing on traditions of Solomonic, hermetic, and Christian ritual magic. Like astrology and geomancy, magical operations could be used to divine things past, present, and to come; unlike the divinatory arts, magic could also be used to effect power over people, objects, and the natural and spiritual worlds. Texts detailing these procedures, deriving from Jewish cabalistic, Arabic, and Christian sources, had circulated amongst clerics in the Middle Ages. Conventionally they outlined a regime of prayer or invocations through which angels or demons (which Forman referred to as spirits) would reveal knowledge.[28] John Dee drew on these texts, extending the remit of revelation to the knowledge of the ends of nature.[29]

Forman had bought a number of magical texts in the 1580s, including a copy of the 1567 Paris edition of Agrippa's *De occulta philosophia*. The suspect books that he took to church in 1587 probably contained magical prayers and images. The following year he first 'began to practice foiygomercy and to calle angells & sprites', and employed John Goodage, then Stephen Mitchel to skry for him.[30] In the spring of 1590 he 'wrote a bocke of nigromanti' and in the autumn he 'entred a cirkell for nicromanticall spells'.[31]

In the 1590s he worried about his lack of aptitude for calling spirits and

27 Ashm. 208, fo. 225.

28 Claire Fanger (ed.), *Conjuring Spirits: Texts and Traditions of Medieval Ritual Magic* (Thrupp, 1998).

29 Harkness, *Dee's Conversations with Angels*. See also Stephen Clucas, 'John Dee's Angelic Conversations and the *Ars Notoria*: Renaissance Magic and Mediaeval Theurgy', in Clucas (ed.), *John Dee: Interdisciplinary Studies in English Renaissance Thought* (Dordrecht, 2006), 231–73; Clulee, *Dee's Natural Philosophy*, 132–9. For other 16th-cent. copies of magical texts see Frank Klaassen, 'English Manuscripts of Magic, 1300–1500: A Preliminary Survey', in Fanger (ed.), *Conjuring Spirits*, 3–31.

30 Ashm. 208, fo. 43^{v}. In his summary of the events of 1587 Forman noted 'I practised magik and had moch strife with divers that I had in suete of Lawe': Ashm. 208, fo. 42^{v}. Throughout 1588 he recorded cryptic notes that might relate to people with whom he practised magic, such as 'Susan Farwell became my daughter' and 'my special frinds and I were set at variance': Ashm. 208, fo. 43^{v}. He wrote the word 'foiygomercy', perhaps in an archaic fashion, in bold, distinct, and upright letters. It might read 'soiygomercy', in which case it probably relates to Dee's pursuit of the 'Book of Soyga', on which see Harkness, *Dee's Conversations with Angels*, esp. pp. 44–5, 161.

31 Ashm. 208, fo. 46^{v}.

looked to the stars to discover whether he would achieve the power of necromancy and to determine the best times for such attempts. Later, in 'Of appoticarie druges', he noted that a skryer's body must be 'purged from evill humours' in order to see the truth in a glass, and listed the variety of spirits and the requirements for calling them.[32] Spirits were simultaneously subtle and elemental; they were made from a celestial substance but had fallen into different levels of the sublunary world. The lowest were utterly damned to the darkness of hell. Others resided either in the fiery region, the airy region, the watery region, or the earthly region. Fiery spirits were the most swift and powerful (second only to the infernal spirits in hell), they could be seen in fire or with light, and were to be called on a fair and still day. Airy spirits, or 'sprites of the ayre', were next in swiftness, caused storms, and were to be called on a fair day. Watery spirits had grosser bodies and were slower, they only had power over watery works, were easier to call and to compel, and could be seen in a glass of water at night or on a rainy day. They had power to effect floods, rainstorms, and tempests, and to bring treasure out of the sea and overturn ships. Earthy spirits were thick and slow in appearance and action, robust and laborious, and were the easiest to see, especially by melancholy men in cold climates. They had to be called in secret and solitary places in a mirror, and they caused earthquakes and fetched treasure. Forman attributed this taxonomy to himself with his name in the margin, though it derives from the classification of demons by Michael Psellus, the eleventh-century Byzantine scholar.[33] An ability to call these spirits, Forman continued, depended on whether one's power came from God, nature, or the church. Some people could bind, loose, and command spirits by nature according to the constellations under which they were born, others, like Moses, received this gift from God, and others, like the Apostles, received the gift from Christ.[34] Forman, it seems, could not call by nature, but he hoped to do so by the grace of God.

Despite Forman's efforts, in September 1591 the spirit would not appear.[35] He continued practising various forms of necromancy. In 1592 he copied the 'Picatrix'.[36] Several years later he left this manuscript out in his study and one Henry Pepper saw it and tried to 'undercrop' him.[37] Early in 1594 he 'made virgun parchment and newe wrote my bock of magickes', probably a procedure to reinvigorate its powers.[38] That year to his habitual tag, 'practizer of phisique and studente of astronomie', he added 'philosophie and naturalle magique

[32] Ashm. 1491, pp. 884, 1127.

[33] For sources that recorded Psellus' scheme, see for instance Clulee, *Dee's Natural Philosophy*, 135, 139.

[34] Ashm. 1491, p. 1127^{r-v}; see also 244, fos. 73^{v}–5.

[35] Lilly, *Life*, 19–22; Ashm. 208, fo. 59^{v}.

[36] Ashm. 244, fo. 97; see also p. 52.

[37] Ashm. 208, fos. 56^{v}, 57.

[38] Ashm. 208, fo. 50.

&c.'[39] In August of that year he dreamt about Christ, incidentally documenting his study of the Solomonic 'Key to knowledge'. Christ showed Forman many things, including

a paper of paste bord halfe a yard long or better & better then a quarter brod, wher on wer drawen round a bout many triangles on joyning to another, and in each triangle was a round ☉. And in the midst of all the triangles was a great randoll [roundel]. And he showed them me pointing them out with a pair of compas & a ruell, and said yt was the ground of all things in the wordle. & him selfe had made yt, and all knowledge did consist therin. And I said ar ther noe more of them but this, & he said ther is but one more of them in the wordle & I waked.[40]

The 'Key to knowledge' portrayed various roundels, or dials like this, along with the prayers that would be invoked over them in order to summon spirits.[41] Forman was also concerned with mirrors and the following day he dreamt that a spirit appeared in three shapes in three different polished glasses and that his three companions could see it but he could not.[42] Four days later he 'drempt I did see in a glas when I did call and that I did heare alsoe & that yt was the first tim that ever I did heare or see & I was annswered directly of all things'.[43] A few years later he again used John Goodage, now referred to as 'a gelded fellowe', as a skryer, noting the following in his casebook:

Glas
Item 1597 the 8 of August ☾ an m at 40 p 9 [Monday, 9.40 a.m.] we began to mak our glase & to praie & Jhon fasted the ☾ ☿ ♀ ♄ befor & the sam dai & bought the glas on ♄ [Saturday] the 6 of Aug, & we drue the circle in vergun parchment.[44]

A couple of months later 'the sprite came and shook the bed for or five times and cast out such a fire and brimstone that it stank mightily and that night he kept much adoe and rored mightily but I saw him not. But I sawe the fire &

[39] This was in 'Grounds of arte': Ashm. 1495, fo. 11.

[40] Ashm. 1472, p. [813] (18 Aug. 1594).

[41] *The key of Solomon the King*, tr. and ed. S. Liddell MacGregor Mathers (1888).

[42] Ashm. 1472, p. [813] (19 Aug. 1594). BL MS Add. 36674, fos. 5–22 is an English version of this work, very similar to many of Forman's MSS but not in his hand.

[43] Ashm. 1472, p. [813] (23 Aug. 1594). The next month Forman dreamt that he was lost on a highway and the archangel Michael appeared to him to show him the way: Ashm. 1472, p. [813] (8 Sept. 1594), though the account is incomplete.

[44] Ashm. 226, fo. 172^{v}. This is probably the same man as 'John Good', who came to live with Forman in 1598, and who later confessed to robbing his study: Ashm. 208, fo. 59^{v}; 392, fo. 136; see also 219, fos. 135, 136. Forman referred to glasses throughout his notes, sometimes meaning scrying mirrors, sometimes distilling containers, and sometimes perhaps ordinary mirrors. For instance, on 4 June 1596 he queried whether to let his man borrow the glass again or not (Ashm. 234, fo. 51^{v}); in June 1596 his alchemical glasses were disrupted (Ashm. 234, fo. 62); and on 6 March 1607 he lost a glass in his study. For the suggestion that this might have been John Ward, the clerk that Forman dreamt about calling spirits in a church in 1599, or John Braddege, who worked for Forman from 1596–1600, see Traister, *Forman*, 221.

then sawe him in a kind of shape but not perfectly.' Two days later it appeared again, this time spitting flames and taking the form of a large black dog.[45] In 1599, the year of the dream with which this chapter began, Forman employed an unnamed seer and dreamt, 'I was sore trobled about hiding of my bocks of papers & I had strange bocks brought me writen w. karacts'.[46] In 1600 he copied a number of books, including the 'Ars notoria', a medieval book of images and orations by which one could achieve knowledge through contemplation, or 'inspection', and prayer instead of study, and Johannes Trithemius' 'Steganographia' (composed in 1499), a manual of cryptography often misread for instructions to summon spirits.[47]

Forman's interest in the 'Ars notoria', which he copied at least three times and illuminated at least twice, marks a shift from his attempts to summon visible spirits to efforts to commune with angels.[48] His version of this text began with an account of the history of how Solomon was selected by God as a recipient of His wisdom, knowledge, and grace. He sent an angel, Panphilius, to Solomon bearing golden tablets inscribed with geometrical images encasing orations or prayers composed of the names of angels in Chaldean, Greek, and Hebrew. Panphilius taught Solomon how to use these tablets, and Solomon thereby obtained all wisdom and knowledge. This art was then passed to Apollonius, a learned doctor and philosopher, who translated the orations into Latin and wrote a commentary on them. He who rehearsed these prayers and contemplated these images (each *notae* was made up of a series of *figurae*) according to the appropriate positions of the moon throughout the month (lunations) and according to the correct regime throughout the day would achieve the understanding of all sciences, a perfect and enduring memory, and the eloquence with which to express such knowledge. This was the first step. The adept could then proceed to the knowledge of the seven liberal sciences,

[45] In another account of the same session Forman recorded that he heard the spirit, but could not see it: Ashm. 354, fos. 236–7.

[46] Ashm. 219, fos. 135–6, 146 (6 Sept. 1599).

[47] Ashm. 208, fo. 62^{v}. On 'Ars notoria' see Clucas, 'Dee's Angelic Conversations and the *Ars Notoria*'; Klaassen, 'English Manuscripts of Magic', esp. pp. 14–19; Page, 'Magic at St. Augustine's'; Thorndike, *Magic and Experimental Science*, ii. 281–3 and *passim*. On Dee's reading of 'Ars notoria', 'Steganographia', and Trithemius' other writings see Clulee, *Dee's Natural Philosophy*, 128–39; Harkness, *Dee's Conversations with Angels*, *passim*. In Nov. 1600 Forman dreamt about borrowing books of magic from a friend, but otherwise he does not specify how he obtained these texts: Ashm. 236, fo. 263.

[48] Bodleian, Jones MS 1; Trinity O.9.7; Jerusalem, National Library, Yahuda MS VAR. 34. For drafts of the drawings owned and labelled by Forman, but I suspect not drawn by him, see Ashm. 820, iii. Forman used Bodley MS 951, an elaborate 15th-cent. copy, and other versions to make his copies. Ashm. 1515 is a translation of Bodley MS 951, without the illustrations, bearing the initials A.C. and probably predating Forman's copies. I am grateful to Julien Veronese, who is preparing the 1st critical edn. of the 'Ars notoria', for advising me about these MSS: private correspondence 29 Oct. 2001. For printed edns. see Cornelius Agrippa von Nettesheim, *Opera Omnia*, ii (Lyons, *c.*1620), 603–60; *Ars notoria*.

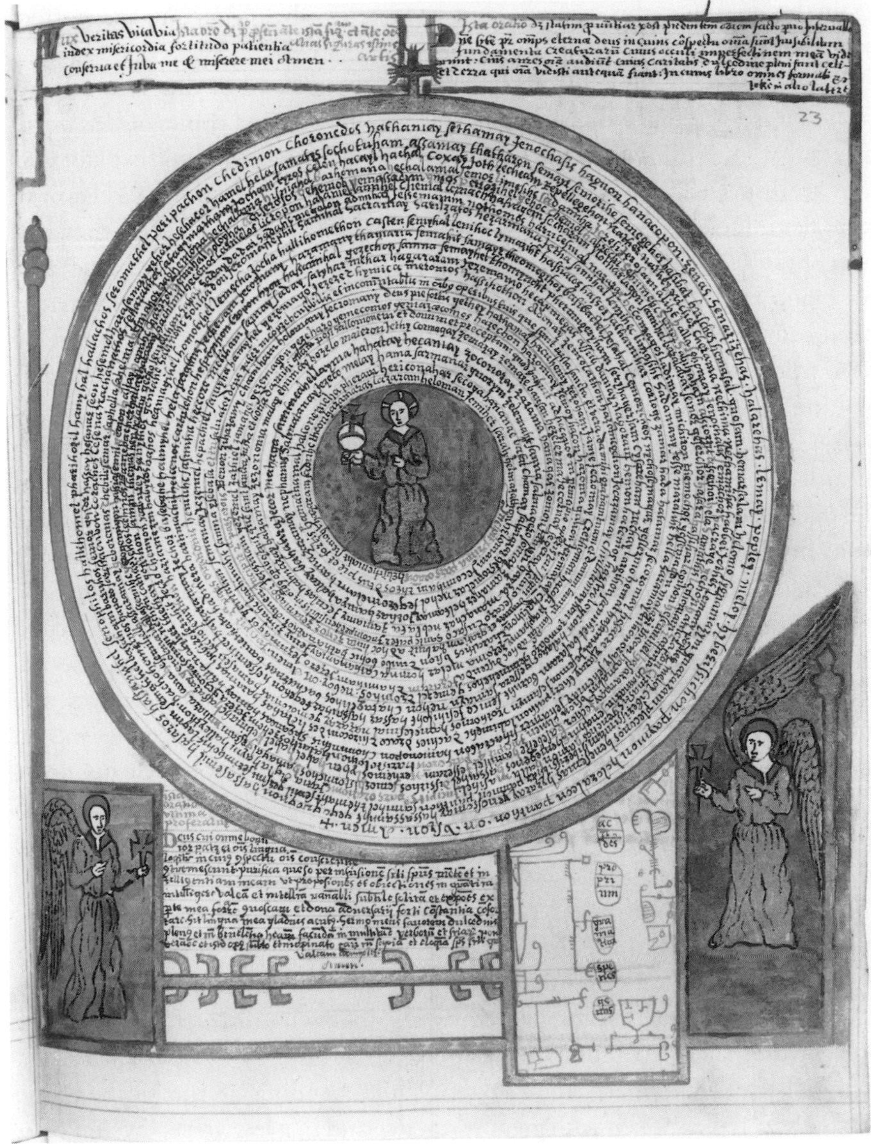

10.1. A page from one of Simon Forman's copies of the 'Ars notoria', Jones 1, fo. 23. By permission of the Bodleian Library, University of Oxford.

again by speaking the orations and inspecting the *figurae* at the correct moments over a period of time.[49]

While Forman's copies of many alchemical texts and of the 'Life' are fair copies, it is uncertain why he made multiple, illuminated copies of 'Ars notoria'. Perhaps he gave them to his friends or sold them, which would explain why they are dispersed from Forman's other papers. One version of this text (now in Jerusalem) included only a single interjection by Forman, a note on the position of the moon, and was probably the most similar to the parent text.[50] His colophon reads 'This booke and al the figures and signs therin contained as youe here find yt was drawen out & written according to the old coppie by Simon Forman gentleman and d. of physick with his own hand 1600 Anno Eliz 42 June.'[51] Two other copies were working texts. The copy now at Trinity College, Cambridge, had no illustrations and was dated 28 June 1600, the same month as the Jerusalem copy. It contained a gloss on the text in English, and at the end Forman added a number of prayers from other texts, including some from printed books, and others that 'I toke out of the other bock that was writen in paper that Mr Conie brought me'.[52] This was George Coney, the friend and client of Forman's from at least the late 1590s with whom he shared an interest in astrology, calling spirits, and books on these topics, though Coney 'was ferfull & timorous in magicalle arte & durst not attempte any more'.[53] The copy of the 'Ars notoria' now in the Jones collection was in progress between 1600 and 1603, and in it Forman incorporated his notes amongst the text. Unlike his annotations to the 'Life', Forman's additions to the 'Ars notoria' were practical, not philosophical, documenting his adherence to a prescribed regime of prayers.

The 'Ars notoria' provides a possible link between Forman's study of magic and his astrological physic, a link perhaps explained by the Neoplatonic origins of the notary tradition. Most of the *notae* represent different arts, and physic is amongst them. This is accompanied by the following instructions, with the precept that these operations were to be done only by someone who had achieved the preliminary knowledge. While standing at the sickbed, the oration was to be spoken with great reverence and in a low voice, 'by and by it shalbe declared to thee and suggested in thy minde by angelical vertues wheather that sicke partie shall recover health or die of that same sickness'.[54]

[49] Ashm. 1515, fo. 23^{v}. [50] Yahuda MS VAR. 34, fo. 8. [51] Yahuda MS VAR. 34, fo. 21.

[52] Trinity MS O.9.7, fos. 107^{v}, 115.

[53] Ashm. 206, fo. 312. This detail is part of Forman's analysis of Coney's nativity and dates from some time after 1602.

[54] Sloane 3822, fo. 175^{r-v}; cf. Ashm. 1515, fo. 34; Jones MS 1, fos. 41–4.

This was the same question for which Forman often sought an answer in the stars. There were further medical uses for this oration. In order to know if a woman was pregnant, the practitioner was to stand in front of her and to utter the prayer. The voices of angels would reveal whether she was with child, and if so, what sex it was. Likewise for the question of a woman's virginity. These were three questions frequently posed to, or by, an astrologer-physician. While the astrologer mapped the heavens at the time of the question and judged the answer according to a set of rules, the Solomonic adept performed the required ritual and was inspired with knowledge directly. The rituals for an astrological interview and a magical action were almost the same.

But Forman did not record whether he practised the notary arts, nor whether he prayed in the consulting room, though a fragment of a work in his hand entitled 'This is the Bocke of cuering and healinge of wondes and diseases in seacrete only by prayer unto god &c' survives.[55] Likewise, though he noted that he began to call angels as well as spirits in 1587, his angelic pursuits were less well documented. He did speak with the angel Raziel, who, as Forman noted in the margins of the 'Life', had given Adam a book of astronomy and magic which was later discovered by Solomon.[56] This was the 'Liber Raziel', a Jewish compilation of esoteric magic, a book that Forman seems to have known and in which he probably found the instructions to summon the angel.[57] They had a conversation about mistletoe in which Raziel explained ('said unto me') that the variety that grew on oak trees

> belongeth to ♃ especially, and ♀ hath a parte therin, and yt oughte to be gathered and administered in hora ♃, betwen ye firste quarter and the full ☾ and beste in Maye. Yt is good againste the dropsie being rubbed theron, and after rub the place with a red cloth.[58]

Forman did not record what else Raziel told him.

Summoning angels and spirits did not necessarily require astrological calculations, but some of these operations included components of Arabic astral magic and relied on the positions of the stars. Such calculations were essential to astral magic, or as Forman sometimes called it, astromagic, the use of

[55] Sloane 3822, fo. 175^{r-v}. See also Ashm. 1495, fo. 38^{v}. Napier did pray in the consulting room: MacDonald, *Mystical Bedlam*, 221–2; Ashm. 240, fos. 130–4; 244, fos. 130–5; 1790, fos. 112–14; 112–25. Cf. Yates, *Bruno*, 151.

[56] Ashm. 802, ii, fos. 3^{v}, 14^{r-v}; see p. 192 above.

[57] Napier also was interested in this book and recorded what Raziel told him: Ashm. 1790, fo. 116; Sloane 3822, fo. 24. Forman seems to have followed Raziel's prescriptions for writings magical books on virgin parchment with special inks: Ashm. 1491, pp. 1303–9.

[58] Ashm. 1491, p. 1278.

magical objects to harness the powers of the stars. These objects 'enclosed som parte of the vertue of heaven and of the plannets according to the tyme that it is stamped caste or engraven or writen in'.[59] Forman documented his pursuit of astral magic above all others. Throughout the 1590s he designed numerous magical objects which he referred to as sigils, laminas, rings, and 'characts', some for his own use, some for his friends and clients, some to cure disease, some to empower their bearer.[60] In 1597 he prescribed Jackemyne Vampena, a Dutch woman married to an English merchant, a series of potions, including one in which a ring engraved with the symbol of Jupiter had been immersed.[61] That year he thought he had lost a gold lamina, flat, metal amulet, which he had worn on his chest, but he found it 'behind my back in my doublet'.[62] In 1598 and 1599 he designed a series of rings and sigils made at the requisite times to capture the desired astral properties.[63] One of these rings had a golden setting holding a large coral stone engraved with the sign of Jupiter, under which was wedged a piece of parchment bearing Forman's name and an inscription of the words and symbols for Virgo and Mercury, the astrological house and its ruling planet at the time of his birth. It was to be worn on the little finger on his left hand, and would protect him against witchcraft and other ills as well as giving 'favour & credit & to mak on famouse in his profession & to overcom enimies'.[64] In 1601 he designed a sigil made under the sign of Scorpio for one Martha Shackleton.[65] In 1609, amongst some notes on Cabala, Forman copied numerous symbols and extensive passages from Agrippa's *De occulta philosophia*, added his revisions, and specified that these symbols could be used in cases of diseases.[66] The following year he designed a golden lamina for Jean Sherly that took four days to make and cost £4. 13*s*.[67] In 1611 he sent Richard

[59] Ashm. 392, fo. 46; see also 390, fo. 30. For more on Forman's magical objects, see my 'Economy of Magic'.

[60] For various laminas see Ashm. 234, fos. 96, 99; 226, fos. 148, 152, 310. For sigils see Ashm. 219, fo. 48; 226, fos. 148, 249^{v}; and examples below. Sloane 3822 is a collection of sigils and texts about them by Forman, Napier, Lilly, and Ashmole.

[61] Ashm. 411, fos. 95, 99^{v}, 115, 118^{v}.

[62] Ashm. 205, fo. 23; 226, fo. 166.

[63] Ashm. 195, fos. 29^{v}, 56^{v}–7^{v}, 58. See Ashm. 219, fo. 48 for details of the timing and costs of a ring and a sigil, and evidence that Forman seems to be paying for these in part in kind with his laminas. One of these was made for Forman's close friend Alice Blague.

[64] Sloane 3822, fo. 11. For Forman's description of how to make an 'imperialle' ring or lamina of gold by inserting a piece of peony, bay, or vervain and images of a lion, ram, and goat and their related astrological symbols on parchment or leather under a ruby, diamond, and heliotrope, then suffumigating it and praying, see Sloane 3822, fo. 77^{v}.

[65] Ashm. 411, fo. 58^{v}. This might be the same Mrs Shackleton whose coat of arms Forman described as having been made for her burial on 7 Jan. 1608: Ashm. 802, fo. 207^{v}. For Forman's account of a sigil of similar design, see Sloane 3822, fo. 96.

[66] Ashm. 244, fos. 6^{v}, 11^{v}.

[67] Sloane, 3822, fos. 13–15. For details of the other rings and sigils that he made that year and the next see Sloane 3822, fos. 16–19.

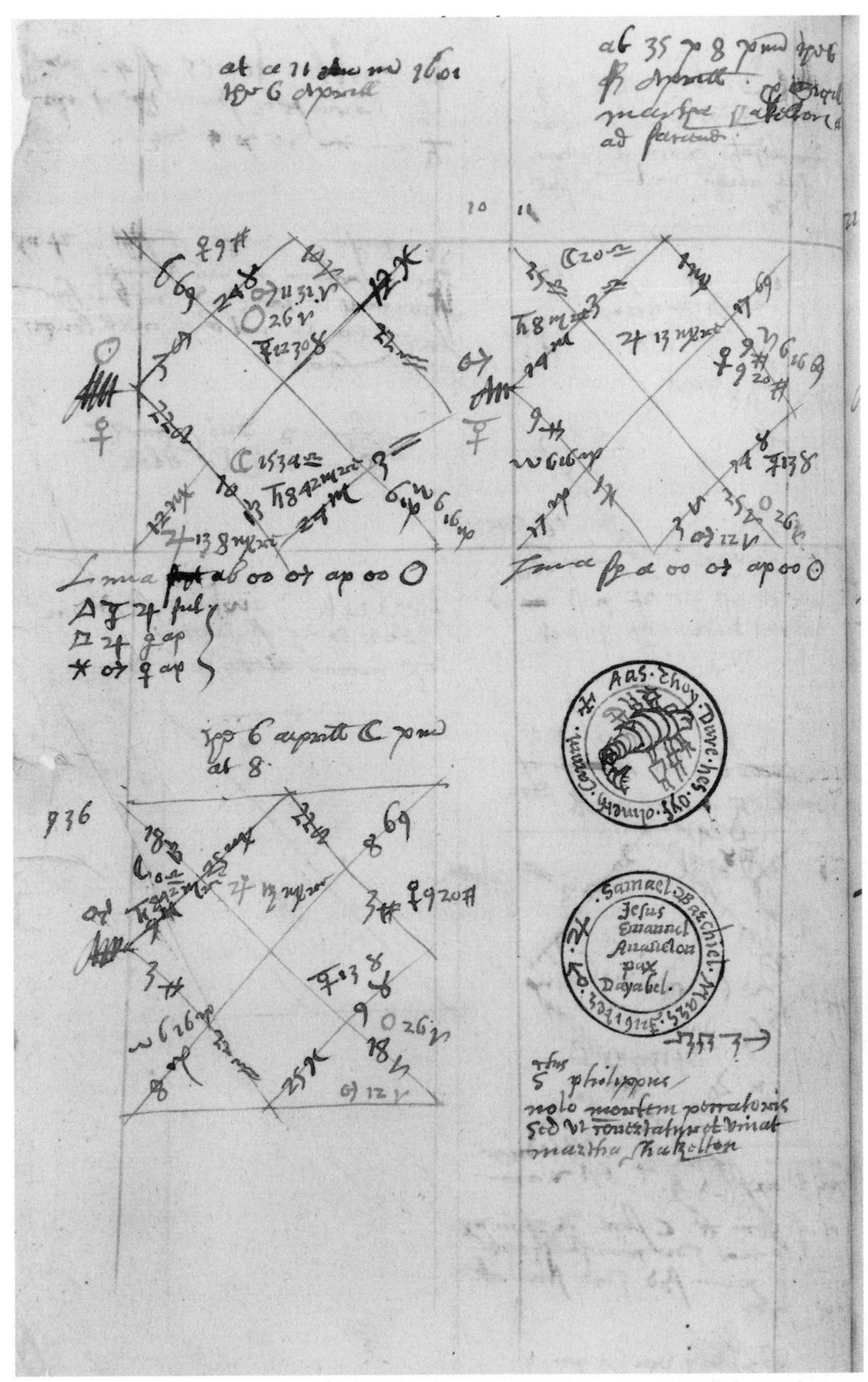

10.2. Calculations for and drawings of the sigil made for Martha Shackelton, 6 April 1601, Ashm. 411, fo. 58^{v}. By permission of the Bodleian Library, University of Oxford.

Napier some brass moulds to make symbols of the planets, and in the accompanying letter noted the following:

> Yf youe have them, and can tell howe to use them youe have a good thinge aswelle for the cueringe of diseases as for divers other purposes to caste therin in mettalle the sigelle of any plannet when he is stronge in the heavens for the effectinge of any purpose or thing pertaining to that plannet or when ther is a conjunction.[68]

Some of these objects became a legacy of Forman's practices after his death.[69]

Astral magic exploited the links between the microcosm and the macrocosm, allowing the magus to draw upon the powers of the stars. Its proponents subscribed to a Neoplatonic and hermetic cosmology, in some cases articulated within a Paracelsian concern for medicine. Natural philosophers, theologians, and demonologists debated whether astral magic worked by nature or by demons, often depending on whether words or images activated the objects. Forman stressed that astral magic was natural. For instance, he described an image that when sunk in a well caused all vessels dipped in it to break, explained that its power was derived from close observations of the planets, and concluded, 'The use of this kind of naturall magick is so lawfull that ther is nothing to be said to the contrary.'[70]

Thoughout 'Of appoticarie druges' Forman discussed astral magic and the production of sigils and rings, and he compiled this commonplace book at the same time as drafting his most sustained treatment of astral magic, his essays on the 'Heavens' (*c.*1606–8).[71] In 'Of appoticarie druges' the entry on 'Magia naturalis' (blank in the Ashmole volumes but complete in the pages now in the Sloane collection) concluded 'And knowe that in all workes which in this wordle ar made The Cause of knowinge, or attayninge to any thinge is done by ymages. And yf youe diligently marke all that we have said and spoken before, youe shall moch proffit to attain to the perfection of this science.'[72] Under the entry for 'Ymage' Forman further described how images worked: 'An ymage is the force of coelestialle bodies flowinge and soe ymages worke by vertue and similitude.'[73] In the entries on 'Sigilla' and 'Amulets' Forman catalogued a series of designs attributed to Paracelsus, Villanova, and other sources for objects to prevent illness, procure wealth, and expel vermin.[74] Sigils with these

68 Ashm. 240, fo. 106. Forman indicated that someone else would have made the sigils.

69 For objects, allegedly made by Forman, brought into the trials in the Overbury case, see the Introduction. For the interest that Lilly and Ashmole took in Forman's sigils, see my 'Economy of Magic'.

70 Ashm. 802, ii, fos. 15ᵛ–16. Forman seems to have drawn this and other examples from a book of magic of Spanish provenance: Ashm. 1494, p. 484; 802, ii, fos. 15ᵛ–16.

71 Ashm. 244, fos. 34–118; see Ch. 2 above for a full discussion of this text.

72 Sloane 3822, fos. 77–8ᵛ, quotation from fo. 77ᵛ.

73 Sloane 3822, fo. 81.

74 Sloane 3822, fos. 6–19, 80ʳ⁻ᵛ, 94–102.

powers were also prominent in the 'Heavens', where Forman explained that magical operations, such as casting sigils, rings, and other objects needed to be conducted according to 'magical hours', the division of a day based on the motions of the eighth heaven.[75]

Forman calculated an astrological or on occasion a geomantical figure for the time at which he was consulted, and read this for the cause of the disease or to foresee its outcome. Sometimes he negotiated his conclusions with the patient or the person who had asked the question. If he judged the disease to be natural or unnatural, he might treat it with herbal or magical remedies, all of which had to be administered at astrologically propitious moments. This was the medical expertise of a self-made magus. Forman had charted the secrets of creation through thousands of texts, across decades of observations and calculations about the motions of the heavens, and in occasional dreams and revelations. He could read the stars and hear the voices of angels. He collected and practised numerous astrological, alchemical, and magical traditions. He was not an inspired magician, an accomplished alchemist, nor an innovative astrologer. His study of these arts was inscribed in his medical practice, the panoply of his persona as an astrologer-physician. For Forman the spiritual pursuits of the magus were grounded in the mundane ambitions of making a living as an astrologer-physician.

[75] Ashm. 244, fos. 48, 91–2. For Ashmole's reading of these notes, see my 'Economy of Magic'.

CONCLUSION

Forman wrote constantly but he almost never finished anything. He read extensively but never articulated a philosophy of medicine. He fashioned himself as a physician while condemning those who earned this title through formal study. He disregarded the voices of his patients but used his astrological judgements to encourage them to be forthright and frank with him. While others promoted a new philosophy, he reinvigorated the study of the occult. Forman's papers preserve these paradoxes. He was a modern magus at work in London, reviving the ancient magical and medical secrets that he read about in books and manuscripts, discovered for himself, and learnt from the friends and associates about whom he recorded little. He used astrology and other divinatory arts to judge whether a disease had natural, unnatural, or supernatural causes. If an affliction was caused by God, then prayer was the best remedy; if it was caused by nature, or by the devil, or a witch working through nature, then the physician could choose from a repertoire of purges or magical interventions. This was not the medicine of learned physicians or empirics. Forman defined himself against them in theory and practice and identified himself with the prophets of old.

Forman's papers are a testament to his perseverance. They are also a testament to a moment when physicians were struggling to establish their authority through a definition of orthodox, Galenic medicine; when medical practitioners were exploring new remedies and beginning to exploit print as producers and consumers of books; and when the wonders of nature became the remit of natural philosophers and physicians who collected curiosities and studied the preternatural. Scholarly books marked these concerns and fuelled new trends. Forman did not contribute to these changes, perhaps because he was too untutored and intellectually disorganized to intervene in these complex debates, perhaps because he framed his aspiration for divine knowledge locally, in terms of his prerogative to practise medicine in London.[1] For Forman, like others, magic had become an elaborate set of skills adapted to suit his own purposes. He called himself the astrologer-physician of Lambeth, domineering, authoritative, perhaps with harsh wit charming his friends and patients into trusting him.

[1] Cf. the noble intentions of many early modern reformers: Clark, *Thinking with Demons*, 222; Webster, *Paracelsus to Newton*, 59.

Notes on his nativity written in 1605 revealed his ambitions and self-perception. In this account, Forman described himself as having four characteristics. First, he had good judgement: 'he shall practice arte with wisemen and with religiouse men and shalbe of greate understange and have a subtille sertching wit and be very politick and of great truth in judgement'. Secondly, he had an aptitude for knowledge, both old and innovative:

> And [he] shall have forsighte and knowledge in many artes and sciences and be apte to learne any thinge and shall give him selfe naturally to astronomi, phisich, and chirurgery and to distillations & making of poticari drugs, and newe inventions of arte and geomantia magick cosmografie philosofie diviniti and in all depe and subtille artes . . .

Thirdly, he instructed people in these arts. Fourthly, he had a sense of justice and civic duty: he 'shall be seen in lawe husbandry and building & shall have great delight to do justice and to maintain the state of a common weal and shall hate opression'. These attributes would be put to three uses: 'He shall be very lucky in marchandiz and in buying and selling of ymovable goods and shalbe a great phisision and astronomer, and in his last years he shall find much treasure by some secret arte or means and shalbe a horder up of gould in his old age.' He would achieve these things, despite much hardship, by his own industry.[2] In the celestial looking glass, Forman saw himself as a magus and as entrepreneur. On the streets of London, he was a successful physician and astrologer, and whether through his medical practice, property speculation, or, less likely, the location of hidden treasure he was worth £1200 at his death.[3] This combination of arrogance and monetary success lent itself to Forman's being branded as a quack, a reputation which, despite his personal shortcomings, does an injustice to his career, to those who sought his services, and to the medical world in which he worked.

Ashmole preserved the legacy of Forman's life and work in London, the written terrain that this study has charted. Like these papers, Forman's reputation has outlived him. He has featured as a charlatan in histories of astrology, alchemy, and medicine in England, but aside from his involvement (albeit hostile) with the mathematical practitioners, he has had no place in histories of the natural sciences. He pursued the occult and wrote in English. He was more interested in operative magic, divinatory techniques, and alchemical

[2] Ashm. 206, fo. 99. For a rare note about Forman's civic duties see Ashm. 219, fo. 135. For astrological questions about property see Ashm. 392, fos. 132–42.

[3] Lilly, *Life*, 23. Ashmole also recorded this figure at the bottom of one of the pages of Forman's diary along with the information that Forman's widow married a Northamptonshire gentleman, Mr Neals, but it is unclear whether he was Lilly's source or vice versa: Ashm. 208, fo. 60^{v}.

preparations than in natural philosophy, systematically recording the results of his procedures and calculations, without, for instance, formulating a theory of matter. I have placed Forman amongst his Elizabethan contemporaries, their books and manuscripts, and their hopes, uncertainties, and diseases. He thought of himself as a magus, overcoming divine trials to make his name and his fortune as an astrologer-physician.

Forman died in 1611, and his death marked not the end of an era in which astrology, alchemy, and magic thrived in London, but the beginning of a period of a more sustained and public pursuit of these subjects. Richard Napier had been Forman's protégé, and he inherited his papers. Napier read through many of Forman's writings, noting astrological rules and good recipes.[4] He also shared them with scholars who visited him, evidently lending a copy of Forman's guide to astrological physic to Matthias Evans and allowing Thomas Robson the opportunity to copy out many of Forman's papers, a process that probably resulted in the hash marks adorning these pages.[5] William Lilly also read some of Forman's papers, probably when he visited Napier throughout 1632–3.[6] In the account of his own life that he wrote at the behest of Ashmole in 1668 Lilly carefully constructed a genealogy of English astrologers, culminating with himself. This story began with Forman. Lilly had moved to London in 1620 as a servant to Gilbert and Margery Wright. Mrs Wright frequently visited cunning or wise men to discover whether her husband would die before her; 'this occasion begot in me [Lilly] a little desire to learn something that way, but wanting money to buy books, I laid aside these notions'.[7] Lilly nursed his mistress through her final illness, and she died in 1624, leaving him a large golden sigil that she had kept hidden with other objects in a scarlet bag in her armpit. This was engraved with prayers and symbols and had been made by Forman in order to ward off a ghost that had haunted Wright's first husband. Lilly recorded its inscriptions 'verbatim' and sold the sigil for 32 shillings. This event marked the beginning of Lilly's independence and the first step in his career as an astrologer.[8]

Before describing how he learnt astrology, Lilly gave an account of Forman's life, based primarily on his life-writings.[9] He praised Forman's astrological integrity. Forman was 'judicious and fortunate' in horary questions such as thefts, and sickness was his 'masterpiece'. He was meticulous and thorough in his calculations and 'had he lived to methodize his own papers, I doubt but that

4 Ashm. 1494, p. 145.

5 For Robson's naming himself in a correction to Forman's notes, see Ashm. 1494, p. 62.

6 Lilly, *Life*, 79. 7 Ibid. 13.

8 Ibid. 15–16. For a fuller account of the history of this sigil, see my 'Economy of Magic'.

9 Lilly, *Life*, 17–23.

he would have advanced the Iatromathematical part thereof very completely'. Despite his calculations, Lilly continued, Forman had difficulty in his pursuit of the philosophers' stone and his own preferment. Whatever Forman's skills, Lilly insinuated that he was an old-fashioned magician. He qualified the reference to the cunning or wise men whom his mistress had consulted with the phrase 'as were then called', not specifying whether these people still existed under a different name or had ceased to practise. He drew attention to Forman's more magical and less respectable activities and distanced himself and his astrology from Forman, though noting his own successes at calling spirits and cavorting with fairies. In Lilly's history, Forman played the part of a cunning man, not an enterprising pioneer of astrological physic.

Eight years after Lilly wrote his *Life*, Ashmole acquired the majority of Forman's papers from Napier's great-nephew, Thomas Napier.[10] A decade later, in a letter to Anthony Wood, Ashmole described Forman as 'a very able Astrologer and Phisitian, as appears by the manuscript bookes he left behinde him, which are now in my possession'.[11] Ashmole had begun to collect books, manuscripts, and objects in the 1640s and by the end of the century he had amassed an extensive collection which included texts on astrology, alchemy, magic, and medicine.[12] He studied these works, dabbled in astral magic in the early 1650s, attempted experiments for the philosophers' stone later that decade, and habitually practised astrology. When he acquired Forman's papers, he compiled lists of titles of Forman's treatises, noted works that he cited, recopied damaged pages, indexed figures that he had cast about the weather and the making of sigils, and sent them to the binder.[13] He soon began practising astral magic again, making dozens of sigils, some to improve his fortune, some to stop his wife from vomiting, most to drive vermin from his house and garden.[14] He systematically annotated the entry on 'Amulets' in 'Of appoticarie druges' with the natural and artificial hours at which they were made.[15]

10 *Ashmole*, ed. Josten, iii. 1208 n; iv. 1454–5.

11 Ibid. iv. 1809.

12 Michael Hunter, *Elias Ashmole, 1617–1692: The Founder of the Ashmolean Museum and his World* (Oxford, 1983), reprinted in Hunter, *Science and the Shape of Orthodoxy: Intellectual Change in Late Seventeenth-Century Britain* (Woodbridge, 1995), 21–44; Josten, *Ashmole*, i. 210; iii. 1208; iv. 1454–5, 1809. Most of these MSS are now in the Ashmole collection in the Bodleian, though it is unclear why some of Ashmole's papers, particularly those containing magical material, are now in the Sloane Collection in the British Library.

13 Ashm. 421, fo. 152; Sloane 3822, fo. 20.

14 *Ashmole*, ed. Josten, ii. 537, 538, 545–9, 567, 578–9, 584, 594, 595, 608, 619; iv. 1508, 1513, 1523, 1533, 1538–40, 1608–32, 1616, 1624, 1629, 1656–7, 1662–3, 1679, 1681, 1688–97, 1738.

15 Sloane 3822, fos. 6–19; *Ashmole*, ed. Josten, iv. 1508. To 'Of appoticarie druges' Ashmole also added a brief entry describing how to make disappearing reappearing ink: Ashm. 1494, p. 552. For Ashmole's annotations see Ashm. 1494, p. 85; Sloane 3822, fo. 84^{v}. Ashmole might also have book-marked items, e.g. the entry on 'Karacters' is presently marked with a slip of paper bearing numbers and astrological houses in Ashmole's hand: Ashm. 1494, p. 586.

He similarly annotated Forman's essays on the 'Heavens', paraphrased them, and checked Forman's figures against other sources, at one point finding Forman's calculations lacking in comparison with those included in Edward Sherbourne's tables in his edition of *The Sphere of M. Manilius* (1675).[16] Ashmole died in 1692, having ensured that Forman's papers were preserved with the rest of his collection of manuscripts, books, and rarities in the newly founded Ashmolean Museum in Oxford.

Forman's death provided a fitting end to his life.[17] Lilly collected rumours about Forman's activities, including his inscription of a book: 'This I made the devil write with his own hand in Lambeth Fields 1596, in June or July as I remember.' Lilly also memorialized Forman's powers by recording the story that his widow, Jean, told him about Forman's final days. In early September 1611, as Jean and Simon ate supper, she began to tease him. She had heard that he could predict whether a husband or wife would die first, and asked which of them would bury the other. He answered that she would bury him within a week. For six days nothing happened, but on the seventh, while he was rowing across the Thames from Lambeth to the City, he fell down, shouted 'An impost, an impost', and died. A wind storm marked the moment, a final tribute to his art.[18]

16 Ashm. 1790, fos. 78–100; 421, fos. 149^{r-v}. For his annotations, see esp. Ashm. 244, fos. 50, 51^{v}, 92, 96–7^{v}, 99^{v}, 107^{v}. Ashmole's final mention of him was in 1680 when he gathered peony roots and fraxinella seeds at a time set 'according to Dr Forman's rule': *Ashmole*, ed. Josten, iv. 1663–4.

17 For Forman's calculations for the moment of his death, see for instance Ashm. 206, fo. 101^{v}.

18 Lilly, *Life*, 22–3. Forman was buried in St Mary's Church, Lambeth on 12 Sept., and if Lilly was correct in saying that Forman died on a Thursday, then Forman died either on 5 or 12 Sept.: cf. Wood, *Athenae Oxonienses*, ii. 104; *DNB*; Rowse, *Forman*, 243, 258. See also Public Record Office, Prob 6/8 (1611), fo. 31.

BIBLIOGRAPHY

The place of publication is London unless otherwise stated.

I. SIMON FORMAN'S PRINCIPAL MANUSCRIPTS

The following is a list of Forman's principal manuscripts by subject, with dates. Unless specified, all items are primarily in Forman's hand, though in the casebooks and alchemical notebooks some passages are in other hands. All manuscripts cited in the footnotes are listed in the Index and many are included in the Chronology. For further bibliographical details see William Black, *A descriptive, analytical and critical catalogue of the manuscripts bequeathed unto the University of Oxford by Elias Ashmole* (Oxford, 1845) and W. D. Macray, *Index to the catalogue of manuscripts of Elias Ashmole* (Oxford, 1866).

Life writings

'The argumente between Forman and deathe in his sickness', 1585, Ashm. 208, fos. 232–48.

'The bocke of the life and generation of Simon . . .', begun 23 Dec. 1600, Ashm. 208, fos. 136–42.

Diary, 1603, Ashm. 208, fos. 1–74.

'Forman his repetition of the troble he had with the doctors of phisick in London and of his delivery in the plague 1592', a psalm, 1604, Ashm. 240, fos. 25–7^{v}; cont. Ashm. 802, fos. 131–3^{v}; see also 802, fos. 123–7.

'Of the name of Forman', Sept. 1605, Ashm. 208, fos. 214–24. The next text is a continuation of this.

'The firste of the Formans . . .', *c.*1605–6, Ashm. 802, fos. 211–15^{v}.

'The issue of Simon Forman', 1606+, Ashm. 208, fos. 225–6.

Forman's nativities, Ashm. 205, fo. 286^{r-v} (perhaps in Napier's hand); 206, fos. 218–25; 208, fo. 12.

Letters to Richard Napier

19 Sept. 1599, Ashm. 240, fo. 103.

31 Jan. [1599 or 1610], Ashm. 240, fos. 104, 111^{v}.

23 July 1611, Ashm. 240, fo. 106.

8 March [year unknown], Ashm. 1488, fo. 89.

Casebooks

Volume I, 17 Mar. 1596–19 Feb. 1597, Ashm. 234, fos. 1–157.
Volume II, 20 Feb. 1597–20 Feb. 1598, Ashm. 226, fos. 1–310^{v}.
Volume III, 20 Feb. 1598–8 Feb. 1599, Ashm. 195, fos. 1–246.
Volume IV, 8 Feb. 1599–31 Dec. 1599, Ashm. 219, fos. 1–229^{v}.
Volume V, 2 Jan. 1600–17 Dec. 1600, Ashm. 236, fos. 1–264^{v}.
Volume VI, 26 Dec. 1600–29 Nov. 1601, Ashm. 411, fos. 1–163^{v}.
Volume VIa, copies of Forman's casebooks in another hand, 11 May–5 Sept. 1603, Ashm. 411, fos. 164–79.

Astrological, medical, and related writings

Guides to geomancy

'De arte geomantica', 1589, Ashm. 354.
Another treatise on geomancy, *c.*1590, revised *c.*1611, Ashm. 392.

Manuals of astrological physic

'The grounds of arte gathered out of diverse authors', 1594–5, Ashm. 1495.
'Liber juditiorum morborum', 1600, Ashm. 355; an exact copy by Thomas Robson, Ashm. 1411.
'The astrologicalle judgmentes of phisick and other questions'.
Version one, *c.*1596–9, copied by Richard Napier, Ashm. 403.
Version two, 1600 with later additions, copied by Sir Richard Napier and Thomas Robson?, Ashm. 363.
Version three, 1606 with later additions, Forman's hand, Ashm. 389.
Partial copy of version two, Sloane 99.
A preface to the above, Richard Napier, 'A treatise touching the defenc of astrologie', Napier's draft, Ashm. 204, fos. 50–63; cont. 240, fos. 137–8. An incomplete transcript, Ashm. 242, fos. 189–96.

Plague tracts

'A discourse of the plague', 1593, Ashm. 208, fos. 110–35.
'Forman's treatise on the plague', *c.*1603–7, Ashm. 1403.
Untitled plague treatise, 1607, Ashm. 1436.
Ashmole's copies of the prefatory materials which are damaged in the above, Ashm. 1790, fo. 102.

Other medical works

'Matrix and paine therof', 1596, Ashm. 390, fos. 175–89.
'The groundes of physique and chirurgerie gathered out of the sayinges of dyvers auncient philosofers', *c.*1589?, Sloane 2550, fos. 1–117^{v}.
'Treatise of purginge', *c.*1589?, Sloane 2550, fos. 118–27^{v}; a copy made by Richard Napier, Oxford, Corpus Christi College MS 169, fos. 1–67 (MSS 168, 170 are companions to this volume in Napier's hand).

'Of the splen or milbe called splen or lien', an incomplete medical tract, Ashm. 244, fos. 160–5.

Miscellaneous astrological, medical, and related papers

'De revolutione mundy', *c.*1603–4?, containing notes on eclipses and the weather, and a draft or copy of an almanac, Ashm. 384.

Notes on judgments for stolen property, pregnancy, prognostications, and other questions, Ashm. 205.

Notes on and calculations of nativities, Ashm. 206; see also 243, fo. 30; 244, fos. 143–5.

Astrological notes and observations on love, lost things, legal disputes, women, and other subjects, Ashm. 390.

Maritime rules and questions, Ashm. 802, fos. 226–75^{v}.

Notes on the planets attributed to Forman, Trinity MS O.2.13, fo. 236.

Notes on Forman's recipes by Josuah Walworth, Forman's son and assistant, 1602–3, Trinity MS O.2.59, 121–49 *passim.*

Astrological, medical, and related texts owned by Forman

A general medical work with some astrological content, inscribed 'September 1611 Docter Formans booke reserved for the use of Clement his sonne', attributed by Black to Forman, but probably owned, not written, by him, Ashm. 1429.

Fifteenth-century astrological extracts owned by Forman, Ashm. 360, iii–v.

A pair of medieval medical texts owned and annotated by Forman, 1574–*c.*1600, King's MS 16.

Three thirteenth- or fourteenth-century astrological and medical manuscripts owned by Forman, Trinity MS O.8.23 (II).

John Cypriano, *A moste strange and wonderfull prophesie upon this troblesome worlde* (1595), with astrological notes by Forman, Ashm. 546.

Alchemical manuscripts

Alchemical commonplace books

'Principles of philosofi', begun 1597, Ashm. 1472.

'Of appoticarie druges', 2 vols., *c.*1607–10, Ashm. 1494, 1491; extracted pages now bound in Sloane 3822, fos. 6–19, 68–102^{v}.

Untitled alchemical commonplace book, *c.*1607+, Ashm. 1430.

Transcriptions of alchemical texts with occasional notes

The following notebooks have been identified. I have followed Black's item numbers. Brackets denote inferred dates, based on hand and format in relation to contiguous dated MSS. Authors and titles identified from incipits are contained in brackets. Many items, especially recipes, contain Napier's marginal approval.

Alchemical notebook I, 1592–3, Ashm. 1490, fos. 28–80

1. [Aegidius du Wes, alias de Vadis], 'A dialoge of Egidius de Vadius betwene nature and the desciple of philosophie of the serchinge out of the philosophors stone', copied 23 Mar. 1592, fos. 28–36^{v}.
2. 'Notes . . . out of Egidius de Vadius', cont. of previous, fo. 38.
3. Experiments, cont. of 2, fo. 39.
4. Notes on Hermes, Geber, Aristotle, Galen, etc., fos. 40–1.
5. 'Frimitor', Robert Frimitor, alias Barker, Friar of Bungay, Suffolk, 'Treasure of treasures', copied 9 Mar. 1592, fos. 42–5.
6. [George Ripley, 'The bost of mercury'], [copied Mar. 1592], fo. 46^{r-v}.
7. 'Versus aros', [copied Mar. 1592], fos. 46^{v}–7.
8. [Richard Carpenter], 'Geber of Spain saith Take the clear lighte . . .', [copied Mar. 1592], fo. 47.
9. 'Arnold of the Newtoune [Villanova] on the great elixar', [copied Mar. 1592], fo. 47.
10. Descriptions of alchemical preparations, [copied *c.*1592?], fos. 49–50^{v}, 52.
11. [Mirer], 'Opus de argento vivo solo . . .', [copied *c.*1592], fos. 53–4^{v}.
12. [Roger Bacon, Epistolae tres ad Johannem Parisiensim or Tractatus trium verborum, epist. III], [copied *c.*1592], fo. 55.
13. 'De rotatione rerum elementat', copied 31 Dec. 1593, fo. 56^{r-v}.
14. Anaxagoras, 'convertionis naturalis', copied 10 Feb. 1593 out of 'Doctor Turners bocke', fos. 57–61^{v} (for notes on this see 18 below).

15–16. Twelve rules and a recipe, [copied Feb. 1593], fo. 62^{r-v}.

17. George Ripley, 'Medulla alkimiae', copied 19 Feb. 1593, fos. 66–74^{v}.
18. 'Notes out of Anaxagoras' (see 14 above), [copied Feb. 1593], fo. 74^{v}.
19. An unfinished glossary of the names of metals, fo. 75.

20–1. Characters used by chemists (cf. Ashm. 1423), fos. 76^{v}–7^{v}.

22. Four chapters, beginning 'To calcine ⊙ and to bring it into ☿ and oylle', fos. 78–80.

Alchemical notebook II, 1585, Ashm. 1490, fos. 81–9^{v}

23. Dialogue between 'Scoller and master', copied 1585, fos. 81–4.
24. Following directly from the previous item. A short instruction beginning 'To all that wilbe perfecte in this scyence, let his medison be gummich and lighte of fusion', copied 1585, fo. 84.
25. 'Termes perteyninge unto the scyence of alkamy here set in order, by the whiche youe shall the more perfectlyer knowe when your worke is finished', copied 1585, fos. 84^{v}–6^{v}.
26. 'Secreta secretorum', notes on medieval alchemical texts, copied 25 July 1585, fo. 87.
27. Notes on the above items, 23–6, fo. 88.
28. Recipes for 'The medison Egiuke Eirueh ∧ 8 ∧ [?] gave to his ffrind', 'To turne ☿ into ☾ good in proffe', and more, [copied 1585?], fo. 89^{r-v}.

Alchemical notebook III, c.1585, Ashm. 1490, fos. 90–153^{v}

29. Recipes, [copied 1585], fos. 90–2.
30. Directions to make twelve kinds of alchemical waters, some attributed to Roger Bacon, others to 'William Fraunces', copied 1585, fo. 92$^{r–v}$.
31. Albertus Magnus, 'Semita recta'[?] (English tr.), [copied *c.*1585–1591], fos. 93, 98–100.
32. Albertus Magnus, 'De sulphere . . .', fo. 101.
33. Directions for blanching copper etc., fo. 101^{v}.

The following is a section of smaller paper, inserted in the midst of the above.

34. Alchemical recipes and procedures, fos. 94–7^{v}.

35–6. Sybiline prophecies, [before 16 Aug. 1591 (see 37)], fos. 102–5, 106$^{r–v}$.

37. Prophecies, added to the above, 16 Aug. 1591, fo. 106^{v}.
38. 'De vitriolo', fo. 107$^{r–v}$.
39. 'A book of the elixir, and of the various substances used by alchemists', [*c.*1584?], fos. 108–9^{v}.
40. Recipes, 'Take red vitriol . . .', [follows from above], fos. 110–11.
41. 'Planetarum nomina . . .', [follows from the above], fo. 111^{v}.
42. 'Off the herbe lunarye', [follows from the above], fo. 111^{v}.
43. Notes on the philosophers' stone excerpted from many authors, fos. 112–13^{v}.
44. [George Ripley, 'Compound of alchemy'], copied 31 Dec. 1584, fos. 114–36^{v}.
45. Notes, fo. 137.
46. 'How thou shalte nip and shut up thi glas . . .', fo. 137.
47. Notes on the four elements extracted from Agrippa, fos. 138–9^{v}.

Items 48–52 seem to have been copied from a single MS or collection.

48. A dialogue, copied from a medieval text, incipit: 'In the name of God Amen. My lovinge child knowe this . . .', [copied Feb. 1585], fos. 140–1.
49. Fragment of Pearce the Black Monk and associated verses, [copied Feb. 1585], fos. 142–3.

50–2. '. . . The great and royall worke of the quintessence of mercury, thorowe the indusinge of Mr Arnold of Newtowne [Villanova]', copied 13 Feb. 1585, fos. 143^{v}–9^{v}.

53–4. An experiment and Forman's notes, based on above, [copied later than Feb. 1585], fo. 150.

55. 'Tractatus quartus de transmutatione metallorum tempore ex Theophrasto . . .', fo. 150^{v}.
56. 'Termina philosophorum', fo. 151$^{r–v}$.
57. Recipes, fo. 152.
58. 'De metallis', fo. 152^{v}.
59. The uses of sandiner, borax, and other substances in the working of metals by goldsmiths and others, fo. 153.
60. Drawings of alchemical instruments, fo. 153^{v}.

Alchemical notebook IV, 1590–1591/1599, Ashm. 1490, fos. 154–98^{v}

61. 'Here followeth the practice of Raymon Lully', 1590, fos. 154–7^{v}.

62. Lully, a circular scheme in Latin, with Forman's English explanations, fo. 161.
63. 'Notes out of the bocke called Semita recta compiled by Raymon Lully', fos. 162–3^{v}.
64. Extracts from Thomas Norton, 'The ordinall of alchemy', fo. 164.
65. Extracts from 'Vincent in his naturall glas', fo. 164.
66. 'The boocke and worke of Sr Roberte Greene totchynge the ph'ors stone', copied 13 Aug. 1591, fos. 165–6.

Items 67–9 are on papers inserted into the notebook.

67–8. [Blomfild's Blossom's], 'The famous worke of Mr Blundeville, of som called Sir William Blundyville or Blomfield', in three parts, copied 14 Aug. 1591; the third part recopied 19 Dec. 1599, fos. 167–70^{v}.
69. Sir Edward Kelly, 'The praies of virtue' (1589), recopied 1599, fo. 171.
70–2. 'Prologus de Johannis de Meduno in cognicione lapidis occulti, quod librum sune studio nequaquam florenti', and related notes and experiments, copied 5 Oct. 1590, fos. 173–8.
73. [Partial copy of the 'Crowning of nature'], cf. Notebook IX: Ashm. 1433, ii, fos. 179–80.
74. [Johannes de Rupescissa, 'Liber de famulatu philosophiae or liber de consideratione quintae essentiae'], copied 4 Oct. 1590, fos. 181–96.
75. 'Est finis de consideratione quinte escentie', written at the end of the above item in the text from which Forman was copying, [4 Oct. 1590], fo. 196.
76–8. Experiments and recipes, fos. 196^{v}–8^{v}.

Alchemical notebook V, 1591/1585, Ashm. 1490, fos. 199–236^{v}

79. Paracelsus, 'The 7 bookes . . . toching the nature of thinges' (1537), copy begun 3 Dec. 1590, finished 8 Feb. 1591, fos. 199–216.
80. Paracelsus, 'Two bockes . . . concerninge the nature of man', copied 10 Feb. 1591, fos. 217–20.
81. [Bernard of Trier], 'The moste excellente and trewe boocke of the reverente doctor Almante and Lord Barnard Erell of March and Trevisan', 1 Oct. 1585, fos. 221–36^{v}.

[81*a*.] Five items of related notes are appended to the above, fos. 236^{v}–40.

Alchemical notebook VI, *c.*1591, Ashm. 1490, fos. 241–89

82. 'The Testament of J. J. [John Jones?], D[octor] of physick' (incomplete), [copied *c.*1590?], fos. 240–76.

82*a*. Forman's incomplete index of the above, fo. 241.

83. Thomas Norton, 'The ordinall of alchemy', copied 23 Mar. 1591, fos. 277–89.

Alchemical notebook VII, *c.*1591, Ashm. 1490, fos. 291–331

84. Humfrey Lock, An alchemical treatise dedicated to Sir William Cecil, Lord Burghley, copied 19 June 1590, fos. 291–325.

[84*a*.] Notes related to the above on preparations and principles, fos. 325^{v}–31^{v}.

Alchemical notebook VIII, 1594/1595/1604, Ashm. 1490, fos. 332–46

85. 'Opus perfectum philosophicum' and other notes, 9 June 1604, fos. 332–5.
86. 'Pater sapientiae', recopied 1599, fos. 336–42.
87. 'Here followeth the opininge of secrets, done by the arte of philosophy', recopied 23 Dec. 1599, fos. 343–5.

Separate items

88. 'A note of the bille and names of the things that Mr [Robert] Parkes was to bwy for [Emery] Mulleneux 1595 the xi March', fo. 350^{v}.
89. 'Forman preface speaking in the bockes behaulfe', a fragment, fo. 352^{v}.

Alchemical notebook IX, 12 Apr. 1608, Ashm. 1433, i, pp. 1–69

St Dunstan (attr.), 'Out of Dunstons practice', 12 Apr. 1608, Ashm. 1433, pp. 1–69.

Alchemical notebook X, 1590–1591/*c.*1606, Ashm. 1433, ii, fos. 1–35

1. Alchemical notes, fos. 1^{v}, 34^{v}, 35 (running concurrently with the next item).
2. 'Hermes Trismegistus on the philosophers stone' and 'The crowing of nature' (for a rough draft see Ashm. 1490, fo. 179), copied 1590, fos. 1–34.
3. 'Consilium conjugii . . .', fos. 1^{v}, 2^{v}, 13^{v}.
4. 'Tabula smaragdina Hermetis Trismegisti', fo. 4^{v}.
5. 'Hortulani philosophi ab hortis maritimis Commentariolus in Tabulam smaragdinam Hermetis Trismegisti', copied 16 Sept. 1591, fos. 4^{v}–10^{v}.
6. Explanations of alchemical terms, fos. 11^{v}, 12^{v}.
7. Extracts from 'Blomfild's Blossoms', fo. 13^{v}.
8. Alchemical processes, fo. 14^{v}.
9. 'Via recta. Thy substaunce and ground of this work for the red elixir is . . .', fo. 15^{v}.
10. Notes on Villanova and Lully, [*c.*1590], fo. 16^{v}.
11. 'Tempus faciendi lapidem', fo. 17^{v}, 18^{v}.
12. 'Ad faciendum ceram rubeam aut viridem . . .', fo. 18^{v}.
13. Simon Forman, 'De lapide philosophico et de transmutatione metallorum' (unfinished), [*c.*1606? (the following is a direct continuation)], fos. 21–32.
14. Notes on procedures, 1606, fos. 30^{v}–2.

Alchemical notebook XI, *c.*1608, Ashm. 1433, iii, pp. 1–31^{v}

1. 'Natura Saturn', pp. 1–4.
2. 'The whole som of the secretes of philosophie in brife gathered by S Forman', begun Aug. 1608, finished 5 Mar. 1609, pp. 5–30.
3. More notes, pp. 30, 31–2 .

Alchemical notebook XII, *c.*1585–1587?/1598, Ashm. 208, fos. 78–107^{v}

1. 'Of cako' [Alexander von Suchten, 'Second treatise on alchemy'], copied 10 Nov. 1598, fos. 78–93^{v}; parts of a rough copy, and parts of another fair copy of this text in Forman's hand are bound in Ashm. 1486, fos. 7–11, 12–20.
2. 'The firste waye to the mineralle stone', copied 6 Dec. 1598, fos. 94–7.
3. 'Opus minerale', copied 9 Dec. 1598, fos. 98–101.
4. 'Of the vegitable Stone', [copied 1598], fos. 102–3.
5. 'But nowe it is com to the laste digestion . . .', copied 3 Mar. 1587, fos. 104–7^{v}.

Alchemical manuscripts owned by Forman

Alchemical tracts and notes, many in the hand of Giovanni Battista Agnello, Ashm. 1490, items A–F, fos. 2–26^{v}, including 'Apocalypsis spiritus secreti', fos. 15–17.

Thomas Digges's alchemical notes, Ashm. 1478, i.

Thomas Moundeford's copies of medieval alchemical tracts, Ashm. 1423, i–iv.

Manuscripts of magic and related subjects

Notes on cabala, 1609/1610, Ashm. 244, fos. 1–22.

'The motion of the 3 superiour heavens', Ashm. 244, *c.*1606–8, fos. 34–118, and related notes, fos. 25–33^{v}.

'Ars notoria', three copies: 1600, Jerusalem, Yahuda MS VAR 34; working text *c.*1600–1, Bodleian, Jones MS 1; working text, *c.*1600, Trinity MS O.9.7; drafts of the illustrations owned by Forman, Ashm. 820, iii.

Artephius, 'Clavis majoris sapientiae', tr. Simon Forman, 1609, Sloane 3822, fos. 103–44.

Manuscripts on biblical and historical themes

'Upon the firste of Genesis', Ashm. 802, fos. 1–12 (misbound and incomplete).

'The life of Adam and Eve', a transcript with additions and annotations *c.*1599, Ashm. 802, ii.

'On Adam and Eve', incomplete, Ashm. 244, fo. 187.

Historical, prophetic, and astrological papers, including a treatise on the Jews, verses on the coming of the antichrist, and accounts of Shakespeare's plays, Ashm. 802.

Notes on giants, 1610, Ashm. 244, fos. 184, 192; 802, fos. 51–9.

'The parlamont and consultation of the devils and their decre about the beginning of Merlin', a romance, Ashm. 802, fos. 66–82.

Notes on the birth of Lucifer, bound with *The Hystory of Kyng Boccus and Sydrake* (1517?), St John's College, Oxford.

II. OTHER PRINCIPAL MANUSCRIPTS CITED

Documents relating to Forman's life

Corporation of London record office: City of London Sheriff's Court Rolls, Box 4, 1610 bundle.

Forman's licence to practise physic and astronomy from the University of Cambridge, Ashm. 1301; see 1763, fo. 44 for Ashmole's copy.

Frances Howard to Forman, a copy of a letter, Dowdson MS 58, fo. 158.

Public Record Office: Stac 5 s. 79/33, Stac 5 s. 12/34, Prob 6/8 1611, fo. 31.

Salisbury, Bishop of Salisbury deposition books, no. 10, fos. 46$^{r–v}$, 57; no. 11, fos. 17$^{r–v}$, 25^{v}, 26.

Other manuscripts

'Ars notoria', Bodleian, Bodley MS 951; Ashm. 1515.

An astrological handbook *c.*1620, owned by Thomas Harley, Folger MS V.b.4.

Edwardus Generosus Anglicus Innominatus, 'The epitome of the treasure of all welth' (1562), Ashm. 1419, fos. 57–82ᵛ; King's, Keynes MS 22; Ferguson MS 199, pp. 19–70; Sloane 2502, fos. 54–69ᵛ, 70–81ᵛ (two copies).

A 1567 book of magic misattributed to Forman, BL Additional MS 36674, fos. 47ᵛ–58.

'The key of Solomon', copied by one of Forman's contemporaries, BL MS Add. 36674, fos. 5–22.

'The life of Adam and Eve', Bodleian, Bodley MS 596; Trinity MS R.3.21, fos. 249–57 (owned by John Stowe); BL Additional MS 35298, fos. 162–5; Oxford, Trinity College MS 57, fo. 157ᵛ.

'Manna', an alchemical treatise, *c.*1600, King's, Keynes MS 33; Glasgow, Glasgow University Library, Ferguson MS 9, fos. 14–24; Ferguson MS 199, pp. 72–8 (partial copy); Sloane 2194, fos. 77–84ᵛ; Sloane 2222, fos. 128ᵛ–36; Sloane 2585, fos. 90–105; Ashm. 1419, fos. 45–56; printed in Houpreght (ed.), *Aurifontina chymica* (1680), 107–43.

Napier, Richard, Extracts from the 'Picatrix', Sloane 3679.

Paddy, William, 'Let closestoole and chamberpot choose out Doctor' [1607], Rawlinson MS poct 160*, fos. 183ᵛ–5.

Royal College of Physicians, Annals Bk. 2, 1581–1608, tr. J. Emberry and S. Heathcote (1953–5).

St Dunstan on the philosophers' stone, Sloane 1744, 1876, 3738, 3757; Oxford, Corpus Christi College MS 128.

'Simon Forman's dream', an alchemical romance, perhaps in Richard Napier's hand, Trinity MS O.8.1, fos. 95–113.

Suchten, Alexander, 'Second treatise on antimony' (1575), Ashm. 1418, iii, fos. 17–30; Ashm. 1459, fos. 136–61ᵛ. Anonymous version under the title 'Of cako', Ashm. 1421, fos. 29–34ᵛ.

Wood, Anthony, Notes on Forman's life, Bodleian, Rawlinson MS D. 912, fo. 643.

III. PRE-1800 PRINTED SOURCES CITED

Agnello (Lambe), Giovanni Battista, *Espositione . . . sopra un libro intitolato Apocalypsis spiritus secreti* (1566).

—— *The revelation of the secret spirit*, tr. R.N.E. (1623).

Agrippa von Nettesheim, Heinrich Cornelius, *De occulta philosophia* (Paris, 1567).

—— *Opera omnia*, ii (Lyons, *c.*1620).

Alexis of Piedmont [Girolamo Ruscelli], *The secretes of the reverende Maister Alexis of Piemont*, tr. William Warde (1558).

Anderson, Anthony, *An approved medicine against the deserved plague* (1593).

Arcandam, *The most excellent, profitable and pleasant book, of the famous doctor and expert astrologian Arcandam of Aleandri*, tr. William Warde (1562).

Ars notoria: The notary art of Solomon, tr. Robert Tanner (1657).

Ashmole, Elias (ed.), *Theatrum chemicum Brtiannicum* (1652).

—— *Elias Ashmole, Autobiographical and Historical Notes, Correspondence, and Other Sources*, ed. C. H. Josten, 5 vols. (Oxford, 1966).

Aubrey, John, *The natural history of Wiltshire*, ed. John Britton (1847).

Babington, Gervase, *Certain plaine, briefe, and comforatable notes, upon every chapter of Genesis* (1596 [1591]).

Bacon, Roger, *Libellus Rogerii Baconi Angli . . . de retardandis senectutis accidentibus* (Oxford, 1590).

—— *The mirror of alchimy* (1597).

—— *Opus maius*, ed. John H. Bridges (Oxford, 1900).

Barrough, Philip, *The methode of physicke* (1583).

Beza, Theodore, *A short learned and pithie treatise of the plague*, tr. John Stockwood (1580).

Blagrave, John, *A mathematical jewel* (1585).

Bonatti, Guido, *De astronomia tractatus X* (Basel, 1550).

Boorde, Andrew, *The breviary of healthe* (1557).

—— *The pryncyples of astronamye* (1547).

B[ostocke], R[ichard], *The difference betwene the auncient phisicke . . . and the latter phisicke* (1585).

Brasbridge, Thomas, *The poor mans jewel* (1592 [1578]).

Bredwell, Stephen, *Physick for the sicknesse, commonly called the plague* (1636).

Bullein, William, *The governement of healthe* (1558).

—— *Bulwarke of defense against all sicknesse, sorenesse, and woundes* (1579 [1562]).

—— *A dialogue bothe pleasaunt and pietifull, against the fever pestilence* (1573).

Carleton, George, *Astrologomania* (1624).

Cattan, Christopher, *The geomancie of Maister Christopher Cattan*, tr. Francis Sparry (1591).

Chamber, John, *Against judicial astrology* (1601).

Cogan, Thomas, *The haven of health* (1584).

Cooke, Francis, *The principles of geometrie, astronomie, and geographie* (1591).

Cortes, Martin, *The arte of navigation*, tr. Richard Eden (1561).

Covell, William, *Polimanteia, or, the meanes lawfull and unlawfull, to judge of the fall of a common-wealth* (Cambridge, 1595).

Croll, Oswald, *Basilica chymica* (Frankfurt, 1609).

—— *Philosophy reformed and improved*, tr. Henry Pinnell (1657).

Cunningham, William, *The cosmographical glasse* (1559).

Cupper, William, *Certain sermons concerning God's late visitation* (1592).

Cypriano, John, *A moste strange and wonderfull prophesie upon this troblesome worlde*, tr. Anthony Holloway (1595).

Dariot, Claude, *A breefe and most easie introduction to the astrologicall judgment of the starres*, tr. Fabian Wither (1583, 1598).

Davis, John, *The seaman's secreats* (1595).

—— *The world's hydrographical description* (1595).

Dee, John, 'Preface' to Euclid, *Elements of geometrie*, tr. Henry Billingsley (1570).

—— *The diaries of John Dee*, ed. Edward Fenton (Charlbury, 1998).

—— *The private diary of Dr. John Dee, and the catalogue of his library and manuscripts*, ed. James Halliwell, Camden Society, 19 (1842).

Dekker, Thomas, *The wonderfull yeare* (1603).

de Medina, Pedro, *Arte of navigation*, tr. John Frampton (1581, 1595).

de Taranta, Valasco, *Tractus de epidemia et peste* (Basel, 1464).

Drouet, Pierre, *A new counsell against the plague*, tr. Thomas Twyne (1578).

Du Bartas, Guillaume de Salluste, *The firste day of the worldes creation*, tr. Josuah Sylvester (1595).

—— *The Workes of Guillaume de Salluste*, ed. Urban T. Holmes, John C. Lyons, and Robert W. Linker (Chapel Hill, NC, 1935–40).

—— *The Divine Weeks and Works of Guillaume de Saluste Sieur du Bartas*, tr. Josuah Sylvester, ed. Susan Snyder (Oxford, 1979).

Duchesne, Joseph (Quercetanus), *The practise of chymicall, and hermeticall physicke, for the preservation of health*, tr. Thomas Tymme (1605).

Eliot, Sir Thomas, *The castelle of helth* (1572).

Evans, John, *The universall medicine* (1635).

Ewich, Johannes, *Of the duetie of the faithful and wise magistrates*, tr. John Stockwood (1583).

Fage, John, *Speculum aegrotorum* (1606).

Ferrier, Auger, *A learned astronomical discourse*, tr. Thomas Kelway (1593).

[Fine, Oronce], *The rules and righte ample documents, toutching the use and practise of the common almanackes, which are named ephemeredes*, tr. Humphrey Baker ([1558]).

Fioravanti, Leonardo, *A joyfull jewell, containing aswell such excellent orders, preservatives and precious practices for the plague*, tr. John Hester (1580).

Forman, Simon, *The groundes of the longitude* (1591).

—— 'Extracts from a manuscript of Dr. Simon Forman', ed. Philip Bliss, *Censura literae*, 8 (1807), 409–13.

—— 'Dr Simon Forman's diary', ed. James Halliwell, *The archæologist, and journal of antiquarian science*, 1 (1841–2), 34–7.

—— *The autobiography and personal diary of Dr Simon Forman*, ed. James Halliwell (1849).

—— '"Matrix and the pain thereof": A Sixteenth-Century Gynaecological Essay', ed. Barbara Traister, *Medical History*, 35 (1991), 436–51.

—— 'Chaos', ed. Robert M. Schuler, *Alchemical Poetry 1575–1700 from Previously Unpublished Manuscripts* (New York, 1995), 49–70.

Fouleweather, Adam, *A wonderfull, strange and miraculous, astrologicall prognostication for this yeer of our Lord God* ([1591]).

Gesner, Conrad, *The treasure of Euonymus*, tr. Peter Morwyng (1559).

Gibbens, Nicholas, *Questions and disputations concerning the holy scripture* (1602).

Goeurot, Jean, *The regiment of life, whereof is added a treatyse of the pestilence with the booke of children newly corrected and enlarged*, tr. Thomas Phayer (1560 [1545?]).

Goodall, Charles, *The Royal College of Physicians of London, and an historical account of the College proceedings against empiricks and unlicensed practicers* (1684).
Harvey, John, *An astrologicall addition* (1583).
——*A discoursive probleme concerning prophecies* (1588).
Harvey, Richard, *An astrological discourse upon the great and notable conjunction of the two superiour planets, Saturne and Jupiter* (1583).
Hermetica: The Greek Corpus Hermeticum *and the Latin* Ascelpius *in a New English Translation with Notes and Introduction*, ed. Brian Copenhaver (Cambridge, 1992).
Heydon, Christopher, *A defense of judicial astrology* (Cambridge, 1603).
——*An astrological discourse with mathematical demonstrations*, ed. Nicholas Fiske (1650).
Holland, Henry, *Spiritual preservatives against the pestilence* (1593).
Hood, Thomas, *The use of both the globes, celestiall, and terrestriall* (1592).
Houllier, Jacques (Hollerius), *De morbus internis libri II* (Frankfurt, 1589).
Houpreght, John Frederick (ed.), *Aurifontina chymica: Or a collection of fourteen small treatises concerning the first matter of philosophers* (1680).
Hues, Robert, *A learned treatise of globes*, tr. John Chimead (1639).
Indagine, John, *Brief introductions*, tr. Fabian Wither (1558).
I.W., *A briefe treatise of the plague* (1603).
I.W., *A coppie of a letter sent by a learned physician to his friend* ([1586]).
Jonson, Ben, *Ben Jonson*, ed. C. H. Herford, P. Simpson, and E. Simpson, 11 vols. (Oxford, 1925–52).
Kellwaye, Simon, *A defensative against the plague* (1593).
The key to unknowne knowledge (1599).
Lambeth Churchwardens' Accounts 1504–1645, and Vestry Book 1610, ed. Charles Drew, iii (1943).
Libavius, Andreas, *Alchemia* (Frankfurt, 1597).
'The Life of Adam and Eve', in R. H. Charles (ed.), *The Apocrypha and Pseudoepigrapha of the Old Testament in English* (Oxford, 1913), 123–54.
——in H. F. D. Sparks (ed.), *The Apocryphal Old Testament* (Oxford, 1984), 141–67.
Lilly, William, *Christian astrology* (1647).
—— *William Lilly's history of his life and times*, ed. Charles Burman (1774).
Lodge, Thomas, *A treatise of the plague* (1603).
Lyson, Daniel, *The environs of London*, iii (1792).
Maplet, John, *A greene forest, or a naturall historie* (1567).
—— *The diall of destiny* (1581).
Melton, John, *Astrologaster or the figure caster* (1620).
N[iccols], R[ichard], 'Sir Thomas Overburies vision' [1616], *The Harleian Miscellany*, 7 (1810), 178–88.
Norton, Thomas, *Thomas Norton's Ordinal of alchemy*, ed. John Reidy, Early English Text Society (Oxford, 1975).
Paracelsus (Theophrast von Hohenheim), *Operum medico-chimicorum sive paradoxorum, tomus genuinus undecimus*, tr. Zacharias Palthen, xi (Frankfurt, 1605).
Paré, Ambrose, *A treatise of the plague*, [tr. T. Johnson] (1630).

Picatrix: The Latin Versions of the Ghayat al-hakim, ed. David Pingree, Studies of the Warburg Institute, 39 (1986).
Plat, Hugh, *The jewell house of art and nature* (1594).
Primrose, James, *The communal antimonial cup wide cast, or a treatise concerning the antimonial cup* (1640).
Recorde, Robert, *The grounde of artes* (1543).
—— *Castle of knowledge* (1556).
Ripley, George, *George Ripley's compound of alchemy*, ed. Stanton J. Linden (Aldershot, 2001).
[Scola Saleritana], *Regimen sanitatis Salerni*, tr. Thomas Paynel (1575).
Schöner, Johannes, *De judiciis nativitatum libri tres* (Nuremberg, 1545).
Scot, Reginald, *Discoverie of witchcraft* (1584).
S.H., *A new treatise of the pestilence* (1603).
Shakespeare, William, *Works of Shakespeare*, ed. James Halliwell (1859).
—— *The Tragedy of Macbeth*, ed. J. Q. Adams (Boston, 1931).
Sidrak and Boccus, *The hystory of Kyng Boccus and Sydrake* (*c.*1537).
—— *Sidrak and Bokkus*, ed. T. L. Burton, 2 vols. (Oxford, 1998).
Smel-knauve, Simon, *The fearefull and lamentable effects of two dangerous comets* ([1591]).
Solomon, *The Key of Solomon the King*, tr. and ed. S. Liddell MacGregor Mathers (1888).
State Papers, *The Complete State Papers Domestic*, 1/5. *1547–1625* (Brighton, 1978), reel 81.
State Trials, *Complete collection of state trials*, ed. T. B. Howell, ii (1816).
Stationers' Company, *A transcript of the registers of the Company of Stationers of London, 1544–1640*, ed. Edward Arber, ii (1875).
Suchten, Alexander von, *Of the secrets of antimony: In two treatises* (1670).
Tanner, Robert, *A briefe treatise for the ready use of the sphere* (1592).
Thayre, Thomas, *A treatise of the pestilence* (1603).
Thornborough, John, *Lithotheorikos, sive, nihil, aliquid, omnia, antiquorum sapientum vivis coloribus depicta, philosophico-theologice* (Oxford, 1621).
Vaughan, Thomas, *Thomas and Rebecca Vaughan's* Aqua Vitae: Non Vitis (*BL MS Sloane 1741*), ed. Donald R. Dickson (Tempe, Ariz., 2001).
Vigo, John, *The whole worke of the famous chirurgion Master John Vigo*, tr. George Baker (1586).
W[eldon], A[nthony], *The court and character of King James* (1650).
[Wilson, Arthur], *The five yeares of King James* (1643).
Wood, Anthony, *Athenae Oxonienses*, ed. Philip Bliss, 5 vols. (1813–20).

IV. POST-1800 PRINTED SOURCES CITED

Aldis, H. G. *et al.* (eds.), *A Dictionary of Printers and Booksellers in England, Scotland and Ireland, and of Foreign Printers of English Books 1557–1640*, gen. ed. R. B. McKerrow (1910).

Allen, D. C., *The Star-Crossed Renaissance: The Quarrel about Astrology and its Influence in England* (New York, 1973 [1951]).

Almond, Philip, *Adam and Eve in Seventeenth Century Thought* (Cambridge, 1999).

Apperson, George L., *English Proverbs and Proverbial Phrases: A Historical Dictionary* (Toronto, 1929).

Appleby, J. H., 'Arthur Dee and Johannes Banfi Hunyades', *Ambix*, 24 (1977), 96–109.

Ash, Eric H., *Power, Knowledge, and Expertise in Elizabethan England* (Baltimore, Md., 2004).

Bamborough, J. B., 'Robert Burton's Astrological Notebooks', *Review of English Studies*, NS 32 (1981), 267–85.

Barry, Jonathan, 'Introduction: Keith Thomas and the Problem of Witchcraft', in Jonathan Barry, Marianne Hester, and Gareth Roberts (eds.), *Witchcraft in Early Modern Europe: Studies in Culture and Belief* (Cambridge, 1996), 1–45.

Barton, Tamsyn, *Power and Knowledge: Astrology, Physiognomics, and Medicine under the Roman Empire* (Ann Arbor, 1994).

Bayer, Penny, 'Women's Alchemical Literature 1560–1616 in Italy, France, the Swiss Cantons and England, and its Diffusion to 1660', Ph.D. thesis, University of Warwick, 2003.

—— 'Lady Margaret Clifford's Alchemical Recipe Book and the John Dee Circle', *Ambix*, 52 (2005), 271–84.

Behringer, Wolfgang, *Shaman of Oberstdorf: Chonrad Stoeckhlin and the Phantoms of the Night*, tr. Erik Midelfort (Charlottesville, Va., 1998).

Bellany, Alistair, *The Politics of Court Scandal in Early Modern England: News Culture and the Overbury Affair, 1603–1660* (Cambridge, 2003).

Bennett, H. S., *English Books and Readers*, 4 vols. (Cambridge, 1965).

Bennett, James A., 'The Mathematicians' Apprenticeship', *British Journal for the History of Science*, 18 (1985), 212–17.

—— 'The Longitude and the New Science', *Vistas in Astronomy*, 28 (1985), 219–25.

—— 'The Mechanics' Philosophy and the Mechanical Philosophy', *History of Science*, 24 (1986), 1–28.

Bianchi, Massimo, 'The Visible and the Invisible: From Alchemy to Paracelsus', in P. Rattansi and A. Clericuzio (eds.), *Alchemy and Chemistry in the Sixteenth and Seventeenth Centuries* (1994), 17–50.

Black, William, *A descriptive, analytical and critical catalogue of the manuscripts bequeathed unto the University of Oxford by Elias Ashmole* (Oxford, 1845).

Bosanquet, E. F., *English Printed Almanacks and Prognostications: A Bibliographical History to the Year 1600* (1917).

—— 'English Printed Almanacs and Prognostications: A Bibliographical History to the Year 1600, Corrigenda and Addenda', *The Library*, 4th ser. 8 (1928), 456–77.

—— 'Notes on Further Addenda to English Printed Almanacks to 1600', *The Library*, 4th ser. 18 (1938), 39–66.

Bowden, Mary, 'The Astrological Revolution of the Seventeenth Century (1558–1686)', Ph.D. thesis, Yale University, 1974.

Brind'Amour, Pierre, *Nostradamus astrophile: Les Astres et l'astrologie dans la vie et l'œuvre de Nostradamus* (Paris, 1993).

Brockliss, Laurence, and Colin Jones, *The Medical World of Early Modern France* (Oxford, 1997).

Burnett, Charles, 'Talismans: Magic as Science? Necromancy among the Seven Liberal Arts', in Burnett, *Magic and Divination in the Middle Ages: Texts and Technicians in the Islamic and Christian Worlds* (Aldershot, 1996), 1–15.

—— 'The Establishment of Medieval Hermeticism', in Peter Linehan and Janet Nelson (eds.), *The Medieval World* (2001), 111–30.

Bynum, Caroline Walker, *Holy Feast, Holy Fast: The Religious Significance of Food to Medieval Women* (Berkeley, Calif., 1987).

Camden, C., 'Astrology in Shakespeare's Day', *Isis*, 55 (1933), 26–73.

Campbell, Anna M., *The Black Death and Men of Learning* (New York, 1966 [1931]).

Capp, Bernard, *Astrology and the Popular Press: English Almanacs 1500–1800* (1979).

Carlson, David, *English Humanist Books: Writers and Patrons, Manuscript and Print, 1475–1525* (Toronto, 1993).

Cerasano, Susan, 'Philip Henslowe, Simon Forman, and the Theatrical Community of the 1590s', *Shakespeare Quarterly*, 44 (1993), 145–58.

Chapman, Allan, 'Astrological Medicine', in C. Webster (ed.), *Health, Medicine and Mortality in the Sixteenth Century* (Cambridge, 1979), 275–300.

Chartier, Roger, *The Order of Books: Readers, Authors and Libraries in Europe between the Fourteenth and the Eighteenth Centuries*, tr. Lydia Cochraine (Cambridge, 1994).

Clark, George N., *A History of the Royal College of Physicians of London*, i (Oxford, 1964).

Clark, Stuart, 'The Scientific Status of Demonology', in B. Vickers (ed.), *Occult and Scientific Mentalities in the Renaissance* (Cambridge, 1984), 351–74.

—— *Thinking with Demons: The Idea of Witchcraft in Early Modern Europe* (Oxford, 1997).

—— 'Demons and Disease: The Disenchantment of the Sick (1500–1700)', in Marijke Gijswijt-Hofstra, Hilary Marland, and Hans de Waardt (eds.), *Illness and Healing Alternatives in Western Europe* (1997), 38–58.

Clifton, Gloria, *Directory of British Scientific Instrument Makers 1550–1851* (1995).

Clucas, Stephen, 'John Dee's Angelic Conversations and the *Ars Notoria*: Renaissance Magic and Mediaeval Theurgy', in Clucas (ed.), *John Dee: Interdisciplinary Studies in English Renaissance Thought* (Dordrecht, 2006), 231–73.

Clulee, Nicholas, *John Dee's Natural Philosophy: Between Science and Religion* (1988).

Cook, Harold, *The Decline of the Old Medical Regime in Stuart London* (Ithaca, NY, 1986).

—— 'The New Philosophy and Medicine in Seventeenth-Century England', in David Lindberg and Robert Westman (eds.), *Reappraisals of the Scientific Revolution* (Cambridge, 1990), 397–436.

—— 'Good Advice and Little Medicine: The Professional Authority of Early Modern English Physicians', *Journal of British Studies*, 33 (1994), 1–31.

Cook, Judith, *Dr Simon Foreman, a Most Notorious Physician* (2001).

Copenhaver, Brian, *Symphorien Champier and the Reception of the Occultist Tradition in Renaissance France* (The Hague, 1978).

—— 'Scholastic Philosophy and Renaissance Magic in the *De vita* of Marsilio Ficino', *Renaissance Quarterly*, 37 (1984), 523–54.

—— 'Astrology and Magic', in Charles Schmitt (ed.), *The Cambridge History of Renaissance Philosophy* (Cambridge, 1988), 264–300.

—— 'Natural Magic, Hermetism, and Occultism in Early Modern Science', in David Lindberg and Robert Westman (eds.), *Reappraisals of the Scientific Revolution* (Cambridge, 1990), 261–301.

—— 'A Tale of Two Fishes: Magical Objects in Natural History from Antiquity through the Scientific Revolution', *Journal of the History of Ideas*, 52 (1991), 373–89.

Crawford, Patricia, 'Attitudes to Menstruation in Seventeenth-Century England', *Past and Present*, 91 (1981), 47–73.

—— 'Women's Dreams in Early Modern England', *History Workshop Journal*, 49 (2000), 129–41.

Curry, Patrick, *Prophecy and Power: Astrology in Early Modern England* (Cambridge, 1989).

Dasent, John, (ed.), *Acts of the Privy Council of England*, xi (1897).

Daston, Lorraine, and Katharine Park, *Wonders and the Order of Nature 1150–1750* (New York, 1998).

Debus, Allen, 'An Elizabethan History of Medical Chemistry', *Annals of Science*, 18 (1962), 1–29.

—— *The English Paracelsians* (1965).

—— *The French Paracelsians: The Chemical Challenge to Medical and Scientific Tradition in Early Modern France* (Cambridge, 1991).

—— and Ingrid Merkel (eds.), *Hermeticism and the Renaissance* (Washington, DC, 1998).

Delany, Paul, *British Autobiography in the Seventeenth Century* (1969).

Dick, Hugh G., 'Students of Physic and Astrology: A Survey of Astrological Medicine in the Age of Science', *Journal of the History of Medicine*, 1–2 (1946), 300–15, 419–33.

Dictionary of National Biography, ed. L. Stephen and S. Lee, 63 vols. (1885–1900), with supplements.

Dixon, Laurinda, *Perilous Chastity: Women and Illness in Pre-Enlightenment Art and Medicine* (Ithaca, NY, 1995).

Dobbs, Betty Jo Teeter, *The Foundations of Newton's Alchemy, or 'The Hunting of the Greene Lyon'* (Cambridge, 1975).

—— *The Janus Faces of Genius: The Role of Alchemy in Newton's Thought* (Cambridge, 1991).

Duden, Barbara, *The Woman beneath the Skin: A Doctor's Patients in Eighteenth-Century Germany*, tr. Thomas Dunlap (Cambridge, Mass., 1991).

Duncan-Jones, Katherine, *Ungentle Shakespeare: Scenes from his Life* (2001).

Dunn, Richard, 'The Status of Astrology in Elizabethan England 1558–1603', Ph.D. thesis, University of Cambridge, 1992.

—— 'The True Place of Astrology among the Mathematical Arts of Late Tudor England', *Annals of Science*, 51 (1994), 151–63.

Eamon, William, *Science and the Secrets of Nature: Books of Secrets in Medieval and Early Modern Culture* (Princeton, 1994).

Edmond, Mary, 'Simon Forman's Vade-Mecum', *Book Collector*, 26 (1977), 44–60.

Emerton, Norma, 'Creation in the Thought of J. B. van Helmont and Robert Fludd', in P. Rattansi and A. Clericuzio (eds.), *Alchemy and Chemistry in the Sixteenth and Seventeenth Centuries* (1994), 85–101.

Fanger, Claire (ed.), *Conjuring Spirits: Texts and Traditions of Medieval Ritual Magic* (Thrupp, 1998).

Feingold, Mordechai, *The Mathematicians' Apprenticeship: Science, Universities and Society in England, 1560–1640* (Cambridge, 1984).

—— 'The Occult Tradition in the English Universities of the Renaissance: A Reassessment', in B. Vickers (ed.), *Occult and Scientific Mentalities in the Renaissance* (Cambridge, 1984), 73–94.

Fissell, Mary, *Patients, Power and the Poor in Eighteenth-Century Bristol* (Cambridge, 1991).

—— 'Readers, Texts, and Contexts: Vernacular Medical Works in Early Modern England', in Roy Porter (ed.), *The Popularisation of Medicine, 1650–1850* (1992), 72–96.

Fleming, Juliet, *Graffiti and the Writing Arts of Early Modern England* (2001).

Fletcher, Anthony, *Gender, Sex and Subordination in England 1500–1800* (New Haven, 1995).

Ganzel, Dewey, *Fortune and Men's Eyes: The Career of John Payne Collier* (Oxford, 1982).

Garin, Eugenio, *Astrology in the Renaissance: The Zodiac of Life*, tr. Carolyn Jackson and June Allen (1983).

Geertz, Hildred, 'An Anthropology of Religion and Magic, 1', *Journal of Interdisciplinary History*, 6 (1975), 71–89.

Geneva, Ann, *Astrology and the Seventeenth Century Mind: William Lilly and the Language of the Stars* (Manchester, 1995).

Gentilcore, David, 'The Fear of Disease and the Disease of Fear', in William Naphy and Penny Roberts (eds.), *Fear in Early Modern Society* (Manchester, 1997), 184–208.

—— *Healers and Healing in Early Modern Italy* (Manchester, 1998).

Getz, Faye, 'Black Death and the Silver Lining: Meaning, Continuity, and Revolutionary Change in Histories of Medieval Plague', *Journal of the History of Biology*, 24 (1991), 265–89.

—— 'To Prolong Life and Promote Health: Baconian Alchemy and Pharmacy in the English Learned Tradition', in Sheila Campbell, Bert Hall, and David Klausner (eds.), *Health, Disease and Healing in Medieval Culture* (New York, 1992), 141–51.

Ginzburg, Carlo, *The Cheese and the Worms: The Cosmos of a Sixteenth-Century Miller*, tr. John and Anne Tedeschi (1980).

Gowing, Laura, *Domestic Dangers: Women, Words, and Sex in Early Modern London* (Oxford, 1996).

Grafton, Anthony, *Commerce with the Classics: Ancient Books and Renaissance Readers* (Ann Arbor, 1997).

—— *Cardano's Cosmos: The Worlds and Works of a Renaissance Astrologer* (Cambridge, Mass., 1999).

—— and Lisa Jardine, '"Studied for Action": How Gabriel Harvey Read his Livy', *Past and Present*, 129 (1990), 30–78.

—— and Nancy Siraisi, 'Between the Election and My Hopes: Girolamo Cardano and Medical Astrology', in W. Newman and A. Grafton (eds.), *Secrets of Nature: Astrology and Alchemy in Early Modern Europe* (Cambridge, Mass., 2001), 69–131.

Grant, Edward, *Planets, Stars, and Orbs: The Medieval Cosmos, 1200–1687* (Cambridge, 1994).

Green, Monica, 'Women's Medical Practice and Medical Care in Medieval Europe', *Signs*, 14 (1989), 434–73.

Greer, Germaine, Jeslyn Medoff, Melinda Sansone, and Susan Hastings (eds.), *Kissing the Rod: An Anthology of Seventeenth Century Women's Verse* (1988).

Grell, Ole, and Andrew Cunningham (eds.), *Religio Medici: Religion and Medicine in Seventeenth Century England* (Aldershot, 1996).

Griffiths, Paul, *Youth and Authority: Formative Experiences in England 1560–1640* (Oxford, 1996).

Grund, Peter, 'In Search of Gold: Towards a Text Edition of an Alchemical Treatise', in Peter J. Lucas and Angela M. Lucas (eds.), *Middle English from Tongue to Text: Selected Papers from the Third International Conference on Middle English* (Frankfurt, 2002), 265–79.

Halbronn, Jacques E., 'The Revealing Process of Translation and Criticism in the History of Astrology', in Patrick Curry (ed.), *Astrology, Science and Society* (Woodbridge, 1987), 197–217.

Halford, M. E. B., 'The Apocryphal Vita Adae et Evae: Some Comments on the Manuscript Tradition', *Neuphilologische Mitteilungen*, 82 (1981), 417–27.

Halleux, Robert, 'Le Mythe de Nicolas Flamel, ou les méchanisms de la pseudépigraphie alchimique', *Archives internationales d'histoire des science*, 33 (1983), 234–55.

Halliwell, James, *A brief description of the ancient and modern manuscripts preserved in the Public Library, Plymouth* (1853).

—— *Outlines of the life of Shakespeare* (Brighton, 1881).

Hannaway, Owen, *The Chemists and the Word: The Didactic Origins of Chemistry* (Baltimore, Md., 1975).

Harkness, Deborah, *John Dee's Conversations with Angels: Cabala, Alchemy, and the End of Nature* (Cambridge, 1999).

—— '"Strange" Ideas and "English" Knowledge: Natural Science Exchange in Elizabethan London', in P. H. Smith and P. Findlen (eds.), *Merchants and Marvels: Commerce, Science, and Art in Early Modern Europe* (New York and London, 2002), 137–60.

Harley, David, 'Rychard Bostok of Tanridge, Surrey (*c.*1530–1605), M.P., Paracelsian Propagandist and Friend of John Dee', *Ambix*, 47 (2000), 29–36.

Heal, Felicity, and Clive Holmes, *The Gentry in England and Wales, 1500–1700* (Basingstoke, 1994).

Heninger, S. K., *The Cosmographical Glass: Renaissance Diagrams of the Universe* (San Marino, Calif., 1977).

Henry, John, 'Occult Qualities and the Experimental Philosophy: Active Principles in Pre-Newtonian Matter Theory', *History of Science*, 24 (1986), 335–81.

—— 'Doctors and Healers: Popular Culture and the Medical Profession', in Stephen Pumfrey, Paolo Rossi, and Maurice Slawinski (eds.), *Science, Culture and Popular Belief in Renaissance Europe* (Manchester, 1991), 191–221.

Hill, Christopher, *Intellectual Origins of the English Revolution* (1972 [1965]).

Howson, Geoffrey, *A History of Mathematical Education in England* (Cambridge, 1982).

Huffman, William, *Robert Fludd and the End of the Renaissance* (1988).

Hunt, R. W., 'The Cataloguing of the Ashmolean Collection of Books and Manuscripts', *Bodleian Library Record*, 4 (1952–3), 161–70.

Hunter, Michael, *Elias Ashmole, 1617–1692: The Founder of the Ashmolean Museum and his World* (Oxford, 1983), reprinted in Hunter, *Science and the Shape of Orthodoxy: Intellectual Change in Late Seventeenth-Century Britain* (Woodbridge, 1995), 21–44.

—— and Annabel Gregory (eds.), *An Astrological Diary of the Seventeenth Century: Samuel Jeake of Rye 1652–1699* (Oxford, 1988).

—— 'Alchemy, Magic and Moralism in the Thought of Robert Boyle', *British Journal for the History of Science*, 23 (1990), 387–410.

Hutchison, Keith, 'What Happened to Occult Qualities in the Scientific Revolution?', *Isis*, 73 (1982), 233–53.

Jardine, Nick, *The Birth of History and Philosophy of Science: Kepler's* A defence of Tycho against Ursus *with Essays on its Provenance and Significance* (Cambridge, 1984),

Jenner, Mark, 'Quackery and Enthusiasm, or Why Drinking Water Cured the Plague', in O. Grell and A. Cunningham (eds.), *Religio Medici: Religion and Medicine in Seventeenth Century England* (Aldershot, 1996), 313–39.

Johnson, Francis R., *Astronomical Thought in Renaissance England* (Baltimore, Md., 1937).

—— 'Thomas Hood's Inaugural Address as a Mathematical Lecturer of the City of London (1588)', *Journal of the History of Ideas*, 3 (1942), 94–106.

Johnston, Stephen, 'Mathematical Practitioners and Instruments in Elizabethan England', *Annals of Science*, 48 (1991), 319–44.

Jones, Colin, 'Plague and its Metaphors in Early Modern France', *Representations*, 53 (1996), 97–127.

Jones, Peter Murray, 'Reading Medicine in Tudor Cambridge', in Vivian Nutton and Roy Porter (eds.), *The History of Medical Education in Britain* (Amsterdam, 1995), 153–83.

Kassell, Lauren, 'Casting Figures for Disease: The Patients of an Astrological Medical Practitioner in London, 1596–1598', M.Sc. dissertation, University of Oxford, 1994.

—— 'Simon Forman's Philosophy of Medicine: Medicine, Astrology and Alchemy in London *c.*1580–1611', D.Phil. thesis, University of Oxford, 1998.

Kassell, Lauren, '"Remember Also the Storri of Cymbalin", or is Simon Forman's "Bocke of Plaies" a Forgery?' (forthcoming).

——'Reading for the Philosophers' Stone', in Marina Frasca-Spada and Nick Jardine (eds.), *History of Science, History of the Book* (Cambridge, 2000), 132–50.

——'The Economy of Magic in Early Modern England', in Margaret Pelling and Scott Mandelbrote (eds.), The Practice of Reform in Health, Medicine, and Science, 1500–2000: Essays for Charles Webster (Aldershot: Ashgate, 2005), 43–57.

Katz, David, 'The Language of Adam in the Seventeenth Century', in Hugh Lloyd-Jones, Valerie Pearl, and Blair Worden (eds.), *History and Imagination: Essays in Honour of H. R. Trevor-Roper* (1981), 132–45.

Kieckhefer, Richard, *Magic in the Middle Ages* (Cambridge, 1989).

——'The Specific Rationality of Medieval Magic', *American Historical Review*, 99 (1994), 813–36.

—— *Forbidden Rites: A Necromancer's Manual of the Fifteenth Century* (Thrupp, 1997).

Kiessling, Nicholas, *The Library of Robert Burton* (Oxford, 1988).

King, Helen, *Hippocrates' Woman: Reading the Female Body in Ancient Greece* (1998).

Klaassen, Frank, 'English Manuscripts of Magic, 1300–1500: A Preliminary Survey' in C. Fanger (ed.), *Conjuring Spirits: Texts and Traditions of Medieval Ritual Magic* (Thrupp, 1998), 3–31.

Kocher, Paul, 'Paracelsian Medicine in England: The First Thirty Years', *Journal of the History of Medicine*, 2 (1947), 451–80.

——'The Idea of God in Elizabethan Medicine', *Journal of the History of Ideas*, 11 (1950), 3–29.

—— *Science and Religion in Elizabethan England* (San Marino, Calif., 1953).

Krausman Ben-Amos, Ilana, *Adolescence and Youth in Early Modern England* (New Haven, 1994).

Laqueur, Thomas, *Making Sex: Body and Gender from the Greeks to Freud* (Cambridge, Mass., 1990).

Laurence, Anne, 'Women's Psychological Disorders in Seventeenth-Century Britain', in Arina Angermen, Geete Biinena, Annemieke Keunen, Velte Poels, and Jacqueline Zikzee (eds.), *Current Issues in Women's History* (1989), 203–19.

Lindley, David, *The Trials of Frances Howard: Fact and Fiction at the Court of King James* (1993).

Long, Pamela O., *Openness, Secrecy, Authorship: Technical Arts and the Culture of Knowledge from Antiquity to the Renaissance* (Baltimore, Md., 2001).

Love, Harold, *Scribal Publication in Seventeenth-Century England* (Oxford, 1993).

McCray Beier, Lucinda, *Sufferers and Healers: The Experience of Illness in Seventeenth-Century England* (1987).

MacDonald, Michael, *Mystical Bedlam: Madness, Anxiety, and Healing in Seventeenth-Century England* (Cambridge, 1981).

—— *Witchcraft and Hysteria in Elizabethan London: Edward Jorden and the Mary Glover Case* (1991).

——'The Career of Astrological Medicine in England', in O. Grell and A. Cunningham (eds.), *Religio Medici: Religion and Medicine in Seventeenth Century England* (Aldershot, 1996), 62–90.

McElwee, William, *The Murder of Sir Thomas Overbury* (1952).

McGuire, J. E., and Piyo Rattansi, 'Newton and the "Pipes of Pan"', *Notes and Records of the Royal Society*, 21 (1966), 108–43.

McKitterick, David, *A History of Cambridge University Press*, i (Cambridge, 1992).

Maclean, Ian, *The Renaissance Notion of Woman: A Study in the Fortunes of Scholasticism and Medical Science in European Intellectual Life* (Cambridge, 1980).

Macray, W. D., *Index to the Catalogue of Manuscripts of Elias Ashmole* (Oxford, 1866).

McVaugh, Michael, *Medicine before the Plague: Practitioners and their Patients in the Crown of Aragon, 1285–1345* (Cambridge, 1993).

Marotti, Arthur, *Manuscripts, Print, and the English Renaissance Lyric* (Ithaca, NY, 1995).

Mascuch, Michael, *Origins of the Individualist Self: Autobiography and Self-Identity in England, 1591–1791* (Cambridge, 1997).

Mayer, Thomas F., and D. R. Woolf (eds.), *The Rhetoric of Life-Writing in Early Modern Europe: Forms of Biography from Cassandra Fédèle to Louis XIV* (Ann Arbor, 1995).

Midelfort, Erik, *A History of Madness in Sixteenth-Century Germany* (Stanford, Calif., 1992).

Moran, Bruce, *The Alchemical World of the German Court: Occult Philosophy and Chemical Medicine in the Circle of Moritz of Hessen (1572–1632)* (Stuttgart, 1991).

Moss, Ann, *Printed Common-Place Books and the Structuring of Renaissance Thought* (Oxford, 1996).

Mozley, J. H., 'The "Vita Adae"', *Journal of Theological Studies*, 30 (1929), 121–49.

Muir, Edward, 'Introduction: Observing Trifles', in Edward Muir and Guido Ruggiero (eds.), *Microhistory and the Lost Peoples of Europe*, tr. Eren Branch (Baltimore, Md., 1991), pp. vii–xxviii.

Multhauf, Robert, 'Medical Chemistry and the Paracelsians', *Bulletin of the History of Medicine*, 28 (1954), 101–25.

Munk, William, *The roll of the Royal College of Physicians of London*, i (1878).

Nance, Brian, *Turquet de Mayerne as Baroque Physician: The Art of Medical Portraiture* (Amsterdam, 2001).

Newman, William R., 'Thomas Vaughan as an Interpreter of Agrippa von Nettesheim', *Ambix*, 29 (1982), 125–40.

—— *Gehennical Fire: The Lives of George Starkey, an American Alchemist in the Scientific Revolution* (Cambridge, Mass., 1994).

—— 'The Philosopher's Egg: Theory and Practice in the Alchemy of Roger Bacon', *Mirologus: Nature, Sciences and Medieval Societies*, 3 (1995), 75–101.

—— and Anthony Grafton, 'Introduction: The Problematic Status of Astrology and Alchemy in Premodern Europe', in W. Newman and A. Grafton (eds.), *Secrets of Nature: Astrology and Alchemy in Early Modern Europe* (Cambridge, Mass., 2001), 1–37.

—— —— (eds.), *Secrets of Nature: Astrology and Alchemy in Early Modern Europe* (Cambridge, Mass., 2001).

—— and Lawrence M. Principe, 'Alchemy vs. Chemistry: The Etymological Origins of a Historiographic Mistake', *Early Science and Medicine*, 3 (1998), 32–65.

—— —— *Alchemy Tried in the Fire: Starkey, Boyle, and the Fate of Helmontian Alchemy* (Chicago, 2002).

Niccoli, Ottavia, *Prophecy and People in Renaissance Italy*, tr. Lydia Cochrane (Princeton, 1990).

North, John, *Horoscopes and History* (1986).

Nutton, Vivian, 'The Seeds of Disease: An Explanation of Contagion and Infection from the Greeks to the Renaissance', *Medical History*, 27 (1983), 1–34.

O'Day, Rosemary, *Education and Society, 1500–1800* (1982).

Oxford English Dictionary <http://dictionary.oed.com/>

Page, Sophie, 'Magic at St. Augustine's, Canterbury, in the Late Middle Ages', Ph.D. thesis, Warburg Institute, University of London, 2000.

—— 'Richard Trewythian and the Uses of Astrology in Late Medieval England', *Journal of the Warburg and Courtauld Institutes*, 64 (2001), 193–228.

Pagel, Walter, *Paracelsus: An Introduction to Philosophical Medicine in the Age of the Renaissance* (Basel, 1982).

Park, Katharine, *Doctors and Medicine in Early Renaissance Florence* (Princeton, 1985).

Partington, J. R., *A History of Chemistry*, ii (1961).

Pelling, Margaret, 'Contagion/Germ Theory/Specificity', in William Bynum and Roy Porter (eds.), *Companion Encyclopedia of the History of Medicine*, i (1993), 309–34.

—— 'Knowledge Common and Acquired: The Education of Unlicensed Medical Practitioners in Early Modern London', in Vivian Nutton and Roy Porter (eds.), *The History of Medical Education in Britain* (Amsterdam, 1995), 250–79.

—— 'Compromised by Gender: The Role of the Male Medical Practitioner in Early Modern England', in Hilary Marland and Margaret Pelling (eds.), *The Task of Healing: Medicine, Religion and Gender in England and the Netherlands, 1450–1800* (Rotterdam, 1996), 101–33.

—— *The Common Lot: Sickness, Medical Occupations and the Urban Poor in Early Modern England* (1998).

—— *Medical Conflicts in Early Modern London: Patronage, Physicians, and Irregular Practitioners 1550–1640* (Oxford, 2003).

—— and Charles Webster, 'Medical Practitioners', in C. Webster (ed.), *Health, Medicine and Mortality in the Sixteenth Century* (Cambridge, 1979), 165–235.

Pereira, Michela, '*Mater Medicinarum*: English Physicians and the Alchemical Elixir in the Fifteenth Century', in Roger French, Jon Arrizabalaga, Andrew Cunningham, and Luis Garcia Ballester (eds.), *Medicine from the Black Death to the French Disease* (Aldershot, 1998), 26–52.

Pollard, A. W., and G. R. Redgrave, *A Short-Title Catalogue of Books Printed in England, Scotland, and Ireland*, 2nd edn. (1986).

Pomata, Gianna, *Contracting a Cure: Patients, Healers, and the Law in Early Modern Bologna* (Baltimore, Md., 1998).

Popper, Nick, 'The English Polydaedali: How Gabriel Harvey Read Late Tudor London', *Journal of the History of Ideas*, 66 (2005), 351–81.

Porter, Dorothy, and Roy Porter, *In Sickness and in Health: The British Experience, 1650–1850* (1988).

Porter, Roy, *Health for Sale: Quackery in England 1660–1850* (Manchester, 1989).

Principe, Lawrence M., *The Aspiring Adept: Robert Boyle and his Alchemical Quest* (Princeton, 1998).

Purkiss, Diane (ed.), *Renaissance Women: The Plays of Elizabeth Carey; the Poems of Aemelia Lanyer* (1994).

Quinn, David B., and John W. Shirley, 'A Contemporary List of Hariot References', *Renaissance Quarterly*, 22 (1969), 9–26.

Race, Sydney, 'Simon Forman's "Bocke of Plaies" Examined', *Notes and Queries* (Jan. 1958), 9–14.

Rappaport, Steve, *Worlds within Worlds: Structures of Life in Sixteenth-Century London* (Cambridge, 1989).

Rattansi, Piyo, and Antonio Clericuzio (eds.), *Alchemy and Chemistry in the Sixteenth and Seventeenth Centuries* (1994).

Read, John, *Prelude to Chemistry: An Outline of Alchemy, its Literature and Relationships* (Cambridge, Mass., 1966 [1936]).

Richardson, Linda Deer, 'The Generation of Disease: Occult Causes and Diseases of the Total Substance', in Andrew Wear, Roger K. French, and I. M. Lonie (eds.), *The Medical Renaissance of the Sixteenth Century* (Cambridge, 1985), 175–94.

Ritson, Joseph, *Bibliographia poetica: a catalogue of Engleish poets* (1802).

Roberts, Julian, and Andrew Watson (eds.), *John Dee's Library Catalogue* (1990).

Roberts, R. S., 'The London Apothecaries and Medical Practice in Tudor and Stuart England', Ph.D. thesis, University of London, 1964.

——'The Personnel and Practice of Medicine in Tudor and Stuart England: Part 2, London', *Medical History*, 8 (1964), 217–29.

Roper, Lyndal, *Oedipus and the Devil: Witchcraft, Sexuality and Religion in Early Modern Europe* (1994).

Rowse, A. L., *Simon Forman: Sex and Society in Shakespeare's Age* (1974).

Ryan, William F., and Charles B. Schmitt (eds.), *Pseudo-Aristotle: The Secret of Secrets: Sources and Influences* (1982).

Sawyer, Ronald, 'Patients, Healers and Disease in the Southeast Midlands, 1597–1634', Ph.D. thesis, University of Wisconsin, 1986.

——' "Strangely Handled in All her Lyms": Witchcraft and Healing in Jacobean England', *Journal of Social History*, 22 (1988–9), 461–85.

Schaffer, Simon, 'Piety, Physic and Prodigious Abstinence', in O. Grell and A. Cunningham (eds.), *Religio Medici: Religion and Medicine in Seventeenth Century England* (Aldershot, 1990), 171–203.

Schiebinger, Londa, *The Mind has no Sex? Woman in the Origins of Modern Science* (Cambridge, Mass., 1989).

Schleiner, Winfried, *Medical Ethics in the Renaissance* (Washington, DC, 1995).

Schoenbaum, Samuel, *Shakespeare and Others* (Washington, DC, 1985).

Schuler, Robert M., 'William Blomfild, Elizabethan Alchemist', *Ambix*, 20 (1973), 75–87.

Scribner, Robert, 'The Reformation, Popular Magic, and the "Disenchantment of the World" ', *Journal of Interdisciplinary History*, 23 (1993), 475–94.

Seaver, Paul, *Wallington's World: A Puritan Artisan in Seventeenth-Century London* (1985).

Sharpe, James A., *Instruments of Darkness: Witchcraft in England, 1550–1750* (1996).

Sharpe, Kevin, *Reading Revolutions: The Politics of Reading in Early Modern England* (New Haven, 2000).

Sherman, William, *John Dee: The Politics of Reading and Writing in the Renaissance* (Amherst, Mass., 1995).

Siebert, F. S., *Freedom of the Press in England 1476–1776: The Rise and Decline of Government Control* (Urbana, Ill., 1952).

Siraisi, Nancy, *Avicenna in Renaissance Italy: The Canon and Medical Teaching in Italian Universities after 1500* (Princeton, 1987).

—— *Medieval and Early Renaissance Medicine: An Introduction to Knowledge and Practice* (Chicago, 1990).

—— 'Girolamo Cardano and the Art of Medical Narrative', *Journal of the History of Ideas*, 52 (1991), 581–602.

—— *The Clock and the Mirror: Girolamo Cardano and Renaissance Medicine* (Princeton, 1997).

Slack, Paul, *The Impact of Plague in Tudor and Stuart England* (Oxford, 1985).

—— 'Mirrors of Health and Treasures of Poor Men: The Uses of the Vernacular Medical Literature of Tudor England', in C. Webster (ed.), *Health, Medicine and Mortality in the Sixteenth Century* (Cambridge, 1979), 237–73.

Smith, Hilda, 'Gynecology and Ideology in Seventeenth-Century England', in B. A. Carroll (ed.), *Liberating Women's History: Theoretical and Critical Essays* (Urbana, Ill., 1976), 99–101.

Smith, Pamela H., and Paula Findlen (eds.), *Merchants and Marvels: Commerce, Science, and Art in Early Modern Europe* (New York and London, 2002).

Smoller, Laura Ackerman, *History, Prophecy and the Stars: The Christian Astrology of Pierre d'Ailly, 1350–1420* (Princeton, 1994).

Sotheby's, *The Collection of J. O. Halliwell*, catalogue for a sale on 21 May 1857.

Stolberg, Michael, 'A Woman down to her Bones: The Anatomy of Sexual Difference in the Sixteenth and Seventeenth Centuries', *Isis*, 94 (2003), 274–99.

Stone, Lawrence, *The Family, Sex and Marriage in England 1500–1800* (1977).

Stone, Michael E., *A History of the Literature of Adam and Eve* (Baltimore, Md., 1994).

Strype, John, *The life and acts of John Whitgift*, ii (Oxford, 1822).

Talbot, C. H., and E. A. Hammond, *The Medical Practitioners in Medieval England: A Biographical Register* (1965).

Tambiah, Stanley, *Magic, Science, Religion, and the Scope of Rationality* (Cambridge, 1990).

Tannenbaum, Samuel, *Shaksperian Scraps, and other Elizabethan Fragments* (New York, 1933).

Taylor, E. G. R., *The Mathematical Practitioners of Tudor and Stuart England* (Cambridge, 1967 [1954]).

Temkin, Owsei, *Galenism: Rise and Decline of a Medical Philosophy* (Ithaca, NY, 1973).

Tester, S. J., *A History of Western Astrology* (Woodbridge, 1987).

Thomas, Keith, *Religion and the Decline of Magic* (Harmondsworth, 1973 [1971]).

——'An Anthropology of Religion and Magic, 2', *Journal of Interdisciplinary History*, 6 (1975), 91–109.

Thompson, C. J. S., *The Quacks of Old London* (New York, 1928).

Thomson, S. Harrison, 'A Fifth Recension of the Latin "Vita Ade et Eve"', *Studi Medievali*, NS 6 (1933), 271–8.

Thorndike, Lynn, *A History of Magic and Experimental Science*, 8 vols. (New York, 1923–41).

——'Robertus Anglicus and the Introduction of Demons and Magic into Commentaries upon the *Sphere* of Sacrobosco', *Speculum*, 21 (1946), 241–3.

—— *The Sphere of Sacrobosco and its Commentators* (Chicago, 1949).

——and Pearl Kibre, *A Catalogue of Incipits of Mediaeval Scientific Writings in Latin* (Cambridge, Mass., 1963).

Tilton, Hereward, *The Quest for the Phoenix: Spiritual Alchemy and Rosicrucianism in the Work of Count Michael Maier (1569–1622)* (Berlin, 2003).

Traister, Barbara, 'New Evidence about Burton's Melancholy', *Renaissance Quarterly*, 24 (1976), 66–70.

——'Medicine and Astrology in Elizabethan England: The Case of Simon Forman', *Transactions and Studies of the College of Physicians of Philadelphia*, 11 (1989), 279–97.

—— *The Notorious Astrological Physician of London: Works and Days of Simon Forman* (Chicago, 2001).

Trevor-Roper, Hugh, 'The Court Physician and Paracelsianism', in Vivian Nutton (ed.), *Medicine at the Courts of Europe* (1990), 79–94.

Turner, Gerard L'E., 'Mathematical Instrument-Making in London in the Sixteenth Century', in Turner, *Scientific Instruments and Experimental Philosophy 1550–1850* (Aldershot, 1990), 93–106.

——*Elizabethan Instrument Makers: The Origins of the London Trade in Precision Instrument Making* (Oxford, 2000).

Venn, John, and J. A. Venn, *Alumni Cantabrigienses, pt. 1. From the Earliest Times to 1751*, 4 vols. (Cambridge, 1922–7).

Vickers, Brian (ed.), *Occult and Scientific Mentalities in the Renaissance* (Cambridge, 1984).

von der Krogt, Peter, *Globi Neerlandici: The Production of Globes in the Low Countries* (Utrecht, 1993).

von Greyerz, Kaspar, 'Religion in the Life of German and Swiss Autobiographers (Sixteenth and Early Seventeenth Centuries)', in von Greyerz (ed.), *Religion and Society in Early Modern Europe 1500–1800* (1984), 223–41.

Walker, D. P., *Spiritual and Demonic Magic from Ficino to Campanella* (1958).

—— *Unclean Spirits: Possession and Exorcism in France and England in the Late Sixteenth and Early Seventeenth Centuries* (1981).

Wallis, Patrick, 'Medicines for London: The Trade, Regulations and Lifecycle of London Apothecaries, *c.*1610–*c.*1670', D.Phil. thesis. University of Oxford, 2002.

——'Plagues, Morality and the Place of Medicine in Early Modern England', *English Historical Review*, 71 (2006), 1–24.

Walsham, Alexandra, *Providence in Early Modern England* (Oxford, 1999).
Waters, David W., 'Nautical Astronomy and the Problem of Longitude', in John G. Burke (ed.), *The Uses of Science in the Age of Newton* (Berkeley, Calif., 1983), 144–69.
Wear, Andrew, *Knowledge and Practice in English Medicine, 1550–1680* (Cambridge, 2000).
Webster, Charles, *The Great Instauration: Science, Medicine and Reform 1626–1660* (1975).
—— (ed.), *Health, Medicine and Mortality in the Sixteenth Century* (Cambridge, 1979).
—— 'Alchemical and Paracelsian Medicine', in C. Webster (ed.), *Health, Medicine and Mortality*, 301–34.
—— *From Paracelsus to Newton: Magic and the Making of Modern Science* (Cambridge, 1980).
Westman, Robert, and J. E. McGuire, *Hermeticism and the Scientific Revolution* (Los Angeles, 1977).
White, Beatrice, *Cast of Ravens: The Strange Case of Sir Thomas Overbury* (1965).
Williams, Arnold, *The Common Expositor: An Account of the Commentaries on Genesis, 1527–1633* (Chapel Hill, NC, 1948).
Williams, Katherine E., 'Hysteria in Seventeenth-Century Case Records and Unpublished Manuscripts', *History of Psychology*, 1 (1990), 383–401.
Wilson, F. P., *The Plague in Shakespeare's London* (Oxford, 1963 [1927]).
Wilson, J. Dover, and R. W. Hunt, 'The Authenticity of Simon Forman's *Bocke of Plaies*', *Review of English Studies*, 23 (1947), 193–200.
Woudhuysen, Henry, *Sir Philip Sidney and the Circulation of Manuscripts, 1558–1640* (Oxford, 1996).
Yates, Frances, *Giordano Bruno and the Hermetic Tradition* (Chicago, 1964).
Zambelli, Paola, *The Speculum astronomiae and its Enigma: Astronomy, Theology and Science in Albertus Magnus and his Contemporaries* (1982).
Ziegler, Joseph, 'Medicine and Immortality in Terrestrial Paradise', in Peter Biller and Joseph Ziegler (eds.), *Religion and Medicine in the Middle Ages* (Woodbridge, 2001), 201–42.

MANUSCRIPT INDEX

GENERAL INDEX